BECOMING
AN OD PRACTITIONER

BECOMING
AN OD PRACTITIONER

ERIC H. NEILSEN

Case Western Reserve University

Prentice-Hall, Inc., *Englewood Cliffs, NJ 07632*

Library of Congress Cataloging in Publication Data

NEILSEN, ERIC H.   (date)
  Becoming an OD practitioner.

  Bibliography: p.
  Includes index.
  1. Organizational change.   I. Title.
HD58.8.N44   1984   658.4'063   83-21147
ISBN   0-13-071555-7

Editorial/production supervision and interior design: Maureen Wilson
Cover design: Lundgren Graphics, Ltd.
Manufacturing buyer: Ed O'Dougherty

© 1984 by Prentice-Hall, Inc., Englewood Cliffs, New Jersey 07632

Printed in the United States of America

10   9   8   7   6   5   4   3   2

ISBN 0-13-071555-7

Prentice-Hall International, Inc., *London*
Prentice-Hall of Australia Pty. Limited, *Sydney*
Editora Prentice-Hall do Brasil, Ltda., *Rio de Janeiro*
Prentice-Hall Canada Inc., *Toronto*
Prentice-Hall of India Private Limited, *New Delhi*
Prentice-Hall of Japan, Inc., *Tokyo*
Prentice-Hall of Southeast Asia Pte. Ltd., *Singapore*
Whitehall Books Limited, *Wellington, New Zealand*

TO
THE MEN AND WOMEN
OF THE MOD PROGRAM

CONTENTS

PREFACE
AND ACKNOWLEDGMENTS

In the fall of 1974, the director of organization development in a large firm headquartered in Cleveland, Ohio, proposed to the faculty of the Department of Organizational Behavior at Case Western Reserve University that it start a Master's Degree Program in Organization Development. The proposer's rationale was that many of his colleagues in the local area had learned some of the techniques of OD through workshops and from collaborating with external consultants (typically Ph.D.s), but few of them felt grounded conceptually in the subject. Such grounding was necessary because more and more companies were shifting from external to internal consultants as their primary source of OD expertise.

I had just come to the department when this event happened, having spent the preceding four years teaching required courses in organizational behavior at the Harvard Business School. I had learned something about management education, strategy oriented consulting, and from my graduate education, organizational sociology and group dynamics. But I had yet to do the kind of collaboration oriented organization development projects that my colleagues at CWRU were known for. I saw the proposal as an opportunity for me to learn the department's ways, since developing a new curriculum would require extensive sharing of ideas. The department already had a well-established Ph.D. program in Organizational Behavior, with a strong OD orientation, had contemplated starting a Master's level counterpart, but had yet to act on this idea. Thus when I took up our proposer's cause my impetus was well-received, and within six months we were recruiting our first class.

This book summarizes much of what I have learned about OD since 1974, both as director of and instructor in the aforementioned program and with my colleagues in the field. Most of the ideas, concepts, and models presented in the book are the byproducts of my attempts to bring into the program what I was learning in the field, and to articulate my learnings in ways that made them useful for the participants' own work lives. In this sense, the book has been a truly collaborative effort, and I would like to acknowledge some of the people whose contributions were especially important.

To begin with, Thomas Cummings and James Waters had a major impact on my thinking about OD long before I began to write this book. The three of us team-taught much of the first round of the program, and my first exposure to what OD was all about at CWRU came largely through our planning meetings and classroom activities. L. David Brown and Robert Kaplan were also helpful in this way at that beginning, and in recent years, William Pasmore, Ronald Fry, and Michelle Spain have played similar roles.

Frank Friedlander, David Kolb, Suresh Srivastva, and Donald Wolfe were our senior faculty who kept us on course and led many of our off-site laboratories and workshops. In particular, Don Wolfe has played a significant role for me both as a dean of many of our labs and as the person who counselled me while I counselled my students.

Suresh Srivastva has also been a pivotal source of support, stimulation, and insight. As chairman of the department, he was my primary backer in getting the program started and has continued to play a major role in buffering the program's innovations from our more traditional academic environment.

The participants in the Master's program, as well as several in our Ph.D. program, have played important roles as colleagues in field projects and as critics of the text itself. Within this group, I owe special thanks to Cathy Spitz who was my primary colleague in the South City project, and to Lorraine Szabo who read and edited early drafts of several chapters. Harlow Cohen, Roy Glenn, Alan Jensen, and Vishal Gujral also were of significant assistance to me in the field, and Constance Savage and David Cooperrider made especially helpful comments on the drafts.

I regret that I cannot also mention by name the large number of clients, spread across half a dozen major projects, and many more smaller ones, who provided me with the opportunity to learn and work with them during this period. The book could not have been written without their cooperation.

My secretary, Darlene Wolfe, and our departmental administrator, Retta Holdorf, performed the arduous task of typing the drafts and doing the necessary administrative work. Lastly, I wish to acknowledge with deepest gratitude the emotional support of my wife, Margaret Osborne Neilsen, and my children, Eric and Lydia.

Though the support, interest, and particularly patience of these many persons have gone into the writing of this book, I am of course solely responsible for the final product.

INTRODUCTION

This book is about becoming an Organization Development (OD) practitioner. It presents a way of thinking about OD and the skills associated with it that is intended to help someone who seriously wants to assume this role. In one sense, this is a kind of cookbook. It presents a series of recipes for finding one's way through the OD process. In another sense, it is an exposition of a particular philosophy and approach to OD.

While numerous procedures are described, often in considerable detail, the underlying emphasis is on providing a way of thinking about OD that emphasizes the field's core values. As an OD consultant, I have frequently had the experience of someone saying to me, "Values are well and good, but I am interested in bottom-line results." This book attempts to show how certain social values, typically associated with the field of OD, are *not* simply well and good. Their pursuit produces long-term bottom-line results.

Values are organizing principles that put particular procedures in perspective and enable both consultants and clients to experiment with and modify organizational routines with an eye toward long-run consequences. To experiment without attention to values is to adopt the fallacy that instrumental organizations are value free; that they are there just to get the job done. The fallacy lies in the fact that choices about what jobs need to be done, by whom, in terms of what priorities, and under what constraints are inevitably determined by the values of an organization's leadership. Moreover, who actually does these jobs, and with what levels of energy, commitment, and care is determined by the values of an organization's membership taken as a whole. There is no such thing as a value free organization.

The values we will be concerned about have to do with the way people manage their relationships at work, their behavior in group settings, and their attempts to lead others. They deal with candidness, self-responsibility, basic equality, holistic relation-ships, organizational commitment, and human potential. As such, they neither rein-force nor challenge broader social values, for instance, about the worth of private en-terprise or professional autonomy. However, they do question the single-minded pur-suit of short-run objectives, when such activities threaten personal and organizational integrity.

The approach we will explore uses these values as guiding principles for decid-ing when to employ any OD procedure or intervention, and how to modify it to fit the demands of a particular situation. The basic concept is to sculpt an OD project in col-laboration with one's clients in ways that model these values and convince clients of their importance. OD procedures, especially those that have been well-tested and rou-tinized, are just as susceptible as other management techniques to misapplication in the service of short-run objectives. This is what we want to avoid.

Using these values as guidelines frees consultants from being trapped in their clients' myopia as well. For clients may view particular techniques, especially those that are currently in vogue, as answers to their problems without realizing the complexity of the particular conditions they are facing. Thinking about the application of a technique in terms of whether it will foster the pursuit of a particular value in the situation at hand puts current fads in perspective and encourages the eclectic use of the whole range of OD technology now available.

Concomitant with our emphasis on values, our approach will involve an ac-tion research orientation. In this orientation, clients' immediate problems serve as starting points for systemic analyses of the surrounding organization. Follow-up inter-ventions are seen as experiments, i.e., as both tests of current understanding and sources of new learnings. Such action research projects provide the arenas in which OD values are modelled for the rest of the organization.

The action research approach is itself consistent with the values we are con-cerned with, because it allows them to be modelled also in the client/consultant rela-tionship. When a project is viewed as a learning effort, blame for past and current mis-takes can be understood in terms of insufficient data and/or understanding. This mini-mizes self-protectiveness and frees up both parties to engage holistically, candidly, self-responsibly, and equally in the learning process.

PLAN OF THE BOOK

The book is divided into three parts. The first part pro-vides an overview of the field. Chapter One defines OD in terms of the values orientation referred to above. Chapter Two is the story of a sample OD project done by the author and his colleagues. Chapter Three reviews this project for the purpose of showing how particular values were modelled in this action research activity. Chapter Four describes the skills a consultant should ideally have in order to do this kind of OD.

The second part explores particular techniques and concepts for designing and executing an organizational analysis and feedback activity. This is a typical first step in an action research project and helps to provide an agenda for subsequent in-novations. We will explore both the procedural details of doing this and ways of ex-ecuting them that embody OD values. Specifically, Chapter Five compares the action research approach with other popular methods of introducing OD to an organization and discusses the merits of action research as the first method for an OD consultant to learn. Chapter Six provides a conceptual roadmap for organizational analysis and guidelines for applying it in an action research context. Chapter Seven reviews the pragmatic details of scouting a prospective client, holding entry meetings, and making contracts. Chapter Eight offers techniques for talking with clients in ways that are both helpful to the client and consistent with our philosophy. Chapter Nine describes techniques for gathering data in an interview/feedback project, with special emphasis on the one-on-one interview. Finally Chapter Ten shows how to prepare data, design and execute feedback meetings, and develop action agendas.

The third part of the book discusses basic techniques for this kind of value oriented action research at the group and individual levels. Chapter Eleven provides guidelines for using this approach in developing task forces and acting as a process consultant to groups at work. Chapter Twelve discusses the theory and technique of role therapy, a personal counselling strategy that enhances our approach.

BECOMING
AN OD PRACTITIONER

CHAPTER ONE

DEFINING THE FIELD
OF
ORGANIZATION DEVELOPMENT

Organization Development is on the verge of becoming a mature field of endeavor, which is to say that a lot of people agree more or less on what it is, but have yet to accept a single written definition. The following attempts, each from different but well-known authors in the field, indicate the current state of convergence:

Organization Development is an effort (1) *planned*, (2) *organization-wide*, and (3) *managed* from the *top*, to (4) *increase organization* effectiveness and *health* through (5) *planned interventions* in the organization's "processes," using behavioral-science knowledge.[1]

Organization Development (OD) is a response to change, a complex educational strategy intended to change the beliefs, attitudes, values, and structure of organizations so that they can better adapt to new technologies, markets, and challenges, and the dizzying rate of change itself.[2]

Organization renewal is the process of initiating, creating, and confronting needed changes so as to make it possible for organizations to become or remain viable, to adapt to new conditions, to solve problems, to learn from experiences, and to move toward greater organizational maturity.[3]

Organization Development can be defined as a planned and sustained effort to apply behavioral science for system improvement, using reflexive, self-analytic methods.[4]

[1]Richard Beckhard, *Organization Development: Strategies and Models* (Reading, Mass.: Addison-Wesley Publishing Co., 1969), p. 9. ©1969. Reprinted with permission.

[2]Warren G. Bennis, *Organization Development: Its Nature, Origins, and Prospects* (Reading, Mass.: Addison-Wesley Publishing Co., 1969), p. 2. ©1969. Reprinted with permission.

[3]Gordon L. Lippit, *Organization Renewal: A Holistic Approach to Organization Development,* 2nd ed. © 1982, p. xiv. Reprinted by permission of Prentice-Hall, Inc.

[4]Richard Schmuck and Matthew Miles, *Organization Development in Schools* (Palo Alto, Calif.: National Press Books, 1971), p. 2.

Organization Development is a process of planned change—change of an organization's culture from one which avoids an examination of social processes (especially decision making, planning and communication) to one which institutionalizes and legitimizes this examination.[5]

In the behavioral science, and perhaps ideal, sense of the term, Organization Development is a long-range effort to improve an organization's problem solving and renewal processes, particularly through a more effective and collaborative management of organization culture—with special emphasis on the culture of formal work teams—with the assistance of a change agent, or catalyst, and the use of the theory and technology of applied behavioral science, including action research.[6]

French et al. (1978), after carefully analyzing these definitions, concluded:

Organization Development is a process of planned, systems change that attempts to make organizations (viewed as socio-technical systems) better able to attain their short and long term objectives. This is achieved by teaching the organization members to manage their organization processes and culture more effectively. Facts, concepts, and theory from the behavioral sciences are utilized to fashion both the process and the content of interventions. A basic belief of OD theorists and practitioners is that for effective, lasting change to take place, the system members must grow in competence to master their own fates.[7]

Today all of these definitions make sense to me, and I find the summary statement above especially well put. I am aware, however, that people who are just entering the field tend to be less impressed. I believe this is because each definition includes several terms which are as unfamiliar to a neophyte as the term Organization Development itself. What is a sociotechnical system? What is meant by organization processes and culture, and so on?

This situation is especially frustrating because people who are interested in entering the field want something clear and simple as a source of orientation. They need it both for themselves and for their friends and colleagues who may want to know where they think they are headed.

One way out of this predicament which I have found especially helpful is to define OD in terms of two values that are readily understood by laymen and practitioners alike:

Organization Development is the attempt to influence the members of an organization to expand their candidness with each other about their views of the organization and their experience in it, and to take greater responsibility for their own actions as organization members. The assumption behind OD is that when people pursue both of these objectives simultaneously, they are likely to discover new ways of working together

[5]W. Warner Burke and Harvey A. Hornstein, *The Social Technology of Organization Development* (Fairfax, Va.: Learning Resources Corporation, 1972), p. xi.

[6]Wendell L. French and Cecil H. Bell, Jr., *Organization Development* (Englewood Cliffs, N.J.: Prentice-Hall, Inc., 1973), p. 15. Adapted by permission of Prentice-Hall, Inc.

[7]Wendell L. French, Cecil H. Bell, Jr., and Robert A. Zawacki, *Organization Development: Theory, Practice, and Research* (Dallas, Tex.: Business Publications, Inc., 1978), p. 7.

that they experience as more effective for achieving their own and their shared (organizational) goals. And that when this does not happen, such activity helps them to understand why and to make meaningful choices about what to do in light of this understanding.

The statement is a long one but the terminology is straightforward. It also sets the stage for explaining the elements in other authors' definitions. For example, people in organizations are by and large not candid with each other about their personal experience of organization life, nor are they adept at taking responsibility for their own behavior in the face of a tradition which says that organizational superiors know what is best for subordinates. Thus, any serious effort at getting people to pursue these values is likely to benefit greatly from careful planning.

Further, an organization-wide approach helps because it minimizes the chances of developing conflicting cultures (the changed and the unchanged) within the same system. Top-down management maximizes the availability of resources for the effort and minimizes the chances of sabotage from above. A long time frame is appropriate, because human values change slowly even under ideal conditions. Behavioral science knowledge is a critical ingredient because the effort focuses on human values. And the presence of a consultant is useful because the enactment of unfamiliar behavior is greatly enhanced by expert support and modeling.

Likewise, organizational processes such as decision making, problem solving, planning, communication, and teamwork can be identified as important targets of OD efforts because they are likely to change in ways that reflect and reinforce changes in values regarding candidness and personal responsibility. As manifestations of these values, these processes are also likely to be identified as points of intervention where consultants can model the value stances they advocate in organizationally relevant ways.

Finally, the notion that system members need to grow in competence to master their own fates goes hand in hand with the value that people should take responsibility for their own behavior.

THE BOUNDARIES OF ORGANIZATION DEVELOPMENT

Using the values of candidness and self-responsibility has the twin advantages of helping to delineate both the boundaries of the field as a whole and the challenges to be dealt with in a given project. With regard to defining the field's boundaries, it clarifies the prescriptive nature of OD and rules out consulting activities that, however effective they might be from a technoeconomic viewpoint, promote either the lack of candor and/or the lack of self-responsibility. On the level of the particular project, this definition fosters continuous inquiry into the current value stances of organization members and sets the stage for understanding the more subtle dynamics of behavior not in line with these values and, therefore, that represent targets for change.

This second advantage was first brought home to me in the early phases of an OD project with a large health care organization. And because this particular feature is central to our further theorizing about the field, a brief digression on this experience and the ideas it produced is worthwhile.

Feeding Back Data at Northern Medical[8]

In the mid-1970s, several of my colleagues and I began a multiyear OD project with a large medical center. While some of the key relationships that made the project possible had been developing for several years, the direct impetus for the project was an invitation to become involved in a program for increasing awareness of patient needs and expectations. Specifically the administrators of this organization (we will call it the Northern Medical Center) had decided that many of their support personnel — that is, people other than physicians — were not treating patients as responsively as they should be. We were asked to develop a training program in interpersonal and patient awareness skills for the support staffs of two outpatient departments. The chairmen of these departments had already volunteered their units as guinea pigs for developing a prototype training program that would hopefully be applied eventually to the rest of the organization.

Because in our experience interpersonal training programs respond more often to the symptoms of important organizational problems, rather than their causes, we asked the administrators whether they were sure that lack of training was the cause of their problems. In particular, had they analyzed these departments or any others thoroughly enough to be convinced that other factors were not equally or more important? For instance, could it be that the support staff knew perfectly well how to treat patients in a courteous, responsive, and efficient manner, but were choosing not to do so because of their feelings about their jobs, their relationships with each other, with the physicians, with the larger institution, and so on? The administrators' answer was no and they and the two chairmen eventually agreed to conduct with us an organizational analysis of their respective departments.

This first involved interviewing a cross-section of their members on topics such as their perceptions of their career progress and aspirations, the nature of their jobs, the quality of their relationships with each other, how the larger institution's structure and policies helped or hindered them from doing their jobs effectively, what changes they would like to make to improve the organization's functioning, what they personally wanted to do more of, keep doing, or stop doing, and what they saw as the most critical problems facing their department.

Each department had a medical staff of eight physicians and other senior professionals and a support group of from twenty to forty people. The latter were comprised of residents, medical attendants, secretaries, nurses, technicians, and desk receptionists. All of the senior professionals and about half of the support people were interviewed in each of the departments.

---

[8]The story of the Northern Medical project and the development of the conceptual model based on it were originally reported in Eric H. Neilsen, "Reading Clients' Values from Their Reactions to an Interview/Feedback Process," in *The Academy of Management Proceedings 1978* (Academy of Management, 1978), pp. 308-12. Parts of the following sections are excerpted from this article.

For each department we broke down the data we gathered into a series of quotations. We then grouped the quotations according to common topics emerging from the data, e.g., perceptions of supervisors, colleagues, subordinates, patients, the institution, technology, the job itself, physical layout, work flow. A document was created for each department in which groups of quotations representing different views on each topic were visually juxtaposed against each other. The authors of the quotations were not identified in these documents, nor were quotations used that identified particular people. The idea was to reveal the nature and variety of viewpoints around frequently referred to issues, rather than to the issues of particular individuals.

The document was then fed back as "a series of snapshots of life in the department," with the hope that it would be used as "a discussion vehicle for identifying important issues for department members to consider in deciding what to do next." In each case the document was first shared with the chairman, then the senior medical staff as a group, and then a series of subgroups that comprised the rest of the department and included as well those who had not been interviewed.

Client Reactions to the Data.   What concerns us here is not the content of the data we fed back. Suffice it to say that for each department it contained a broad mix of positive and negative views that revealed training as only a partial solution to the problems at hand. Rather, our focus is on the way in which various subgroups reacted to the data and the interview/feedback activity itself, for this is where values regarding candidness and self-responsibility came into play.

To begin with, different subsets of our client groups displayed four basic kinds of reactions to the process. Figure 1-1 contains some representative quotations for each kind of reaction. The comments suggesting interest in the process and inquiry into the data were essentially what we were striving for. For the most part we managed to develop dialogue along these lines in each of the groups we fed back to. Rarely, however, did other people make attempts to deal with the data in this way until we modeled such behavior and actively encouraged this approach. The more spontaneous reactions covered the other three categories.

Moreover, while there were some comments of every variety in each group, different groups tended to specialize in particular categories. The senior professionals in Department A focused more on platitudes toward the process and attacks on imagined authors of derogatory comments that they thought might apply to themselves. The support staff in Department A, on the other hand, expressed a considerable amount of skepticism and apathy. The senior professionals in Department B emphasized two kinds of responses: vacillating between outrage and denial, on the one hand, and apathy and skepticism on the other. The support staff in Department B expressed more outrage and denial than any other group.

These differing reactions, moreover, were indicative of the kinds of issues we found most important to deal with in our subsequent work with each of these groups. The senior people in Department A continued to welcome our procedures and then would use them as opportunities for competing with each other and attacking other groups. For instance, a series of weekly problem-solving sessions designed to treat

FIGURE 1-1
Types of Reaction
to Feedback Data

OUTRAGE TOWARD THE PROCESS;
DENIAL OF THE DATA

"I think this is dangerous."
"You should never have printed things like this."
"Why wasn't I told to my face?"
"We don't really have any problems."
"There are just a few complainers here."

APATHY ABOUT THE PROCESS;
SKEPTICISM ABOUT THE DATA

"I could have said more but I didn't think it was worth it."
"Everyone knows this already."
"Just watch, nothing will happen."
"Are they really going to act on this?"

INTEREST IN THE PROCESS;
INQUIRY INTO THE DATA

"It's useful to have the quotes without authors; any of us could have said this."
"The comment about . . . was something I never thought of."
"I don't agree with the statement that . . ."
"Can someone help me understand why someone would say . . . ?"

PLATITUDES TOWARD THE PROCESS;
ATTACKS ON IMAGINED QUOTERS

"Glad to have things out on the table."
"We needed this."
"What they need is a good stiff kick in . . ."
"Most of this is . . .'s own fault."

Source: Adapted from Eric H. Neilsen, "Reading Clients' Values from Their Reactions to an Interview/ Feedback Process," in *The Academy of Management Proceedings 1978* (Academy of Management, 1978), p. 309.

issues raised in the feedback process suffered continuously from verbal jousting, lack of candor, scapegoating of people who were not present to defend themselves, and a refusal to make action commitments.

The support staff in Department A (the subordinates of the group referred to above) maintained their skeptical posture in a series of vertical group meetings. The meetings were designed to develop closer, more supportive relationships between each senior professional and this person's support team. The critical difficulty for us as consultants was to get each team to see the activity as having any hope of success.

True to their initial outrage and denial, many of the senior and support staff in Department B avoided interaction with us for several months. Work proceeded with those who were interested, but major progress was made only when some of our allies confronted their colleages and showed their commitment to take action on problems revealed in the feedback data. This happened initially with the support staff and only much later with the senior professionals. The latter had to overcome some apathy as well. Reports of success from the other department, plus our own confrontation with them over their failure to meet mutually agreed to deadlines seemed to contribute to their eventual involvement.

Client Reactions and Group Orientations. The events described above remind one of the truism in psychotherapy that the opening comments of the patient hold the key to the cure. The problem, of course, is how to interpret the comments so that the key is revealed. While we as OD consultants did not see ourselves as therapists, but rather as advocates of a particular approach to managing, one can argue that the clients' reactions to the interview/feedback process contained important messages about the issues we would have to deal with in order to accomplish our objectives. In particular, they turned out to be indicative of more general patterns of behavior in each group that were consistent with different combinations of the two core OD values and their opposites.

A little theory building here is necessary to bring this point out. Juxtaposed against people who value the sharing of personally meaningful data on their organizational lives are those who think it should be held back. Juxtaposed against those who value taking personal responsibility for their actions are people who prefer that others take this responsibility for them. If one assumes that individuals can hold any combination of positions on these two issues, it is possible to derive four separate stances.

Each of these combinations in turn can be viewed as a set of underlying values for justifying a different style of face-to-face interaction—what one might call a group orientation. But only one of these is completely consistent with the underlying values of OD. The other three represent important contrasts to the ideal orientation.

Figure 1-2 identifies the four group orientations in relation to the possible combinations of choices people can make about candidness and self-responsibility. In the following paragraphs we will first elaborate on each orientation with respect to how the members of a group that follows the values associated with it might communicate with each other and make decisions. Then we will relate each orientation back to a particular client group at Northern Medical, its reactions to our activities, and some additional data about its members.

FIGURE 1-2
Group Orientations
and OD-Related Values

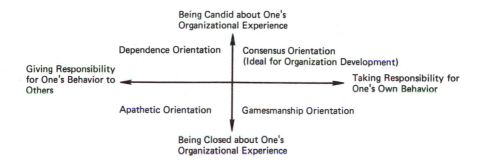

Source: Adapted from Eric H. Neilsen, "Reading Clients' Values . . . ," p. 310.

The Consensus Orientation

The *consensus orientation* indicated in the upper right hand corner of Figure 1-2 refers to the kind of group behavior that is ideal in terms of organization development values. As the figure implies, such behavior is justified by a commitment to be candid with others about one's organizational experience and to take responsibility for one's own behavior as an organization member. These values ideally pervade every aspect of group life. For purposes of comparison with the other orientations, let us consider two especially important features: communication and decision making.

Communication.   Members continuously share their perceptions, assumptions, and feelings with each other regarding both their own fulfillment and the effectiveness of the organization. The degree of sharing depends largely upon how closely one works with another. Personal viewpoints about both self and organization are seen as relevant to organization tasks and are expressed in most meetings.

Decision Making.   Decisions are made through the sharing of viewpoints, mutual recognition of differences, negotiation around substantive issues, and the development of a consensus with respect to issues where unanimity is not critical.

Following Schein (1969), consensus is achieved when a disagreeing member can say: "I understand what most of you would like to do. I personally would not do that but I feel that you understand what my alternative would be. I have had sufficient opportunity to sway you to my point of view but clearly have not been able to do so. Therefore I will gladly go along with what most of you wish to do."[9] Note that this process involves both sharing of data and the maintenance of responsibility for one's own actions. The speaker above is voluntarily going along with the group and is not putting responsibility on anyone else.

The Gamesmanship Orientation

Members of groups that follow a *gamesmanship orientation* share one of the values underlying OD: taking personal responsibility for one's own behavior. However, they differ with OD values regarding candidness and take the alternative stance of keeping their personal experience of organization life to themselves. This has major consequences for the overall tone of their group activities.

Communication.   Members keep their true ideas about self-fulfillment and organizational effectiveness to themselves. The assumption is held that sharing data on these issues can threaten personally desired outcomes. A major task of organization life is to guess other people's positions from their public, task-related behavior, and to take these hypotheses into account in fashioning one's own posture.

Decision Making.   Each member makes his/her own decisions on how to behave. This may include the choice to conform outwardly to any decision-making

---

[9]Edgar H. Schein, *Process Consultation: Its Role in Organization Development* (Reading, Mass.: Addison-Wesley Publishing Co., 1969), p. 56. ©1969. **Reprinted with permission.**

procedure while simultaneously manufacturing and manipulating data strategically to keep unilateral control over one's choices and facilitate personally desired outcomes. Conflict is dealt with in any procedure by inferring positions from others' strategic behavior so that metaconversations occur based on mutual recognition of data manipulation strategies, while the fantasy is maintained that the publicly stated procedure is being followed.

In essence, group life in the context of this orientation is a strategic game. Each person strives for personal gain, potentially at others' expense, and all words spoken, norms established, structures created, and so forth, are treated in this light.

The Dependence Orientation

Group members who follow a *dependence orientation* in their dealings with each other also share one value in common with organization development ideals and embrace the polar opposite of the other value. Only in this case their positions are the reverse of those who follow a gamesmanship orientation. Candidness is stressed but taking responsibility for one's actions is foregone in favor of giving this to someone else. The result is a very hierarchically oriented pattern of behavior that leaves little doubt about who is in charge but also places a major burden on leaders for expertise and information handling.

Communication. Sharing of perceptions, assumptions, and feelings about self-fulfillment and organizational effectiveness takes place between a limited number of members and the rest of the membership. The criterion used to determine with whom to share is perceived ability to make choices, in behalf of the self, that are better than one's own. "Tell me what to do; I trust your judgment."

Decision Making. Decisions are made by the chosen others according to the procedures these persons prefer. The procedures may involve a consensus oriented format, but in such cases the followers are looking for cues from their leaders. Such cues are sought no matter what procedure is followed. In the extreme form the chosen others themselves rely on a still smaller cadre, until there is one person at the center who speaks to the divine.

The Apathetic Orientation

Members of groups that possess an *apathetic orientation* pursue the polar opposites of both OD values. Responsibility for one's personal behavior is given to others and candidness is seen as inconsequential or even threatening. This results in the lack of both energy and autonomy.

Communication. Members keep their true ideas about self-fulfillment and organizational effectiveness to themselves. Here the assumption is held that sharing these data will not make any difference, so why bother.

Decision Making. In the extreme form, members who follow this mode refuse to think they can make decisions that will affect their personal fulfillment and/or organizational effectiveness. They simply do as they are told by others who seem to be doing as they are told. Technically, therefore, they are making the decision to conform, but the point is that this decision is seen only as a means to survival. It does not involve the proactive pursuit of anything beyond this. In the event of conflicting demands, members either wait for new orders, often without declaring the need for them, or follow routines they have already established, regardless of their relevance to current conditions.

Applying the Model to the Two Departments

The group orientation model helped to explain both the different kinds of reactions people had to the feedback activity and our subsequent experience with each group. Further data on the individuals involved also supported the model's logic. Those individuals in each department who were the first to view the process with interest and to inquire into the data in a problem-solving manner were also the strongest followers of the consensus orientation. They were the most candid about their experience in general, talked about themselves as being fully in charge of their own lives and responsible for their own choices, and showed a natural propensity toward consensus decision making even when they were not aware of our definition of the term.

Those who responded with platitudes toward the process while attacking imagined quoters showed a gamesmanship orientation in other ways as well. For instance, the senior professionals in Department A who responded most strongly in this way were strong self-starters, highly competitive in general, and committed primarily to their own professional enhancement. Most of them had been working together for about six years, were specialists with major reputations, and led very full professional lives that extended beyond departmental duties, a condition which encouraged internal competition for resources.

A major task of our work with them was to get them to see how their interpersonal competitiveness had prevented them from developing a candid working climate with their large and highly interdependent support staff. Simultaneously, mutual recognition of our commonly held value regarding the need to take personal responsibility for one's actions, helped us to form meaningful relationships where the value of candidness could be given a fair test.

The behavior of their subordinates who had reacted to the interview/feedback process primarily with skepticism and apathy was generally understandable in terms of the apathetic mode. Lack of consistent leadership, training, and others' caring for their development had led to high turnover, loss of pride, and a strong commonly held sentiment that our activities were too little and too late to be of much use. Only those physicians who demonstrated a renewed commitment to their welfare by actively responding to their feedback, inviting more of it, and being candid about their own views, were able to secure stable involvement in the vertical groups we helped to set up.

The dependence orientation enlightened the outrage and denial of many of the members of Department B and was clearly evident from this unit's history. This had been a very small department until a year before our entry. At that time a new, dynamic chairman had been appointed and the department had mushroomed overnight. The department exuded an aura of enthusiasm under the new chairman's charismatic leadership. Most members were extremely busy in developing the roles that they had been assigned and were highly dependent on both chairman and the other senior professionals (themselves young and enthusiastic) for support and encouragement.

The feedback data had revealed the first signs of strain for all to see. They indicated that some people thought others were not pulling their own weight, or were incompetent or uncooperative. While these comments were few in comparison to a great many positive statements in the document, they ran against the publicly shared image of the department as a smooth running and harmonious system in which the leaders were looking after everyone's welfare. It was much easier to deny the data and avoid the consultants than to examine the strengths and weaknesses of the dependence mode.

Real progress was made only when certain members assumed responsibility for acting on their own and established a consensus model for problem solving that represented a viable alternative to running to their leaders whenever difficulties arose. Moreover, in this process candidness between those who acted and us, the consultants, regarding our respective hopes and concerns for the department, appeared to be an important force in making things happen.

The additional skepticism among several of the senior professionals in this department appeared to be tied largely to space problems. The group was clearly overcrowded and the politics of the larger institution indicated that little would be done to alleviate the problem for at least a couple of years. It was easy to attribute many of the problems in the feedback data as due at least in part to these conditions. The physicians who were skeptical saw an increase in space as the overriding solution. Since nothing could be done about it in the near future, they saw little reason to explore the data further. Luckily, reports of success from the other department, our confrontation regarding their lack of involvement, and strong support for the project from the chairman eventually led to some promising new activities.

Caveats to Pursuing a Consensus Orientation

In light of the foregoing discussion of the Northern Medical project, one can see that OD not only embodies a call for candor and self-responsibility, but also a logical derivative of these values — what we have called a consensus orientation. Simultaneously, OD is against gamesmanship, apathy, and dependence orientations as ideal states for organization members to pursue because these orientations are supported by one or more contrasting values.

Note, however, that we are talking about ideal states, visions which are intended to guide people's energy and learning. As we see it, OD does not advocate the consensus orientation as the only appropriate way to interact in an organization at any point in time. It is the target to strive for, but not necessarily the most appropriate response to a given situation. What stands in the way of such an all-encompassing prescription is a reverence in the field for yet another set of values, those dealing with a humanistic posture toward life.

OD strives for candidness and personal responsibility, but it does so while attempting to provide ongoing and satisfying responses to people's needs for safety, security, and self-confidence. A person who does not experience psychological safety and at least a reasonable level of job security in his or her organizational life, is likely to find the pursuit of candidness threatening. For being candid can make one vulnerable to manipulation by other actors in the system. Likewise, to attempt to take responsibility for one's own behavior when one does not feel confident to make decisions in one's own best interests is only adding insult to injury.

Much of what happens in the early stages of OD projects centers around the identification of where these more basic needs are not being met and the development of strategies for doing something about it. A considerable amount of work often needs to be done to garner support from powerful actors in the system, to secure agreements around job security and the appropriate use of data, and to develop supportive relationships with key actors who are already feeling insecure, unconfident, and threatened in their jobs. These issues need to be responded to before any meaningful pursuit of OD values can take place. They remain alive, moreover, as any project unfolds, and success depends heavily on their successful treatment with respect to any OD activity.

An important implication of this is that orientations that are not consistent with OD values—for example, gamesmanship, apathy, and dependence—need to be accepted as legitimate responses to people's needs to protect themselves in many situations. When people feel competent but experience candidness as threatening, the gamesmanship orientation makes sense. When they feel significantly less competent than others but also safe in confiding with at least some of the latter, dependence makes sense. When they feel incompetent and view candidness as unsafe, apathy is a logical response. These orientations, together with the consensus mode, comprise the reality of organization life.

Organization Development practitioners recognize this reality and appreciate both its logic and its implications. Moreover, they spend much of their time helping their clients to do the same. But they do so with a mission in mind. This is to work with their clients to create conditions under which candidness and self-responsibility make sense. They also do so while recognizing that, at best, their goals will only be achieved partially.

OD VALUES AT THE RELATIONSHIP LEVEL

Thus far we have tried to articulate the core values of OD in terms of their implications for group or general face-to-face interaction. This seems appropriate because, as French et al. (1973) have noted, the primary emphasis in OD to date has been on enhancing the cultures of formal work teams. To engage in OD successfully, however, one cannot focus on the group level alone. Work group cultures are affected, on the one hand, by the more intense relationships particular members have with each other and, on the other hand, by the structure and operating policies of the formal organization. Consequently, OD activities need to focus on these levels as well.

Being candid about one's organizational experience and taking responsibility for one's own actions not only promotes the consensus orientation in group work, but also encourages interpersonal relationships that are characterized by a shared sense of equality and a willingness to relate as whole individuals.

These individual postures in turn promote a way of relating interpersonally that we would characterize as colleagueship. And just as the consensus orientation in group work is only one of several ways to participate that organization members are capable of enacting, colleagueship is only one form of relationship that one can find in any organization. Once again, some contrasting styles of relating can be identified by juxtaposing the polar opposites of its underlying values (see Figure 1–3).

FIGURE 1-3
Types of Relationships and OD- Related Values

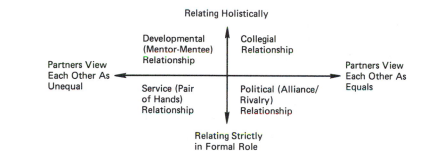

The Collegial Relationship

A *collegial relationship* is one in which people share a mutual concern for each other's development and experience themselves as having both the right and the responsibility to play an active role in helping such development take place. This involves sharing one's aspirations for the other, confronting and yet respecting differences in opinion around these aspirations, actively attempting to influence the other's development in day-to-day affairs, and providing wise counsel and emotional support in times of stress.

Both parties experience themselves as basically equal to each other along dimensions such as competence in their professional specialties, social maturity, and human worth, and in their own feelings of anxiety about the basic existential choices that they face as human beings and organizational participants. This makes mutual give and take possible, with a minimum of concern for whether one should or should not say something to the other because of differences in personal status.

The parties also treat each other holistically in the sense that their mutual concerns are for each other as unique individuals and not just as incumbents of particular roles. For instance, as your colleague, I may be concerned with your current and future welfare independent of the organization to which we both belong, and I would expect you to do the same with respect to me. This makes it possible for me to share a problem with you that may not even be relevant to our role relationship, although your skills might be helpful nonetheless. Were our relationship strictly defined by our roles, I might think that sharing such a problem would be out of place, and lose the help you might give me as a result.

Our assumption here is that equality and relating holistically breed colleague-ship. The experience of equality also enhances one's sense of responsibility for one's own actions, and vice versa. Relating holistically enhances candidness, and vice versa. Thus, colleagueship resonates with the consensus orientation in broader patterns of in-teraction. One does not necessarily have to have both at the same time, but the tension to develop both is there. For the OD specialist, this suggests the inducement of one as a pathway to inducing the other. For those who choose not to pursue OD values, it sug-gests that fears about following the OD approach at one level may stem from concerns about particular problems on the other. It will soon become apparent that the same kinds of dynamics are at work with respect to the other kinds of orientations and their corresponding relationship types.

The Political Relationship

In what we are calling *political relationships*, the partners view each other as equals but relate to each other personally primarily in terms of their formal roles. This leads to a situation in which each partner views the other as a potential instrument or obstruction to his or her own ends and conducts his or her relationship with the other based on this premise.

Suppose, for instance, that I am the production manager and you are the marketing manager of a particular business. We are structurally equals in this com-pany and consider ourselves roughly equal on other dimensions as well. We have chosen to relate to each other largely in terms of our formal roles. Therefore, I neither know or am concerned about you as an individual outside of this role, and vice versa.

Suppose, further, that you come to me with a rush order for a customer who happens to be important to you personally but whom I do not view as much different from any other customer in terms of the responsiveness that production should give to him or her. One option I have is to go by the book and respond to your request accord-ing to the priorities laid down in the company policies. But since we are equals in the amount of discretion and de facto power we have, I also may experience some desire to suggest a bargain with you. For instance, I might suggest that I give this order top priority in return for your siding with me on a request for a new piece of equipment in an upcoming policy meeting. I may not say this overtly, but I let you know indirectly what I have in mind, and find you giving signals to suggest that you are willing to co-operate. If you do not help me when the time comes, I go back to playing strictly by the rules, or perhaps find a way to get even with you through an informal trade with some-one else.

The assumption here is that the lack of a more holistic relationship heightens attention to people's mutual use of each other as objects. When this is combined with the perception of the other as roughly equal and thus both potentially valuable and not unduly threatening, political ways of relating are encouraged.

Note further how political relationships resonate with the gamesmanship orientation. Equality heightens personal responsibility. Relating strictly on a role-to-role basis facilitates the keeping of one's personal experience close to the chest. As in the example above, gamesmanship around communication and decision making resonates with political behavior.

The Service Relationship

In a *service relationship* the parties relate to each other in role only and recognize some level of inequality, at least in their overt behavior if not privately. Thus, one party controls the other as a role player, presumably in the context of some organizationally sanctioned mission.

The result of this condition, as we have observed it in our work, is that the weaker party experiences himself or herself as "just a pair of hands." The relationship is largely devoid of affect. There is little initiation on the part of the weaker party. Following orders is all that counts. The weaker party, moreover, is likely to behave self-protectively whenever his or her welfare is not protected by organization policy. Apparent gestures of good will by the more powerful party are typically viewed as paternalism by the other, and if the relationship is stable, are not generally expected.

Such relationships are clearly not ideal from a humanistic perspective and yet they also need to be recognized as both viable and agreeable to both parties in many situations. They are institutionalized in many union–management relationships and are typical of situations where people choose to work simply for the extrinsic rewards.

Service relationships resonate with the apathetic orientation in group life. Acceptance of one party as more valuable than the other, at least as it relates to the organization's concerns, facilitates the giving up of personal responsibility for one's own behavior by the less valuable party and the assumption of this responsibility by others. Once again, staying in role facilitates refraining from disclosing one's personal experience of organization life.

The Developmental Relationship

A *developmental relationship* arises when two parties recognize each other as unequal along some important dimensions such as skill, knowledge, maturity, and experience, and yet still choose to relate to each other holistically. This situation parallels a parent–child relationship, and we assume that, more often than not, it leads to a mutual attempt to develop important qualities of the less equal party. For instance, mentor–mentee relationships in organizations have these qualities.

Relating holistically facilitates and is facilitated by the more valued party's sharing of his or her experience, wisdom, and so on, and provides the other party with a more complete role model to follow. The acceptance of inequality provides a sense of legitimacy for one party following the advice of the other and helps both parties deal with feelings of counterdependence that are likely to develop in the learner due to the pervasiveness of the relationship.

Thus, developmental relationships also resonate with the dependence orientation, at least in the short run. Over the long run, if such relationships are successful, they are likely to lead to some other way of relating and a different group orientation to go with it.

Caveats to Pursuing a Collegial Relationship

We noted earlier that orientations which are not consistent with OD values — for example, gamesmanship, apathy, and dependence — need to be accepted as legitimate ways of behaving by people who use them to cope with the experience of insecurity, unsafeness, and incompetence. Thus, these conditions have to be responded to in order for the consensus orientation to make sense. Two other legitimizing conditions need to be addressed at the interpersonal relationship level if a collegial way of relating is to be justified as well. These are the need for an individual's development of a clear and integrated identity and for the development of a basic sense of competence.

Identity development is critical as a precursor to relating holistically. Studies have indicated that people who do not have a comfortable sense of who they are can lose what sense of identity they do have in the attempt to relate holistically to others.[10] Staying securely within the boundaries of one's formally defined role or relying heavily on mentors for emerging role definitions are important coping devices for such people. Thus, OD practitioners who choose to work at the interpersonal level need to be helpful in this regard.

While most of the people encountered in OD projects have already secure identities as mature adults, there are at least two forces at work that require attention. First, identity development as we have come to understand it is a lifelong process.[11] As people rise through the hierarchies of their organizations, or simply continue their maturation as adults, they encounter new situations for which their present identities are inadequate. All of us are, in some degree, continuously unlearning and relearning who we are. Particularly difficult situations either in private or public life, moreover, may require extended periods of time for people to adjust to. Thus, the identity issue is never completely resolved, and this places boundaries around the appropriate pursuit of completely holistic ways of relating.

Second, the OD process itself often causes people to reexamine their identities and the assumptions around which they have built them. This is part and parcel of the change process that we will discuss in later chapters. Some identity change is likely to be very beneficial in the course of experimenting with the OD approach. At the same time, practitioners need to be aware that they cannot do everything at once. A developmental relationship with the client is often a necessary first step in reestablishing a secure sense of self.

In modern Western society, a sense of competence consistent with one's age and social status is in the same vein a precursor to the experience of basic equality with

---

[10]Erik H. Erickson, *Childhood and Society* (New York: W. W. Norton Co., 1950), pp. 263-66.

[11]*Ibid.*, pp. 269-73.

others.[12] Like identity, the process of developing a sense of competence begins early in life, but it can also be derailed at any point in time. Once again, the sheer process of growing up organizationally and personally requires continuous new learning. And the OD process, likewise, can bring people's attention to their flat sides and throw them into a temporary state of feeling inferior. Thus, practitioners who work at the interpersonal level need not only to attend to identity issues but also to the process of teaching their clients new skills and helping them reaffirm the many strengths they have already acquired.

OD VALUES AT THE ORGANIZATIONAL LEVEL

The Organization Development philosophy which we are espousing also has important implications for organization-wide structure and policy. Just as the two basic OD values resonate with particular choices about how to relate to others on a personal basis, they also resonate with particular views of top managers about organization members in general. These, in turn, justify the creation and maintenance of different types of structure and policy, which we will call different organizational forms. The critical dimensions here deal with assumptions about people's intent and their value to the organization (see Figure 1–4).

FIGURE 1-4
Organizational Forms That Go with Particular Assumptions about Organization Members

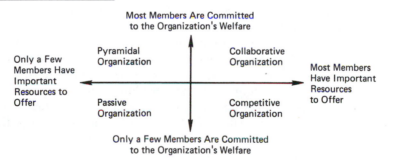

Collaborative Organization

Collaborative organization derives from a situation in which the top managers of an organization — that is, those with the most economic and legal control over its operations — are operating under the assumption that most members are basically committed to the organization's welfare and that most of the latter also have important resources to offer for the organization's successful operation. When these assumptions are in effect, the stage is set for developing structures and policies where coordination is achieved through the broad sharing of organization-wide plans, the use of collective

---

[12]*Ibid.*, p. 260.

rewards and punishments, and decentralized formal control over important functions and processes.

Specifically, the assumption of common interest and commitment justifies sharing plans and rewards. The assumption that most members control important resources—for example, expertise, interest, and energy—justifies broad patterns of delegation in order to ensure cooperation and maximize the use of formal authority where it makes the most sense technically.

The component policies and their underlying assumptions also reinforce one another. Working together through a shared plan and under a shared fate facilitates the further discovery of the diverse resources people do have when everyone is pulling together. Broad delegation makes sharing plans critical for effective coordination and facilitates multiple inputs that help to make the plan maximally effective, when people are convinced that they do have unique resources to offer.

Collaborative organization, in turn, resonates with the consensus orientation toward decision making in group interaction. Common access to formal plans directs candidness to issues that are clearly important to the organization. General candidness facilitates the creation of plans that address what people think is really important. Broad delegation affirms the need to take responsibility for one's own actions. The willingness to take such responsibility facilitates delegation. Consensus decision making is an ideal vehicle for creating plans and delegating tasks under collaborative structures and policies.

Competitive Organization

Competitive organization derives from a situation in which top managers assume that many people have important resources to offer but are also convinced that many members may not be committed to the organization's welfare. Consequently, they decentralize formal control over important functions and tasks to meet the reality of a de facto decentralized pattern of resource control. At the same time, however, they create structures and policies for coordination that limit knowledge of strategic plans and objectives to the people they think they can trust and provide other resource holders only with the data they think will help the latter to accomplish the objectives that they, the top managers, want them to pursue. This is accompanied by reward systems that focus on those specific objectives and thereby justify the lack of access to data relevant to other organizational concerns.

An important consequence of this top management posture, however, is that the people on the receiving end of these attempts at unilateral control soon learn to use their own resources to play the same game in return. The organization becomes an arena for tests of personal or subgroup power. People compete for control over the formal organization by testing how far others are willing to bend in order to obtain the resources and cooperation they, the testers, have to offer.

Competitive organization resonates with the gamesmanship orientation in group life. The metaconversations that go on in the context of the latter, with their implied threats and inducements masked by superficial conformity, provide an important vehicle for testing boundaries without having to actually take action. In essence, if by what I can imply in a conversation I can either get you anxious enough about what I might do if you do not comply with my wishes, or get you interested enough in what I could do personally for you were you to comply, I might get my way without actually having to act. Thus, social order is maintained in the short run. Major power plays are saved for critical threats or opportunities where gamesmanship does not work. They are more palatable, because gamesmanship prevents them from occurring so often that the system's integrity is threatened.

Gamesmanship, in turn, encourages the development of a competitive organization. Lack of candor combined with superficial conformity, on the one hand, and strategic deviance, on the other, justify strategic, unilateral coordination by those with ultimate economic and legal control. The major tests of strength and the reorganizations that follow are based on logical responses to situations in which people have learned not to take each other's words at face value. Simultaneously, they make gamesmanship in the future all the more important and do not require organization members to develop other ways of relating to each other.

Passive Organization

Passive organization evolves when top managers hold assumptions that are completely antithetical to those consistent with OD values. Here they assume that relatively few members of the organization control important resources that are critical to the latter's success and, simultaneously, that only they and their closest associates are committed to the organization's welfare. Under these conditions formal control over all important functions and tasks is centralized, and coordination, as with competitive organization, is achieved through the strategic manipulation of information and rewards.

The consequence of this organizational pattern is that people below the first few levels in the hierarchy learn to approach organization life in a passive manner. The lack of information about how the larger organization operates and where it is going reduces the incentive to be an active contributor in any area but one's own specialized task. Lack of formal authority over all but minor functions makes it difficult to engage in power games typical of the competitive form. Those retaliatory activities that do occur tend to take on a passive aggressive quality—for example, restriction of output, apathy, absenteeism.

While those who do have formal control are conversely free to do whatever they want, they too must live with the fact that the rest of the system, which they have at their command, is passive. It does what it is told to do in a behavioral sense, but it cannot help them discover unforeseen contingencies or new ways to achieve objectives, or new resources for doing so. This may be exactly what the leadership wants. The costs, however, need to be recognized.

Passive bureaucracy resonates with the apathetic orientation at the group level. The position that one's ideas and desires do not make a difference justifies following orders blindly. The failure in actual behavior to share ideas and to take responsibility for one's behavior only encourages those in control to maintain their unilateral style of coordination and to refrain from decentralizing control over resources.

Pyramidal Organization

In the case of the *pyramidal* form of *organization*, top managers are willing to assume that the bulk of the membership is committed to the organization's welfare, but that relatively few people have control over important resources that can determine the organization's success. This results in a pattern of organization that facilitates the broad sharing of plans and objectives, but one that is characterized by a clear hierarchy. The latter ensures that all important decisions are made at the top and encourages one to think of the organization as a pyramid. Imagine, for instance, a small manufacturing firm in a low-technology industry.

Resistance to the logic of the hierarchy is dealt with through the allocation of successfully greater amounts of formal authority to successively higher levels in the pyramid. Members are induced to contribute to the overall plan by the tying of rewards to the success of the total task. They are deterred from deviating from the plan, in turn, by the threats of sanctions from others who have access to more resources than they do.

While differences in formal control over the organization's resources are important for maintaining behavioral compliance, the simultaneous use of collective rewards to induce people to think in behalf of the organization's goals is what guides the development of this organizational form over time. Work flows, divisions of labor, roles, and responsibilities change as top leadership learns what activities are most likely to create the income necessary to fuel the reward system. Clearly, top management cannot provide these rewards continuously from its own resources without eventually depleting the latter. This would encurge it either to develop a more collaborative form of organization if shared plans and rewards were maintained, or to create a passive bureaucracy if legal rights or sheer force were resorted to as the primary means of coordination.

Pyramidal organization resonates with the dependence orientation at the group level because both paradigms involve the acceptance of other people's right to determine one's own choices and to share data relevant to task objectives. The only difference is that at the group level these are responses to personal values, they are ends in themselves, while at the organizational level they are means to an end.

A major problem with this form is that people do not always choose others to depend on who are appropriately placed in the formal hierarchy and distribution of labor. Thus, "informal" organizations develop that compete for control with the formal. This makes it all the more important for top leadership to provide a continuous stream of rewards that are responsive to members' needs.

Caveats to Pursuing Collaborative Organization

It should be abundantly clear to any reader familiar with modern organization life that there are major drawbacks to fostering collaborative organization as a general norm. The difficulties fall neatly into two categories, empirical reality and ideology. Most people in modern societies have *not* been raised to make the welfare of the particular organizations they are working for an extremely high priority. Such loyalty comes more often through positive experience over a long period. One might not expect this to occur much beyond the upper ranks of management in rapidly developing industries where firm membership is changing rapidly or in types of jobs that have a short life span by their nature—for example, project engineering and computer work. In the professions, there even appears to be a shift toward greater emphasis on personal career management at the expense of any particular organization.

Likewise, there are many organizations in which the distribution of control over important resources is highly skewed. While one can argue on a basic level that every human being has much to offer any organization by nature of his or her energy, intellect, and especially human capacity to learn, such factors as socioeconomic background and status, as well as formal training and education, almost guarantee a skewed distribution of resource control. In the fight for organizational survival, managers are often obliged to take advantage of this situation and tailor their control and reward systems to keep and attract those who already possess important resources.

Consequently, it is not surprising that many managers would balk at instituting a uniformly collaborative form for their organization. Pyramidal, passive, and especially competitive paradigms often make much more sense. By the same token, there are probably few moderate to large organizations where at least some subunits do not exist whose conditions are appropriate for collaborative management. Higher levels of management in general, stable professional groups such as those we will discuss in the next chapter, and stable work groups at lower levels, tend to face a reality that embodies both high commitment to the organization's welfare and de facto decentralized resource control with respect to a wide range of important tasks. A major task of the OD specialist is to identify where these pockets exist and focus his or her efforts on them. Part of these efforts may indeed involve helping the client to identify such groups and to accept the need for other forms of management in other parts of the organization.

Even when the objective conditions are right, however, another barrier can stand in the way. This is the ideology of one's key clients and the rest of the organization's management. Few OD projects ever get off the ground unless the primary client and a good number of this person's colleagues possess a basically humanistic orientation. A general preference for participative management and an interest in developing people's talents seem to be critical for developing a sound OD project in the first place and for actually getting something out of it. OD consultants need to determine very quickly whether their prospective clients fit this mode and bow out gracefully when they do not, regardless of the client's overt interest in a project or the incentives he or she may offer. Having encountered an ideal client, moreover, a consultant needs to determine whether the person has sufficient support from colleagues as well as whether the objective conditions discussed above are right.

CONCLUSION

We have defined Organization Development at its most basic level as the attempt to influence the members of an organization to expand their candidness with each other about their views of their organization, and their experience in it, and to take greater responsibility for their own actions as organization members. Individuals who pursue these values, we believe, find themselves involved in a continuous process of both personal learning and organizational renewal. Their organizations change and grow in response to membership needs, rather than become cages in which people play self-defeating games with each other or allow themselves to be used as objects, or accept dependence relationships that stifle personal growth and greater organizational contribution.

On a broader level, we have argued that following these core values in day-to-day interaction has major implications for people's personal relationships with each other and for the character of the organization as a whole. In essence, they represent entry points into a distinct world view. This particular world view is relatively new to modern society. However, it is consistent with current theories of ideal individual health. And it also resonates with a mode of organization that acknowledges the contributions and value of the individual, on the one hand, and collective needs and goals, on the other.

We have also listed a number of cautions that need to be considered before attempting to influence people to assume OD values. Being candid with others about one's organizational experience is difficult when people do not experience psychological safety and at least a modest degree of job security. Taking responsibility for one's actions is difficult if one does not have a basic sense of self-confidence. Relating holistically to others can be threatening if one does not possess a secure identity. Viewing others as equals in some basic sense requires an equally basic sense of competence. Trying to decentralize formal control over resources does not make sense unless the de facto pattern of control is roughly complementary or can easily be made so. And promoting coordination through shared plans and rewards needs to be supported by an underlying commitment to the organization's welfare. Finally, both of the latter require an ideological commitment, however nascent, to humanistic management. These conditions suggest a great deal about when OD is most likely to succeed. In essence, it works best with organizations whose members are mature, psychologically healthy adults, who are committed to the organization's welfare and who have important resources to offer, and whose leaders are willing to risk experimentation to enhance individual and organizational health. Many of today's organizations, or at least major parts thereof, fit these criteria to a considerable degree. Thus, while there are constraints on where OD can work, they are not overpowering. They simply need to be recognized and dealt with realistically.

In the next chapter, we will see the kind of work that can be done through OD when the conditions are favorable.

CHAPTER TWO

DOING OD:
A CONSULTANT'S DIARY

In Chapter One we discussed the goals of Organization Development and set the stage for describing what actually happens in an OD project. This chapter describes one such project in considerable detail. Since this book is about becoming an OD practitioner, we will describe the project from the consultant's viewpoint. Beyond the obvious objective of providing you with a concrete example of what doing OD is like, we want to demystify OD as a process.

This, of course, assumes that OD attracts mystical attributions. In my experience, it does, for both managers and other consultants. There are three major reasons why this happens. First, as you may have already noticed, the goals of OD are rather idealistic. We are in the business of either influencing the basic values of an organization or of helping people articulate their values in terms of behaviors that may initially seem nonsensical or self-destructive, given "the hard facts of the real world." This is different from more technical management consulting and tends to be riskier and therefore more prone to failure. As a result, OD people are likely to be seen as a "little out of the ordinary" as well.

Second, OD requires consultants to develop relationships with their clients that are more emotional than typical business relationships. A manager who may not even know your name one day may after a few days or weeks be sharing important issues with you that he or she rarely discusses with anyone, much less an outsider. The client is often unaware of how this happens. Thus, it is easy for one to be seen as a kind of magician, hopefully a benign one, but a magician nonetheless.

Finally, doing OD frequently involves saying the unsayable in group meetings and proving that the world does not come to a crashing halt as a result. It also involves suggesting courses of action that lead to desirable results, although many clients cannot figure out how or why . Thus, the process itself may become mysterious.

The truth is that OD is like genius—"one percent inspiration and ninety-nine percent perspiration" (Thomas A. Edison). To be sure, there is a uniqueness to it: a series of ideas, technologies, and sentiments that are out of the ordinary, difficult for nonpractitioners to understand, and that produce unusual effects. Using them well takes commitment, training, and experience. But the rest is much like any consulting and/or staff activity in a large organization.

A typical OD activity is shaped in terms of a project. Someone has to initiate it. It has to be sanctioned by the powers that be. This usually requires that it be tied to a fairly specific set of goals, and that it be bounded in such a way that it will not interfere with higher priority tasks. The component activities need to be defined beforehand to indicate who will be involved, in what ways, and for what period of time. Results or evaluations of progress need to be scheduled at critical intervals.

Like most staff work, OD also involves some rational problem-solving phases. After a relationship has been established and some objectives set, data need to be gathered and analyzed, interpretations fed back, and action steps planned and implemented. Many of the techniques OD practitioners use to do this are not typical. For instance, collaboration, personal modeling, and attention to the experience of doing the task itself are stressed. Nonetheless, the basic format is traditional.

In fact, it is this marked contrast between strict adherence to a traditional format and using this format as a vehicle for introducing innovative ways of thinking that helps OD succeed. Following basic procedures that are familiar to the organization's members helps OD make sense to them. Departure from the usual or expected becomes a point of interest and inquiry: "These people seem to know what they are doing; I don't know what is happening now but perhaps I should try to understand." The less credibility one has established as a competent consultant/staff worker in the eyes of clients before departing from the norm, the greater the risk of being discounted before being given a fair hearing. We will say much more about this in later chapters.

The particular project we will describe needs to be put into perspective in two ways. First, it is intended to provide a sampling of OD activities, not a generalizable example of all that OD involves. No single project can do the latter. In the chapter to follow, we will show how this project fits into a broader conceptualization of OD activities in general. Second, the project was conducted by a team of external consultants. Thus, it does not treat the special problems that internal consultants face in doing OD.

This may be seen as a drawback for many readers who envision themselves as internal practitioners. For the purpose of introducing the subject, however, this should not be a major difficulty. The basic activities are the same. I have chosen an externally conducted project because this comes from my experience as a university professor.

GETTING STARTED AT SOUTH CITY CHEMICAL

My work with South City Chemical[1] began in the fall of 1978. One of my OD students referred me to one of this organization's managers at a conference for research managers in the chemical industry. The manager was a member of South City's research and development division. He had asked

---

[1]Disguised name for a large high-technology producer of chemical products.

my student for names of OD practitioners who might be interested in conducting an analysis of his division to identify barriers to and opportunities for the division's further development. I had been working with a large health care organization for the preceding three years and was definitely interested in getting back to an industrial setting where I had received the bulk of my behavioral science training.

A few days later the South City manager called me. Noting my interest, he invited me to visit him and several of his colleagues to discuss my particular approach. He told me I was one of four consultants they were considering and that I would meet with a four-man task force assigned the job of selecting a consultant for the analysis.

I learned a number of other things about South City Chemical during this conversation and another where we ironed out the details of my upcoming visit. First, the project would deal specifically with the research and development division of the company. This was a 250-person operation whose function was product innovation, starting from the conception of new products and proceeding to the point of customer approval. At this point, various marketing and production functions took over.

The division was subdivided into four major product groups plus a facilities management section that was to oversee various services—analytical, pilot plant, library, report writing, building maintenance, personnel, and labor relations for the division. About 100 of the division's members were professionals with varying degrees of research and marketing expertise; the rest were secretaries, administrators, and technicians.

The structure of the division was relatively flat in terms of reporting relationships (see Figure 2–1). A single manager directed 15 to 25 professionals in each product group. The facilities management section had a second tier of managers who headed up the various departments and reported to the facilities manager. The facilities manager and the four product group heads reported to the division manager.

About one-third of the technicians worked in a pool and provided services for a wide variety of activities. Another group worked in the pilot plant. And the rest assisted individual professionals.

FIGURE 2–1
Abbreviated Organization Chart
of the Research and
Development Laboratory
at South City Chemical

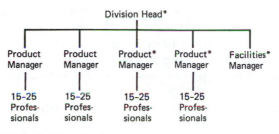

*Selection Team Members

Coordination of individual professional activities was achieved through a complex MBO (management by objectives) process that each product group manager conducted. Coordination of product development activities was achieved through task forces whose membership changed according to the stage of the project's development and that were headed by project leaders. No additional authority was given to the project leaders, who changed as the project developed. Commitments to particular projects were negotiated in terms of segments of a professional's time during the year and coordinated through the MBO process.

The MBO activities and project objectives were aligned through yearly business plans and budgets which were, in turn, integrated into an overall plan for the entire corporation. Division-wide operations were handled by a top management team comprised of the division head, product group heads, facilities manager, and five senior professionals who performed various advisory functions for the division and, in some cases, for other parts of the organization.

Regarding the project itself, there were no burning issues creating the impetus for analysis. The top management team simply decided that the internal state of the division needed some attention. It had been several years since any activity along these lines had taken place. Various managers noted that a wide variety of seemingly unrelated issues were creating "unrest" in the division; therefore, some internal development activity seemed appropriate at the time.

The group assigned the task of selecting a consultant included the division manager, facilities manager, and two product group managers. My contact was one of the product managers. Prior to my first visit, this person sent me: (1) the company's annual report; (2) the division organization chart; (3) a chart showing how the division's resources were apportioned to the various phases of product development; and (4) photocopies of slides the group had used to present the analysis proposal to the top management team.

MEETING THE SELECTION TEAM

My first visit to South City took place over an evening and most of the following day. It began with dinner with all four members of the selection team at a local restaurant. Luckily, I was the first consultant to visit. Thus, they had no immediate reference point for comparison and I could set the stage in any way I wanted. Looking back, I think I essentially won the contract during our first encounter.

After a round of introductions and pleasantries, I found it easy to describe the analyses I had been doing recently in other organizations, and they enlightened me on how their project started. The division had been created by the merger of a more basic research-oriented group and a technical marketing group. Corporate management had done this in an effort to tighten coordination between the two groups at a time when their relations were especially poor. The division had been in its current state for several years.

The division operated on a very tight budget throughout the years following the merger. People's roles had evolved in many unique ways that seemed to have maximized the use of their individual talents. At the same time there had been relatively little upward mobility within the division, and little attention had been given to career development or pathing.

In the years immediately following the merger, people had been quite happy just to hold their own and prove that they and the division could make useful contributions to the organization. But now, many professionals had held the same jobs for five or six years. There were few new people to train to replace them, and there was little idea of how they could rise from where they were. In particular, some marketing personnel were frustrated over not having the power and visibility in the larger organization that they thought their experience now deserved. There was frustration over the lack of additional authority for the project manager role. Some researchers seemed to be dissatisfied with their own career prospects. And there were bits and pieces of other complaints popping up.

None of these complaints had been expressed with great intensity or politicking; but it was clear that there was enough uneasiness to make an analysis worthwhile. The members of the team were also convinced that such an analysis needed to be broad enough to capture the variety of concerns that people might have. They seemed to be saying, *If we are going to do this, let's be thorough about it.*

What I said in return was eventually transformed into a memo (to be discussed in a later section). The basic approach I had recently used while working with a large health care organization (the Northern Medical Center project referred to in Chapter One) seemed to fit their needs very well. It was broad-based and maximized the opportunity for people to speak for themselves. And it could be applied to the entire division.

We also began to get to know each other as individuals in this meeting. Perhaps most interesting to me was the fact that the division manager was familiar with Organization Development. He had participated in a major OD project in another division in the early 1970s that had met with mixed results. Now I understood why, until this moment, no one had mentioned the words "Organization Development." This was to be an "analysis." The idea was officially borne out of the experiences of the two product group heads who had heard about large-scale analyses being undertaken at other chemical firms from their conversations at recent research association conferences. No one flinched when I began to describe myself as an OD consultant, but it was clear that officially we were not doing "OD."

I was a little concerned at first about this message. While I knew the initial request was for an analysis, I was hoping that the door would be open to a variety of OD interventions based on the results of this activity. I became more comfortable, however, as I discovered that the division manager was very interested in behavioral issues, had built his reputation as a manager's manager, and had worked for long periods with other behaviorally oriented consultants around a number of interesting development activities. This was clearly to be an analysis to start with, but there was nothing immediately apparent to prevent it from becoming a lot more. On the contrary, having a primary client with a behavioral orientation suggested that much more might be done.

One other important fact came out of this meeting. The foursome I was dealing with were not totally supported in this endeavor by the rest of their colleagues on the top management team. There had been no overt resistance but some of the other managers had been skeptical about whether an analysis was either necessary, worth the time and attention it might require, or worth the effort that might be required on issues it raised. If I got past the hurdle of being selected by this group, I would still have to convince the rest of the top management team.

The following morning involved two activities. First, I met with the selection team, minus the division manager, to review what we had discussed before and to explore further details of what I was proposing. An interview format that they planned to give other candidates as well is included in Figure 2-2.

This meeting went very smoothly. I had answered most of these questions the night before. The next four hours were spent in interviews with each of the team members, ending with the division manager. Each meeting provided me with new data about the division, and I used it to find out more about each manager's own world—his career, job, concerns, aspirations, hopes for the analysis. We had a very brief meeting as a group following lunch and I went home.

In retrospect, I have not had a better entry experience. I got along well on a personal basis with all four individuals. All four showed a lively interest in my work, and I found them interesting in turn. I felt as if they had been candid about my potential involvement without sacrificing the process they had set up. And they seemed willing to state their own concerns and objectives without worrying about conforming to a "party" line.

Equally important, the setting looked promising. Even under tight budget constraints, the division appeared to be run through a very broad pattern of resource control, and tight coordination was achieved through shared planning. I noted that

FIGURE 2-2
Questions for Consultants

Tell us about organizational analysis.
What is your view of what an analysis is?
What options do we have: (1) paper and pencil, and (2) small group?
What are the pros and cons of different kinds of analyses?
What is the value/danger of an analysis to the organization?

TRACK RECORD

How many analyses conducted?
What types of organizations?
Which companies?

COMPETITION

How do you rate our other candidates?
Why should we choose you over the others?

FINAL QUESTIONS

How would you conduct an analysis? Time scale/costs.
How would you advise communication to the division?

some groups seemed to be rewarded more than others, but the overall ethos was that the division as a whole survived or failed based on everyone's contribution. Thus, the underlying conditions that can make OD work seemed to be there.

Finally, I had been treated in an efficient and professional manner. It was clear that this group was used to working with consultants and that they ran their affairs through tight scheduling, open dialogue, and a commitment to shared goals and procedures. In essence, what I had experienced was consistent with what they told me about how the organization was run.

A MEETING WITH THE TOP MANAGEMENT TEAM

A few weeks later my original contact phoned me to tell me that the team had chosen me as the most suitable consultant. The task now was to convince the rest of the top management team. Though all four selectors would support me, the bulk of the task was mine. We set a date for my next visit and a letter from the clients soon followed (see Figure 2–3).

My next meeting was over dinner with the selection team. We dealt with four issues at this time. First, we went over the points in their letter. There was little controversy here since I either agreed with or was sympathetic to most of the issues they had raised. I did convince them that, since the questions I had proposed were so general in nature, it was really not necessary to "work in phases for different groups of people for different questions." My experience was that these questions would reveal relevant differences across different groups if they existed. When the division manager stressed that he wanted us to interview every person in the division onsite, we also agreed that the scope of this task was sufficiently large to put off consideration of outsiders' views of the division (item 7) and of the views of people officially within the division who were working at other sites (item 8). Both options could be considered after the first phase of the study had been completed.

Second, the clients elaborated on the rest of the management group's concerns about the release of forces they could not control. We decided we could cope with this by making it clear to all involved at the beginning that no changes in response to the study were guaranteed. Management's obligation would be to acknowledge the concerns and desires that were raised by the analysis and to say whether they would act on each issue and if so, in what way, within what time frame, and with what priority. Thus, the study was to be framed as a sensing device where acknowledgment of what was learned would be forthcoming but particular actions not promised. Beyond this, the division manager said he definitely wanted management to respond in constructive ways to as many issues as the division could, given its resources and operating priorities. The study would be a flop if no constructive actions could be taken.

We also discussed each of the other managers in the top management group—their roles, personal styles, priorities, and any hidden agendas they might have. I found these descriptions especially helpful. I would have more confidence going into the next day's meeting with some idea of what to expect.

Third, the division manager made a point of discussing the future of the selection team. He had a lot of experience working with task forces and wanted to make sure

FIGURE 2-3
Excerpts from Client's Letter

We have heard from experts on organizational analysis and have developed from that certain views. Perhaps I should list them:

1. The general idea of the analysis process you described at our meeting is appealing, that is:
   a. Interviews with x people over several days
   b. Digest information, feed back to management group
   c. Management input
   d. Feedback to whole group

2. We may decide to work in phases for different groups of people for different questions.

3. We have become very sensitized to the need for the management group's "ownership" of the process. We must have pretty solid consensus as to the approach and questions among this group for the analysis to be successful.

4. We have also become very sensitized to the great care and attention needed to explain the analysis to the division as a whole. This is to prevent false expectations.

5. The role of our "informal organization" and how it interacts with the formal organization has excited our interest.

6. We have confirmed our initial view that this audit must be, and must be seen to be, directed at achieving specific results (divisionwide effectiveness), rather than at general factors such as morale.

7. We are generally sympathetic to probing outside the division where external influences pose problems or opportunities—for example, it may be smart for the analysis to include people in our production or sales areas if these interfaces cause problems. It is rather suspect to extend this to include customers.

8. We have not yet debated whether to include certain subsidiary research centers in the company in the analysis. We might discuss this (at quite low priority) at our next meeting.

9. I believe some of our management group have concerns about whether an analysis will release forces we cannot control. Perhaps you could briefly discuss how to contain this risk.

Please compose a short writing for us that outlines your proposed project in more detail. We would like to distribute this in preparation for the top management team meeting when we would like to discuss the above and various other issues.

I sent the requested statement in my next letter (see Figure 2-4).

The approach that my colleagues and I use begins on a general level and moves toward specific issues through a series of interviews, feedback presentations and discussions, and problem-solving sessions. The total design of the program is continuously open to critique and modification. A typical sequence of activities might involve the following:

1.   Presentation of the study objectives and methods to the people who will be directly involved.

2.   Individual interviews with the sample selected.

The interviews inquire into such topics as: (a) how people define their job priorities; (b) their expectations of the others with whom they work most closely; (c) their perceptions of others' expectations of them; (d) their perceptions regarding the current effectiveness of these relationships; (e) perceptions of how current division policies help and hinder them from performing effectively; (f) what they would like the division and their subgroups to do more, the same, or less of; (g) what they personally would like to do more, the same, or less of; (h) particular problem areas they would like to raise for attention; (i) personal aspirations for the study. A brief written questionnaire can also be administered to tap opinions or issues of particular interest to top management.

3.   The next step is for my colleagues and me to digest these data and feed them back. The specifics of the design are usually worked out with a planning committee before being implemented. There are some base-line principles we work under, however. First, every person interviewed must be fed back to in some form. This maintains the integrity of the process. Second, the data are presented in a form that does not identify *particular* individuals either as the authors of particular perceptions or as the recipients thereof. This both contributes to the integrity of the process and encourages people to focus on *what* are the problems or opportunities facing the division and not *who* are the problems or opportunities. A partial exception to this might occur when an individual manager wants feedback on others' perceptions of his/her performance. In this case, we might present relevant data to this person privately but not to other managers and do so without identifying particular authors. Third, data are fed back only to those people to whom it has been agreed to beforehand are relevant. Thus, data fed back to the top management group as a whole would pertain to issues facing the division as a whole, while data relevant only to a particular department's concerns would be fed back only to that department. It would be up to the manager of that department to decide whether he or she wanted to share them more broadly thereafter. Fourth, managers of particular subunits are given the data relevant to their subunits first. After discussing the data with the consultants, they decide if any adjustments should be made before the data are forwarded to subordinates. Fifth, a consultant is present whenever data are fed back for the first time in order to facilitate discussion, clarify the intent of the design, and help individuals deal with important issues.

We have found that operating within these guidelines minimizes problems in confidentiality and use of the data for evaluating individuals (which is not our intent), and it maximizes attention to systemic issues that can be treated in subsequent problem-solving sessions. The guidelines also permit flexibility in feedback methods to be used.

FIGURE 2-4 *Continued*

The form of the data fed back can be as open-ended as a package of anonymous quotations that reveal the variety of viewpoints within the division on important issues, to a series of specific interpretations by the consultants that are backed up by quotations. The sequence used in feeding back the data starts from top management and moves downward so that there are no surprises for superiors in what subordinates will hear. At the same time we make every effort to get the people who receive the data to discuss their reactions to them, elaborating on particular ideas, discounting others, and so on, so that everyone is satisfied that the data actually reflect the thinking of people within the organization.

4.   Once the data are fed back and people have discussed their reactions to them on a general level, the time is ripe for at least one long (all-day) problem-solving session with the top management group. The purpose of this activity is: (a) to come to some consensus about the current state of the division; (b) to draw a picture of an ideal state for this unit; (c) to identify discrepancies between the current state and the ideal; (d) to prioritize the issues to be worked on; and (e) to devise action plans for dealing with each issue.

that one particular phenomenon he had found common to them would not occur. This was that the task force would become permanently identified with the project and other members of the top management team would see it as the selection team's project and not their own. The division manager, on the contrary, wanted to do everything he could to make sure that this became the top management team's project and not just the selection team's. He said if all went well on the following day he would disband the selection team. The facilities manager would become my primary contact. I, and whoever assisted me, would be expected to get to know all top management team members equally well. And in the immediate future, my visits would involve dinners and lunches with the other members to facilitate this. I agreed that this was a wise move. However, I was disappointed at having to reduce my contact with this particular group, which I was just getting to know and finding quite enjoyable.

Finally, I talked about the people whom I was thinking of inviting to work with me on the analysis. Although I wanted to select my own staff, I also wanted the team to know something about them and their skills. I had three people in mind, all graduate students in my department, Organizational Behavior at Case Western Reserve University. Two of them, Alan Jensen and Cathy Spitz, were third-year Ph.D. students and had held summer internships doing OD in large research organizations. Additionally, I had worked with Alan for over a year in another OD project and had been Cathy's advisor. The third student, Vishal Gujral, was a second-year Ph.D. student and my advisee. This would be his first field experience. I thought he would be an attractive participant because he had a B.S. in physics and a firm appreciation for the hard sciences, the world of our clients. The team seemed pleased with these people's backgrounds and was quite happy to go ahead with them.

The next day we met in one of the division's conference rooms. Twelve of us sat at a square table, I to the right of the division manager and the three selection team members interspersed among the other managers. The division manager began the meeting by reviewing the activities of the selection team from the time they were asked to select a consultant. He introduced me next and said that the bulk of the meeting would be devoted to a discussion between the rest of the group and me. He ended his opening speech by saying that he wanted this to be a candid discussion of people's concerns about and hopes for the analysis: "People should speak now or forever hold their peace, because once the meeting is over we will be in this together." I felt grateful for his support but at the same time a little anxious that he might be forcing the project on some of those present.

I was then given the floor and proceeded to say a little more about myself. A few eyes lit up when I mentioned that this would be my fourth project with large R&D organizations, one of which had integrated its marketing functions with research in similar ways. I also talked about my department at Case Western Reserve University and the kinds of work we did in general. I ended by going over the memorandum that had been distributed to the group, which dwelt in particular on dealing with raised expectations as a result of the analysis.

We spent the following two hours patiently going over everything the selection team and I had done. We went over the selection procedures to clarify why a local university had not been selected for this study. Some members described an analysis conducted just prior to the creation of the division. This analysis had not been fruitful and critics accused its principals of singling out certain people who were fired during the merger of the marketing and research groups. People wanted assurance that the current project would be qualitatively different from the previous one; I assured them it would. Certain managers spoke of particular expectations they would not want to deal with if they came out of the study, and we discussed how to respond to them by being up front about them from the beginning. I discussed the prospective members of the team. People were intrigued by the idea of working with a woman consultant in this male-dominated organization, and thought that Vishal's Indian background would be an asset, since a number of the division's professionals were also from Eurasian and Asian countries. The division manager helped bring out individual concerns and ensured inputs from all present. Twenty minutes before the appointed end of the meeting, he made a final request for major concerns. There were none, so we discussed what to do next.

We made two decisions in these final minutes. First, we decided that I would bring my team on the next visit and, second, that we would begin the project by interviewing the top management team. I also suggested that the analysis be introduced to a dozen other people whom the managers saw as important opinion leaders in the division, even though they were not on the top management team. These people would also be interviewed on our next visit and would be enlisted along with the top management team to introduce the analysis to the rest of the professional staff.

Equally important, someone raised the issue of clearing the project with the union to which all of the technicians belonged. Everyone agreed that as many hourly personnel as possible should be interviewed and that the union's support was critical. The division manager would contact the union administration to discuss the project before our next visit.

My visit ended with a dialogue with the division manager. We reviewed the events of the meeting and agreed that things had gone well. We also agreed I would write a contract and send it to him in plenty of time for a formal response, and thus a firm agreement, before the next visit. The letter that served as our contract for the following year is repeated with only minor disguises in Figure 2–5.

Beyond the business of the contract, the only other noteworthy item we discussed was the problem of gaining approval from the union. The division manager thought the union would support the project since they had agreed to similar activities in other parts of the organization. He was also aware, however, that he had yet to discuss the project with union personnel. He was wondering how they would respond, knowing that considerable momentum within the management ranks had already developed.

FIGURE 2–5
The Contract Letter

January 19, ____

Dear Client:

Pursuant to my conversations with you and your management team on December 15, ____ , I am proposing the following guidelines for an analysis of the division:

1.   The basic objective of the analysis will be to collect, share, and study information from the professional and technical staff that will allow this group to identify opportunities for and barriers to improving the effectiveness of the division.

2.   The general character and sequence of the activities to be undertaken to achieve this objective and the ethical considerations to be subscribed to during this process are outlined in the memorandum I presented to your management team in preparation for our meeting on December 15, ____ (relevant sections of which are attached).

3.   The details of particular activities proposed in the aforementioned memorandum will be established collaboratively among you, your management team, myself, and my colleagues.

4.   While it may not be necessary to interview each and every member of the division, our focus will be on the division as a whole, and we will attempt to tap the perspectives of every major group within its boundaries.

5.   Fees (confidential).

6.   In regard to the nature of South City Chemical's business and the extent to which I and my colleagues would be privy to information of a product, productivity, product cost, technological and employee nature, I and my colleagues would agree not to directly or indirectly, disclose or use, either during or after the life of this project, any secret or confidential information, knowledge of data of South City Chemical, without prior written consent of South City Chemical, subject to the following understanding: A subsidiary objective of our work with you is to gain knowledge and experience that will enable us to contribute to the art or science of Organization Development. The contribution may well take several forms—doctoral theses, recognized behavioral sci-

FIGURE 2-5 *Continued*

ence journals, formal books of a text nature that may be references to practitioners in the applied behavioral sciences, and professional papers delivered at meetings of the profession. To this end we would agree to submit material, proposed for publication, to you and your management team well in advance of a publication date. Written material, thus submitted, which did not meet, in your opinion, the criterion of saving you, your colleagues, or South City Chemical from embarrassment or damage, would be jointly revised to the mutual satisfaction of the parties.

There might, of course, be cases in which we would draw on experiences with you in the context of general writings and where the project itself was not identified. In such cases we would not be obliged to consult with you. We would consult with you, however, whenever it was clear that we were writing about our work in a large R&D division.

7. Case Western Reserve University cannot enforce any Security Undertaking that you might ask us to sign. While we would agree to sign such a document, subject to the constraints noted above, it would be up to each of us as individuals to abide by this agreement.

Using the following assumptions, it looks as if the data gathering phase will cost roughly \$_____.

1. Pairs of us interview the 18–22 most significant professionals at a rate of four per day.

2. One-on-one interviews with each of the other 60 professionals at a rate of four per day per interviewer.

3. A representative sample of 50 technical personnel are interviewed one-on-one at a rate of 8 per day.

The remainder of the proposed budget should be sufficient to conduct personal feedback sessions with you regarding data from each of your areas; to hold group feedback sessions with eight to ten people at a time covering the entire division, and to hold an all-day session with the management team to review the data and begin to plan how to respond to it.

I will be working with three graduate assistants (Vishal Gujral, Alan Jensen, and Cathy Spitz). Provided we can fill our schedules appropriately, it will take nine days to do the interviewing. I propose that we make three two-day visits beyond the initial three days planned for February 7, 8, and 9. If we did this at biweekly intervals, we would be done with the data collection phase by the end of March. I will be unavailable during the first two weeks in April but could start the feedback sessions in the latter part of that month. A reasonable target data for completing the project as proposed would be the end of May.

Regarding our upcoming visit, my understanding is that the bulk of our time will be spent interviewing the 18–22 (you pick the exact number) most influential people in the division. We might meet with you on the evening of the 6th to work out any issues of concern to you in this letter; then have a joint meeting with the people to be interviewed on Wednesday morning to answer questions about the process and proceed from there to the interviews. Each of our pairs could do three on Wednesday, four on

FIGURE 2-5 *Continued*

Thursday, and four on Friday. This adds up to 22 potential interviews with pairs of us. If you have a smaller number in mind for the most potent group, we can split pairs and interview other professionals one-on-one in the time remaining.

I have also enclosed a draft of a memo which you might pass on to _____ for introducing the project to those to be interviewed who are not part of the management team. I will call _____ to work out the details of this.

I trust you had a pleasant holiday season and look forward to seeing you on the 7th. If there are any issues you want to discuss immediately, please call me at _____.

With warmest regards,

Eric H. Neilsen
Associate Professor

MORE ENTRY MEETINGS

We had three more introductory meetings between the time of the events described above and the start of the interviews. The first was a cocktail/dinner party to introduce the top management team to my colleagues, Alan, Cathy, and Vishal. This meeting went well for reasons beyond our control. Enroute to the dinner, our car had a flat tire in a deserted area. We arrived almost two hours late, hungry and tired but also embarrassed and eager to please. The management team members had had time for a couple of cocktails each and were quite happy to listen to our tale of woe. Needless to say, breaking the ice was easy; formal introductions were kept to a minimum. We went to bed with little or no anxiety about the formal meeting to be held the following morning.

The second meeting, the reader will remember, was intended to introduce the project to a dozen other opinion leaders in the division in the presence of both the top management group and the analysis team. We began by meeting for a few minutes with the top management group to make sure we all knew each other. Then the other managers joined us and the meeting began in earnest.

Once again the division manager introduced the analysis, this time by retelling the history of the selection procedure. He ended by saying that we had been selected because we seemed to know more about research organizations than our competitors. Also, his rationale for using an external consulting team was that we could be more objective, like people from Mars who could assess the division with a minimum of political interests and biases.

My teammates and I introduced ourselves and I went over the analysis plan once again. The question-and-answer session that followed was very similar to the one I had had with the management team. Similar questions were asked. The only difference was that now I had reinforcers on both sides. When I did not understand a question or respond to it effectively, either one of my colleagues or the members of the top management team would chime in. I remember feeling more like an orchestra conductor than a player at this time.

The new participants asked two novel questions. First, one person found it hard to believe that we were being brought in if the division manager did not think he had a problem; therefore, what *was* the problem? In response to this, I simply reiterated what I had been told, adding that organizations, like people, had "seven-year itches" and needed a periodic assessment of their health as a matter of preventive maintenance.

Second, the division manager was asked why he did not do the analysis himself instead of asking outsiders to do it. After all, was it not his responsibility to know what people were thinking? The division manager reiterated what he had said at the beginning of the meeting: An external analysis would be more objective.

Somehow I was not sure that our answers were convincing. The slight tension I was experiencing would have to be resolved through our future behavior.

As soon as this meeting was over, we were whisked into another for which we were considerably less prepared. This one was with two senior union personnel with no one from management present. The division manager had called me the week before to say that such a meeting might take place. We had agreed that it could be a useful step in gaining the union's approval that, as of yet, had neither been given nor denied. However, as the division manager was on his way out the door, having introduced us to each other, I suddenly realized that I had given little thought to exactly what I would say. The four of us had simply agreed the night before that we would be candid and let the chips fall where they might. By contrast, it soon became clear that the union people knew exactly what they were up to.

It was not long before I found myself describing the history of the project to date, the nature of our approach to analyzing organizations, and the various steps in our proposal. The division manager had followed our posture of being candid to the point of sharing our contract letter and the preceding note on our approach with these people. Thus, what I said was not new, but it was no doubt just as good a way for us to present ourselves to them as it had been with the managers. Many of the usual questions followed. I had the feeling I was reciting catechism.

With these preliminaries over, we got down to brass tacks. One of the union managers, who was responsible for the plant site, did most of the talking. He told us that the union was concerned about several things.

Union–management relations were currently quite good, but had taken years to develop. A decade before, the company had been very paternalistic. The tenor of relations had gradually shifted to a legalistic nature and only recently had reached the point where a spirit of collaboration was evident around certain projects. In light of this, the union wanted nothing to happen that would jeopardize current relations. In particular, it was important that the analysis would treat union personnel on an equal footing with management in terms of feedback provided. Moreover, as the more talkative union man put it: "There is no doubt that, at the end of the analysis, management will foot your bill. But it is not at all certain that we will be any better off."

I asked how the union or its members might be hurt by the analysis. This launched us into a discussion of the division's previous OD experience. It had occurred just prior to the merger of the marketing and research groups. People had been asked to state their views candidly about each other and their work during the project; and not long after, a sizeable number of research and marketing managers had been let go. Although the union personnel had been protected by their contract during this purge, many were convinced they had unwittingly played a role in these dismissals. They were afraid this might happen again. Moreover, our union representative told us that, although the current division manager was respected by the union, he was afraid that people's memories of the previous effort might "poison" our data.

Another reservation centered around the collaborative activities that union and management had recently developed. These activities had the same behaviorally oriented flavor to them—for example, more informal, face-to-face discussions of work hours, worker health and safety, and so on—and had taken a long time to get going. The union was surprised that the union–management group that had sanctioned these efforts had not been consulted about our analysis and had not been invited to join the activity from the beginning.

In spite of these issues, the meeting seemed to go well interpersonally. We found a few things in common to chat about in terms of our personal backgrounds and interests. Alan, whose father had been a union member, established an easy rapport from the beginning. We left the meeting not knowing whether the union would support the analysis, but felt we had done a good job of presenting our case. The union people had shown us that they could behave as professionally as anyone else.

This combination of uncertainty over support, plus pleasant interpersonal relations, was also evident in the last introductory meeting that took place on the evening of the same day at a nearby motel. We met with the facilities manager, who was standing in for the division head, the two union administrators we had met with earlier, and six union stewards who represented the various work groups within the division. We followed the same format as in the previous meetings and ended with dinner, where we interspersed ourselves among the stewards around a large table.

As dinner progressed and tongues loosened with the wine and pleasant surroundings, the stewards became intrigued by our proposed activities. We would have little trouble working with them if they agreed to do so. However, the conversations we engaged in returned again and again to the earlier OD project. We had been assured in the meantime that the project had not been a significant factor either in precipitating the merger of the marketing and research groups or in the selection of those to be dismissed. Nonetheless, there was no way of proving this point. As outsiders, we had to take both management and the union at face value. Both sides knew it, and there was little we could do other than await the outcome of their respective deliberations.

A couple of weeks later, the union agreed to take a neutral stance toward the analysis. Management would publicize the project among the union members within the division. Union members who were willing to be interviewed would be allowed to do so with no interference from the union. However, the union would not push the project; if a union member asked the advice of a steward, he would be told to make up his own mind. In return, some union administrators would have access to the data to be fed back to the division management, receive it when the top management team did, and participate in some of the feedback sessions where union personnel were present.

Both we and the division manager had hoped for more. Only one-fourth of the union personnel signed up for interviews. This led to some interesting dynamics in the feedback sessions (to be discussed later) that almost all of the union people attended.

CONDUCTING THE INTERVIEWS

Interviews began on the afternoon of the day when the meetings just discussed took place. As suggested in our contract letter (Figure 2–5), we interviewed the 24 most potent people in the division in three days, working in pairs. Each interview lasted about two hours and addressed at a minimum the following questions:

1.   Tell me about your job. What do you do from day to day, regardless of whether it is in your job description?

2.   How would you prioritize the various aspects of your job?

3.   Whom do you work with most closely (3–5 people)?

4.   What do you expect from each of these people?

5.   What do you think they expect from you?

6.   How well are these expectations being met?

7.   How do the current structure and policies of the division help or hinder you from doing your job effectively?

8.   In what ways have things been changing, remaining the same, in the division over the past several years?

9.   Suppose you had three magic wishes, how would you use them to make the division more effective?

10.   What would you personally like to do more of, the same, and less of?

11.   What problems in particular should our analysis bring the division's attention to?

12.   What are your personal aspirations for this study?

We interviewed in pairs to start for a number of reasons. First, we wanted to maximize our exposure as a group to each of these important people, so we would get to know each other as rapidly as possible. Second, doubling up increased the probability that at least one friendship with an interviewee would develop and lay the groundwork for more significant collaboration later on.

Third, this tactic allowed us to "calibrate" our interviewing styles. While our personal styles would inevitably influence the data we gathered, it was important to establish some uniformity in our probing on particular questions. We also switched off with each other so that all possible pairs could interview together several times. We also benefited by observing each other in an interview setting.

Fourth, doubling up spread the work load of typing these especially important conversations and provided opportunities for cross-checking our observations. The latter helped us assess the less tangible aspects of the interviews (the emotional tone of the encounter and significant nonverbal behaviors) and enhanced our understanding of the interviewees' responses to particular questions.

Finally, by continuously changing pairs, we developed rapidly as a group. We each had something in common to talk about with each other at the end of three days. And no one was inequitably left out of important interviews or stuck with the less exciting encounters.

To make sure we were on board with each other, we typed these interviews as soon as we returned from this visit, and read and critiqued each other's material. We interviewed alone thereafter, and covered the rest of the division's 100 professionals plus 34 union members during the next six weeks.

Most of our comments about the interview process will be covered in Chapter Nine. Likewise, significant interview content will be reviewed in later sections of this chapter. However, there were some unique aspects of the study worth mentioning here.

To begin with, our respondents (outside of the first 24) varied immensely in their depth of knowledge about the study. We had provided a sample memo for senior managers to introduce the activity to their staffs. However, some respondents heard only that their manager had introduced the project at a meeting, which they happened to have missed; others had been given photocopies of our contract letter. In any case, it was almost always necessary to review the project with whomever we interviewed.

At first, I was a little annoyed at this need for continuous rehashing. Later, however, I realized that this behavior was consistent with the way the division worked in general. It was a byproduct, in all likelihood, of work life in a very flatly structured organization. Every manager or professional was involved in a myriad of activities with overlapping groups. Consequently, there was little work history that was shared in the same way by everyone involved. A great many meetings required historical recitations to get everyone on board. We found that most of the staff were quite good at this; by the end of the interviewing we had become quite adept at it, too.

Even though our respondents showed an interest in us as individuals and in our work, they were skeptical that the analysis would lead to any useful results. Many of our interviews were stimulating. Almost everyone cooperated and rapport was easily established. People were extremely candid and took delight in spinning theories with us on why the division operated the way it did and what the consequences were.

At the same time, people's predictions of outcomes for the study and their criteria for success were extremely modest. Generally, people thought the study would be successful if a few noticeable policy changes resulted. The changes did not necessarily have to be successful in the long run if they were logical and deliberate responses to the data and showed that top management was listening.

This feature is worth pointing out because it revealed that the system was ready for change and experimentation long before the study data were fed back. What had been missing was the sanction for such activity, not the energy to carry it through.

Last, it is important to note that we used the interview process as an opportunity for mutual education. While we tried to make sure that our respondents had plenty of time to answer our questions and to direct the discussion to things they wanted to talk about, we also made a conscious effort to let them get to know us, our department, our conceptual approaches, and so on. Often we would take a half-baked theory into an interview, and after our respondent had a chance to offer unbiased data, we would share our theory and ask for opinions. The resulting discussion would lead to an altered theory to be taken to the next interview, and so on.

We have no doubt that as the days went by, people talked about us and our ideas and this affected the data we subsequently gathered. This was fair game from our viewpoint, however. We were not scientists looking for unbiased data but collaborative analysts looking for ways to be biased that reflected the understanding and concerns of the members of the division.

ANALYZING THE INTERVIEW DATA

Our interviews yielded approximately 500 pages of typewritten notes. The procedure we used to digest these data and prepare various feedback documents is reviewed in Figure 2–6. This is the introduction to the division-wide feedback document, copies of which were made available to all division members prior to the feedback sessions.

FIGURE 2–6
Introduction to the Feedback Document

MEMORANDUM   May 9, _____

To: Members of the Development Division

From: Professor Eric Neilsen, Cathy Spitz, Vishal Gujral, Gervase Bushe,*
                and Alan Jensen

Subj: Organizational Analysis of the Division

This is the master document for our analysis of the division. We created it from our interviews with 134 of you, covering all members of the salaried staff and a sample of hourly personnel. It is long (you said a great deal), and since the format may be unfamiliar to you, we would like to start with an explanation of how we put it together and how we think it might best be used.

How We Analyzed the Data

We started by transcribing each of the interviews and looking for common topics that people seemed to dwell on. Some of these, of course, stemmed from the kinds of questions we asked, while others emerged from your choices as to what to focus on as our conversations progressed. Armed with these topics, we then went back through each interview and gathered the quotations related to each topic, creating new topic categories in the process or restating initial ones in order to cover as many issues that were raised by more than a few people that we could identify.

The next step was to group the quotations under each topic in terms of common themes, positions taken, or opposite views of the same issue. We then arranged these

*During the interview process, Alan Jensen had to leave the project to respond to another commitment. Gervase Bushe, a second-year graduate student, filled in for him.

FIGURE 2-6   *Continued*

clusters of quotations (separated by asterisks) in a sequence that seemed palatable for reading, alternating positive views with negative observations with action suggestions, and so on.

Next, we "cleaned" the data in the sense that we omitted potentially offensive language, occasionally rewrote a phrase so that a particular person could not be identified, and generally saw to it that we had followed the principle of anonymity in terms of particular authors and targets of personal comments.

Finally, we wrote a summary statement for each topic, reviewing the kinds of views expressed under it. In the document that follows these are grouped together in an initial statement, as well as stated separately at the beginning of the sections of quotations related to them.

Please bear in mind that except for some very general observations, these summary statements are not intended to convey a reading of either the intensity of particular views or the number of people who voiced them. Our intent in this document is to share with you the diversity of the issues you discussed and the diversity of the ideas you expressed regarding them. We invite you to think of the document as a series of snapshots of life in the division, taken from many different angles.

How to Use the Document

The most thorough approach we have in mind would be as follows:

1.   Read the summary statement at the beginning to get a feel for the data.

2.   Read each section to get an idea of the ways people actually talked about the issues.

3.   Are there important views we have left out? Are your views included in some way under each topic?

4.   Of all the topics discussed, which are the most important to you personally (make a list)?

5.   Under each topic on your list, which views would you like to discuss with the people you work with; either because you do not understand them or because you want to explore their intensity, or because you think action should be taken in response to them?

Over the next few weeks a series of meetings will be held to discuss the data. Your manager and a consultant will be present at the one you attend. Leaders of major groups will attend meetings with their colleagues and superiors as well as with their subordinates. We hope to use these meetings for three purposes:

1.   As a vehicle for confirming, discounting, restating, elaborating the data;

2.   As an opportunity to appreciate the division for what it is today and to expand your awareness of its functioning; and

3.   As a tool for identifying where your concerns and energies lie regarding problems to be resolved and opportunities for improving the way the division operates.

The next step will be for your leadership to use their experiences in these meetings to develop appropriate responses to your concerns and energies.

Two other types of documents are being prepared. One deals with issues of particular concern to each major group. The other one contains feedback for particular managers who requested it. Both will follow similar formats and the same constraints on anonymity for quoters. You should have access to your group document before your feedback meeting. This goes only to your group. Each personal feedback document will go only to the particular person being discussed in it.

It has been an interesting task thus far, and we look forward to the feedback sessions.

Table of Contents

A.   People's Perceptions of Their Jobs and What It Is Like to Work in the Division

B.   People's Perceptions of the Division's Work Philosophy

C.   The Quality of Relationships with Peers

D.   Quality of Relationships with Superiors

E.   Relationships with Subordinates

F.   Division Identity

G.   On the Present Structure of the Division

H.   Consequences of a Flat Organization

I.   Diversity of Groups in the Division: Autonomy Versus Uniformity

J.   Status Differences Among Major Job Groupings

K.   Project Leadership: A Controversial Activity

L.   MBO: The Instrument and Its Use

M.   Ability to Advance in the Division/South City Chemical

N.   Rewards in the Division

O.   Skill Development (Learning Opportunities)

P.   Union–Management Relations

Q.   Information Meetings

R.   The Division's Relationship to South City Chemical and Its Environment

S.   Stability Versus Change

T.   Interests, Desires, Expectations, Concerns, Motivations Surrounding the Analysis

FEEDING BACK THE DATA

The feedback sessions themselves were planned in the sequence agreed to in the contract letter. After we had analyzed the data for several weeks, we called the division manager and suggested the formats we eventually used. Once we obtained approval, we worked up a complete draft of the division-wide document and sent it to him for more detailed comments. These were discussed during a day-long visit where we also developed a schedule of feedback meetings for the rest of the division.

While it was only natural for us to spend part of this day discussing the content of the interview results, we devoted the bulk of the time to strategizing around the feedback process itself. Regardless of what the data said, we wanted to enlist the division manager's help as a collaborator in the feedback process. For instance, we wanted to make certain that the format was palatable, that the meetings were sequenced logically, that the appropriate people were attending each meeting, that the general format for conducting the group meetings was not too much a departure from the way meetings were normally run, and that the division manager would be behind what we were doing because he had indeed helped to plan it.

This visit went without incident. We spent the next week polishing the division document and preparing the individual and group feedback documents as well. We sent 15 copies of the finished division document for distribution to the top management team and union representatives a week prior to our first meeting to discuss the data from this group. Figure 2–7 shows the schedule we followed thereafter.

Some readers may find these details boring. I have included them to emphasize that a great deal of the OD process is administrative dog-work. Involvement in administrative detail can contribute to the higher goals of a project, however. For instance, in this study we really got to know what it was like to work with the division manager during this period, and vice versa. We also discovered that we shared a concern for efficient, professional preparation. This gave us credibility in each other's eyes at a time when mutual support was especially important.

Space constraints make it impossible to discuss in detail the 50 hours of meetings that followed over the next two weeks. I do, however, want to comment on the general character of what we did. To begin with, we tried to use the meetings to do more than simply feed back data. The meetings were also used for gathering further data to test our interpretations of the interviews, and simultaneously, as opportunities for collaborative problem solving around the issues recognized and agreed to be important. We invited this strategy implicitly in the introduction to the feedback data, and designed individual and group meetings to encourage this as well.

FIGURE 2-7
South City Chemical
New Products Division

To: Division Managers/Advisors   Date: May 15, _____

From: Divison Managers   Revision #2

Re: Neilsen and Associates Analysis Feedback

For group feedback sessions the consultants will work in pairs so that two teams can meet simultaneously. Group meetings will take place in Conference Rooms 1 and 2. Personal feedback sessions will take place in the individual's office.

DATE

May 14	9:00–11:00	Consultants discuss division document plus personal feedback document with division manager.
	2:00–?	Management team plus union representative review document as a group with the consultants (document distributed

FIGURE 2-7   *Continued*

beforehand). Individual managers will receive their group and personal feedback documents at the end of this meeting but will not discuss them on this day.

May 16	8:00–9:30	Consultants meet with Mr. A to discuss division, group, and personal feedback data.
	9:30–11:00	Consultants meet with Mr. B to discuss division, group, and personal feedback data.
	1:00–2:30	Consultants meet with Mr. C to discuss division, group, and personal feedback data.
	2:30–4:30	Consultants meet with Mr. D to discuss division, group and personal feedback data.
May 17	8:30–10:30	Consultants meet with Mr. E to discuss division, group, and personal feedback data.
	10:30–12:30	Consultants meet with Mr. F to discuss division, group, and personal feedback data.
	1:00–3:00	Consultants meet with Mr. G to discuss division, group, and personal feedback data.
	3:00–5:00	Consultants meet with Mr. H to discuss division, group, and personal feedback data.
May 22	8:00–9:30	Consultants meet with Mr. I to discuss division, group, and personal feedback data.
	9:30–12:00	Mr. A plus group Mr. B plus group and other division personnel
	1:00–4:30	Mr. E plus rest of Analytical Group Mr. F plus rest of group
May 24	8:30–12:00	Mr. G plus half of group Mr. H plus half of group
	1:00–4:30	Mr. G plus rest of group Mr. H plus rest of group
May 28	8:30	Mr. I plus half of his group
	12:00	Mr. B plus pilot plant group
	1:00	Mr. I plus rest of his group
	4:30	Mr. I plus Technical Publications Group
May 29	8:00–10:00	Management Group feedback
	10:00–6:00	All-day Management Team–Open Systems Planning Session (lunch provided)

We usually began the meetings with individual managers by asking for their gut responses to the data. Well before this meeting, each manager would have received his individual feedback data (3 to 10 pages), a document of similar length with themes and quotations specific to his group, plus the division-wide document. We would ask him to start anywhere he wanted to, including his thoughts about the process itself.

Most people felt that we had produced an almost overwhelming amount of material to digest thoroughly. They also recognized, however, that the individual and group documents focused on what was relevant for a particular person or group in the division-wide document. The latter, in turn, could be used to put any particular person or group situation in a broader perspective. Thus, although there were not quantitative indices to help people compare themselves or their groups with others, or for interpreting the data quickly, there were clearly qualitative methods available for doing this.

Most managers responded to our opening gambit in a fairly predictable pattern. They usually informed us that there were few, if any, surprises in what they had read. We tended to respond to this with enthusiasm, since the documents were intended to reflect the reality of life in the division as people actually experienced it. Thus, someone who saw no surprises was clearly in touch with the current culture. Logically, this would then set the stage for action-oriented problem solving around particular issues. Often this is what happened, with the manager picking an issue that was quite remote from what the data suggested might be of immediate concern to him.

In most cases, especially if we had established good rapport, the conversation would gradually drift back to issues that were closer to home—for example, a particular theme in the personal feedback data, a pressing problem in the group document, or a controversial issue in the division-wide document that the manager in question had already taken a strong stand on. Up until this point in the meeting, our role would have been simply to draw out the manager by trying to help him state his ideas clearly and appreciating what he had to say. We continued to do this around the more sensitive issues if we were asked. On occasion, we offered our own ideas as well.

How articulate we were about our own ideas depended, in turn, on how well we had interpreted the data. On the evening before each interview we would go over a manager's data plus our experiences of this person, trying to predict how he might respond to the documents and, therefore, what issues we might be facing together at this point in the conversation. We would think about conceptual inputs that might be helpful to him, things we wanted to say about relevant aspects of our own experience, what we would do under the same conditions, useful ways to assess the situation further before taking action, and so on. We would also decide how important it was to us personally and to the project to confront the manager in question on particular issues, and sometimes even how we might get the conversation started around these issues if it did not occur naturally.

Our predictions never worked perfectly, but preparing this way was clearly helpful. It gave us a starting place and often provided bits and pieces of ideas that were useful in ways and in contexts we had not anticipated. Our clients seemed to appreciate it because it indicated we had given some thought to them as individuals. It was a way of not only analyzing data together, but trying to do something meaningful in response to them.

The last 45 minutes of each feedback meeting was set aside to prepare for the group meeting(s) that we and the manager had scheduled with his subordinates. We offered the same basic format to everyone and then encouraged modifications to fit each manager's preferences and the particular conditions he faced. We asked the manager to imagine how his group would respond; and using these data plus the group document, we would prepare for the meeting together in much the same way we had prepared for our meeting with the manager on the night before.

The basic group format was as follows. The meeting started with the manager asking each person to offer one reaction to the group and division documents. It could be a statement about the process, an addition to/subtraction from/query about the data, a request to the group to pay attention to a particular issue, or a statement out of the blue. The intent of this activity was to generate an agenda for the next three hours' discussion. Summaries of what was said were put on flipcharts and, going around the room, people could offer as many ideas as they wanted to. Since this was introduced as an agenda-setting activity, people usually commented only once and rarely more than twice. (A typical variation on this procedure was to give each person five minutes of air time to comment on the data in whatever way he or she thought was relevant.)

The group then addressed topics from this list that were agreeable to everyone. As in the case of individual interviews, the first ones picked were usually the least important, and discussion would once again shift gradually into more critical issues. Likewise, sometimes we and the manager were well prepared for what turned out to be critical and sometimes we were not.

The last 45 minutes of these meetings were devoted to preparing the manager to take the group's outputs to the division-wide planning session, where the responses to the feedback activities would be reviewed and division-wide action considered. Here the typical procedure was to ask each person to take the chalk or magic marker and check three issues recorded during the meeting that he or she thought needed the most attention from division-wide management. The activity often began with an air of nonchalance, but frequently ended with a touch of solemnity, as if an important symbolic ritual were being enacted, that is, the group voice was being invoked.

The checks were tallied and occasionally some issues restated or clarified. The meeting would typically end with the manager restating his own hopes and his understanding of what was being said.

We followed this format quite closely in about two-thirds of our group feedback meetings. Most of the managers proved to be quite skillful at drawing out and listening to their subordinates' viewpoints. This was consistent with the feedback data on superior–subordinate relations. The latter suggested that communication, when it occurred, was good. If there was a shared problem in this area, it was that there was simply not enough vertical communication. This, in turn, suggested why most of these meetings went so well; they were opportunities to communicate about a great many issues that were often given short shrift in the rush to complete technical tasks.

Not all of the meetings went as expected. However, those that did not were easy to understand in retrospect. They almost always involved union personnel who had not volunteered to be interviewed but who had agreed to come to the feedback meetings. We had set up each meeting to include the union personnel who worked most closely with the professionals present. Occasionally, the proportion of noninterviewed union people in a meeting was quite high. When this happened, we were faced with a subgroup whom we knew less well, who had not contributed to the data in the feedback documents, and who had already voiced their distrust in the project by having rejected the initial invitation to participate.

As a result, the feedback documents per se became less relevant. The conversation almost invariably turned to questions about management's intent, the viability of the study, the likelihood of any meaningful results, and so on. We usually had to begin at the beginning.

These events themselves represented meaningful data. For while many viewed union–management relations as friendly, the message here was that many others saw them as distant. Why was management seeking the opinions of union personnel systematically for the first time in over seven years? Would history repeat itself and another debacle follow? Was management just showing good form or was it seriously interested in addressing issues of concern to union people?

Luckily, these questions were answered positively as managers and professionals responded to the union men's questions. They listened and discussed their own concerns candidly. Sometimes this led to a group interview until union people were more "on board." In a couple of cases, however, an uncomfortable silence from the union personnel suggested that some important work needed to be done at this interface.

Finally, there were a couple of meetings involving a manager and a group of union people where the feedback data pointed unambiguously to some specific problems. In these instances, we confirmed problems in a straightforward manner and spent the bulk of the meeting identifying a more preferable state of affairs and what steps might be taken to get there.

THE DAY-LONG PLANNING SESSION

A day-long planning session designed to recapitulate the feedback activities and to shift the focus to action planning was held immediately after the last feedback session. The top management team, several other managers who had held group feedback meetings, and two union representatives attended. The latter two, incidentally, had between them attended all of the group feedback meetings and were now as knowledgeable about the project as anyone in the division.

The session began with each manager presenting his group's concerns and priorities. Presentations varied from fairly detailed lectures, complete with overhead transparencies, to terse readings of group summary statements. We took notes on flipcharts and had papered the walls with them by noon when the initial presentations were over. Clearly, there was a bulky mass of data to digest. What was on the flipcharts addressed considerably less than what was in the original feedback documents, but each group seemed to have gone its own way and the task of consolidating group outputs looked overwhelming.

After lunch, however, we tried an intervention that got off to a rocky start but ended up creating a semblance of order out of all the chaos. It occurred to us during the feedback sessions that, while each group was developing a slightly different set of issues and priorities, the same kinds of statements were coming from people with the same functional orientations, regardless of what groups they were in.

Thus, people with important marketing tasks would almost always bring up issues regarding project leadership, technical marketing authority, marketing career paths, and so on. By the same token, people heavily involved in research would point to the difficulties of getting promoted without entering the management ranks, lack of technical innovation projects, desire combined with anxiety around doing long-range work, and so on. Likewise, the union personnel and the secretarial work force had their own issues. Since all of the work groups were cross-functional, so were the feedback meetings. And, therefore, these functionally based commonalities might not have been common knowledge within the division.

We began the afternoon by recognizing the enormity of the task of synthesizing the group data and suggesting it might be simplified by doing one more analysis activity, that is, creating lists of what people with different functional orientations were saying. We related our general observations (as noted above) to support this strategy but offered only the barest specific examples. We wanted the managers to discover the major commonalities for themselves and were convinced they could do it with relatively little effort.

They rebelled within 20 minutes. People were already overwhelmed. Why generate even more data? When would the data generating stop and problem solving begin? We held to our position that this final strategy would simplify the data immensely; but finally agreed to present our own detailed interpretations to the group.

This worked. By the time we were halfway through the first list (for what we had called "market facers"), various managers had caught on to the logic of our strategy and were busy adding to and correcting what we were saying. We started off each of the other lists in the same manner and were done within two hours.

We then made a list of "everyone's issues," that is, those germane to all groups. Finally, we went back over the flipcharts on the walls from the morning's presentations and made a list of issues not included in the five sets of messages just created. The final list contained about a dozen items, all of them specific to particular projects. Thus, 16 group-specific lists that overlapped in a host of ways and were simultaneously difficult to compare due to differences in language, frameworks, and priorities had been reduced to six. And these six were mutually exclusive and easily understood by everyone present. It had been an exhausting group effort but we were quite pleased with ourselves.

The final task of the day was to formulate some initial action steps in response to the data. No one offered immediate solutions to particular problems, but many agreed on the idea of creating task forces to respond to each of the functional lists.

The division manager was amenable to this strategy with respect to the marketing and technician lists. Task force members would be recruited from people having the relevant functional backgrounds. Each task force would be given several months to formulate an action program to respond to the issues on its list. It would be expected to consult widely with other members of the division and to make its proposals as concrete and realistic as possible. Both groups would report to the division manager. We would be available as consultants to their problem-solving processes, but they would work on their own to the limits of their ability.

Rather than create task forces, the division manager delegated responsibility for responding to the secretarial and research facers lists to, respectively, the facilities manager and the division's most respected scientist. Both men could proceed in any way they wished, although it was understood that following the task force guidelines seemed to make the most sense.

The list containing "everyone's issues" and the project-specific list, on the other hand, would be dealt with by some form of the top management team. It was impossible to say what the exact composition of this group would be, since the feedback session for the current top management team had ended with a resolution to reorganize.

In any case, everyone agreed that all six lists should be responded to, and that the rest of the division should be informed of the day's deliberations as quickly as possible. This was done over the next week through a memorandum that we prepared with the division manager. Shortly after it was circulated each manager met with his subordinates to discuss the planning session from his own perspective, get their response to the proposed actions, and answer any questions. The membership's response to both the new framework and the proposed action was favorable and the task forces were organized shortly thereafter.

FOLLOW-UP ACTIVITIES

The planning session marked the official completion of our initial contract and the beginning of a more eclectic relationship with the division. We now shared a common picture of the problems and opportunities facing the division and had developed helping relationships with particular managers, including the division head, which ensured us a role in the follow-up to the analysis. The following sections indicate the kinds of activities we engaged in during the following year.

Further Analysis and Dissemination of the Study Results. Throughout our analysis of the feedback data and the feedback sessions, we had kept our own opinions about the division as a whole to a minimum. Quite frankly, this was because we had yet to develop a cogent position that we felt confident about. It had been hard enough to organize the data for presentations and to provide helpful formulations to particular groups and individuals. The division manager spotted this, however, and asked us to prepare a personal statement. We agreed to do so as part of a project review session that the division manager had also asked us to hold a month after the planning session. This session was for the benefit of the division head's superior and this person's staff and was thus something of a special occasion.

For this session, we wanted to highlight the strengths and weaknesses of the division in a thought-provoking perspective that did not invite defensiveness. We listed division strengths around a particular theme as "achievements" and related weaknesses as "unintended consequences." The causal link implied in this format made sense in terms of the data. Figure 2–8 summarizes this part of our presentation. Besides exemplifying the format, this figure also describes our view of the overall situation we had encountered.

FIGURE 2-8
The Consultants' Assessment
of the Organization

The Division Has a Very Strong Task Orientation

Achievements:

- Little bureaucracy, red tape, or power politics
- Well organized to respond to moderate/short-term opportunities
- Successful integration of marketing and research
- High autonomy, intrinsically rewarding work

Unintended Consequences:

- Lack of attention to functional career development
- Failure to recognize multiple worlds in the division, e.g., those of marketers, researchers, etc.
- Concerns around equity — grass-is-greener sentiments

Action:

- Task forces to explore differential responses to particular groups while maintaining flat, integrated project-oriented structure

*   *   *

A Sophisticated, Autonomous Work Force Managed Largely Through Personal Plans and Business Plans

Achievements:

- MBO (Management by Objectives) and business plans have nurtured autonomy, goal orientation, sophistication around innovation, how to work the system, recognition and use of talents in others, openness, self-confidence, realism, ability to state goals in terms of business plans and to collaborate with colleagues in the same group

Unintended Consequences:

- Greater attachment to jobs and immediate work groups than to the division or corporation

FIGURE 2-8 *Continued*

- Preoccupation with MBO process leads to lack of attention to bigger picture, problems in resolving work priorities
- No sense of mission for division as a whole
- Feeling uninformed despite high interaction levels

Action:

- Division management team collaboration around long-term innovation
- Inclusion of analytical, service groups in business planning activities to manage upcoming work load proactively
- More sharing of plans/MBO outputs among groups to enhance communication

*   *   *

A Lean, Competent, Business-Oriented Management

Achievements:

- Business orientation balanced between marketing and research
- Management of professionals through delegation and MBO
- Responsiveness to business plans, budgets, efficiency
- Concerned with selling the division to rest of the corporation
- Generally competent—no deadwood in leadership functions
- Good interpersonal, organizing skills

Unintended Consequences:

- Managers seen as managers, not mentors for research or marketing types—leads to personal distance
- External concern leads to lots of time on the road, heightens disconnectedness, "Where is he when I need him?"
- A large staff makes access difficult
- Preoccupation with selling the division to the corporation leads to lack of selling the corporation to the division
- Product group leaders manage as centers of star systems

Action:

- Clarification of mutual needs/expectations regarding leadership
- Alternative mechanisms for getting help/guidance/advice
- More feedback from the corporation to the division

*   *   *

A Work Force That Is Growing Wiser but Older Every Day

Achievements:

- High level of job skills
- Maximum use of unique personal talents
- Lower training costs
- Efficient use of material resources due to long experience
- General capacity to run a very lean organization to meet tight budget constraints

Unintended Consequences:

- Lack of new blood for ideas and support
- Little room for error—a small number of personnel changes may have major impact
- Naiveté and energy are key components of innovation
- Loss of incentive for mobility within the division, increased desire to move out
- Being resolved to undesirable conditions rather than risk change

Action:

- Add staff in both research and market facing roles

*   *   *

A Budget Conscious Operation

Strengths:

- Obvious

Unintended Consequences:

- Mild sense of deprivation especially for hourly and secretaries
- Pilot plant problem
- X project
- Annoying production/shipping development roles
- Heightens short-term, conservative orientation within research

Action:

- Decisions regarding pilot plant, X project
- Facilities improvement
- Budget in longer term development projects to keep research spirit—long-term orientation

This presentation was so well received that we eventually gave it to the division top management team, the entire division, and the president's council of the corporation. Ironically, its preparation, once we had gotten around to digesting the data, had taken little more time than the time it had taken to prepare for one of the feedback sessions.

Development Work with the Top Management Team.   As was mentioned earlier, one outcome of the feedback session on the operation of the division's top management team was the decision to reorganize. The feedback indicated that the team's two major functions, division administration and policy making around product innovations, tended to get in the way of each other. Some members of the team had skills, responsibilities, and interests that related to one function and not to the other. Nonetheless, they were obliged to attend all of the group's meetings. Often, this meant saying little for hours at a time because the function being discussed was not relevant to them. At the same time, their presence under these conditions made it cumbersome to add other members of the division to the team whose roles were more relevant to this particular function.

Beyond this, decision making around administrative issues tended to drive out discussions regarding product innovation. Consequently, there was less division-wide coordination around the latter than the team thought advisable.

These and other reasons led the team to agree to reorganize into two separate groups, one for each function. Such a reorganization, moreover, would pave the way for responding to another widely held perception that the division manager was trying to fulfill too many responsibilities. The result was a lack of accessibility to him or other administrative decision makers on matters requiring division-wide approval. Splitting the top management team in two and making one responsible for administration would make it easier for the division manager to delegate many administrative tasks without sacrificing a division-wide perspective.

We became involved in these changes initially through our presence in the feedback discussions. We followed this up through a number of discussions with the division head and other team members. Perhaps our most significant contribution to the process was a weekend workshop with the new administrative management team, that is, the subgroup of the top management team now assigned to administrative tasks and expanded to include other administrative personnel.

This workshop served three purposes. First, it was a vehicle for bringing the new members of the team on board. Second, it was the occasion on which the division head confirmed his decision to delegate major administrative tasks to this team and discussed how this might best be done. Finally, it was an important opportunity for us to share our ideas about effective teamwork and colleagueship.

We were responsible for designing and running the workshop at a nearby motel. We combined experiential exercises with conceptual inputs and applications of same to the development of the team as an ongoing work unit. Incidentally, this was our first occasion to share the paradigms described in Chapter One with a large group of the division. The atmosphere finally seemed right for discussing our OD philosophy on a conceptual level. Up until this time, most division members viewed our activity as simply an organizational analysis. The workshop went well and we continued our involvement in this particular change activity for several weeks by attending team meetings and consulting with members.

Role Negotiation at the Pilot Plant. A problem reaching crisis proportions just as we began the analysis had to do with the hourly work force in the division's pilot plant. The pilot plant was a small-scale (20-person) production operation designed to take the bugs out of the manufacture of new products from the laboratory prior to commercialization.

Major morale problems had been created by a series of reductions in the pilot plant's work force due to a reduced need for this kind of work. The reductions resulted in an antagonistic relationship between management and the rank and file. The group's feedback data were negative, to say the least. Demand for the plant's services was continuing to fall, in part due to the products being developed and in part due to the plant's worsening reputation. The pilot plant manager was on the verge of recommending that it be shut down. The union personnel, all well protected through many years of seniority, were on the verge of not caring.

In the feedback meeting, however, we challenged both sides to try cooperating with each other. Both agreed that the present situation was fulfilling to no one. A ray of hope developed when the manager promised to do his best to get more work for the group and the hourlies promised to increase their productivity in areas where everyone knew they were restricting output. One of the conditions of this agreement, however, was our continued involvement in meetings between the work force and the manager.

Shortly after this event, the pilot plant manager was promoted. One of the first things we did with his successor (a scientist from the division) was to bring him up to date regarding what had happened. We held an open meeting with the new manager and hourlies in which we (1) confirmed what had happened and the promises involved, and (2) engaged in a systematic exchange of expectations between the new manager and the workers. The new leader got off to a good start by finding an agreeable answer to a problem that the work force had been complaining about for several months. Productivity and climate improved markedly thereafter.

Personal Counseling. A wide variety of one-on-one counseling activities that were often followed by small group problem-solving sessions also evolved out of the analysis. Many of these activities involved the task forces organized to respond to the feedback from various functional groups. For example, the scientist in charge of responding to the research facers list replicated our feedback meeting methodology to come up with a series of action suggestions and used us as consultants to his consulting.

CONCLUSION

A year later we were in the mature stage of an OD project relationship. We knew the division and its people and they knew us as individuals, our philosophy, and our potential as resources to them. For the six months thereafter, however, we had no further contact with the division. By the time these months had passed, the work of the task forces had been completed, and the division manager invited us to do a major evaluation both of how the division had changed and what its members thought about the project as a whole. Besides documenting concrete changes in policy, this involved another interviewing activity with a cross-section of 45 division members, the development, administration, and analysis of a questionnaire based on these interviews, that was filled out by all of the members, and yet another round of reports.

While a description of this second study is beyond the scope of this book, it can be noted that the results were highly positive. The list of concrete improvements that were attributed at least in part to the project covered over fifty items, and Likert scale assessments of our approach and the study's general value to the division averaged over 4 on a 5 point scale (1 = poor to 5 = excellent).

CHAPTER THREE

OD AS
AN INFLUENCE PROCESS

How do OD consultants influence people to pursue OD values? The answer to this question may not be immediately apparent from the description in the preceding chapter and yet it is central to understanding what OD is all about. For OD values are advanced only in part by OD consultants communicating their logic through words. For instance, it was not until quite late in the South City project, at the administrative management workshop, that we first shared the conceptual schemes noted in Chapter One with our clients. OD values, rather, are advanced by the totality of the OD consultants' behaviors, that is, by how they write, as well as how they speak, how they interact, and the roles they create for themselves and others in project activities. If one reads Chapter Two from this viewpoint, one can begin to see the varieties of tactics we used to advance OD values, and that there is at least some evidence that we succeeded.

I will review some of the things my colleagues and I did in the South City project in this chapter in order to demonstrate how the OD influence process takes place. First, however, I will present a framework for thinking about the influence process that I have found helpful in this kind of work.

CONTENT, PROCESS, AND CONTEXT

The activity of influencing others has been widely discussed in the behavioral sciences.[1] The focus has generally been on the various behavioral strategies available (forcing, trading, evangelizing, creating perceptions of dependence and

[1] A classic in the field is John R. P. French and Bertram Raven, "The Bases of Social Power," in *Group Dynamics*, 3rd ed., eds. Dorwin Cartwright and Alvin Zander (New York: Harper and Row), pp. 259-69. A current treatment for managers can be found in John P. Kotter, *Power in Management* (New York: AMACOM, 1979). A more exhaustive analysis can be found in Jeffrey Pfeffer, *Power in Organizations* (Marshfield, Mass.: Pitman Publishing, Inc., 1981).

obligation), the conditions under which particular strategies are most likely to succeed (types of organizational goals, cultures, the number and nature of constituent groups, and their interdependencies with the organization), and the resources necessary to implement a particular strategy (arms, scarce goods, charisma, information). However, for the OD specialist, a somewhat different perspective is useful, one that highlights the ways influence attempts are orchestrated as well as the influence messages themselves. This is because OD consultants usually operate with small amounts of many different types of influence (the power of the pen, one's choice of words in a conversation, very short-term control over the use of time and space, and over meeting activities). In order to use these resources with maximum efficiency and effect, an OD specialist needs to understand their interdependencies and make them highly congruent with one another. For if the same message is sent in several ways simultaneously—for example, the written word, visual imagery, the spoken word, affect-laden intonation, what one is sitting on, whom one is sitting next to, and how one is moving among people—the impact of the total message can be amplified greatly regardless of the weakness of each message taken alone.

In line with this approach, I have found it useful to think about three ways of communicating a message intended to influence another's behavior.

1. Content—the subject matter to which one brings another's attention.

2. Process—how one interacts with another in the course of addressing a particular subject.

3. Context—the conditions under which one interacts with another around a particular subject.

Each way can be used to communicate parts or all of a given message. When used in concert with each other, they can have a very powerful total effect. Indeed, I have found that many individuals who are in the business of influencing others under conditions where the value of their resources is initially questionable—for example, organization consultants in general—use all three ways with consummate skill.

For example, in an MBA course on the management consulting industry, I invited on separate days a senior partner from each of three major types of consulting firms to spend an afternoon with the class. My purpose was to give the students a feel for the cultures of these different firms. The payoff for my guests, of course, was the opportunity to publicize their organizations and to look over potential job candidates. To these ends, we met in a comfortable lounge with a small blackboard and established a very loose agenda that would allow the guest to steer the conversation in any way he wanted.

The first guest was a senior partner from a major consulting firm that specialized in corporate strategy. He arrived in a black, pinstriped, three-piece suit, remained standing bolt upright with a stoic expression on his face while I introduced him, and proceeded immediately to the blackboard once my introduction was over. There he wrote a large, neat T on the board and said, "As I see it, there are two kinds of management consulting. There is the kind that deals with organizational processes [puts the word 'process' under one side of the T]. And there is the kind that deals with corporate strategy [puts 'corporate strategy' under the other side of the T]. We deal strictly with corporate strategy [puts a big X across the word 'process'].''

We spent the rest of the afternoon talking about corporate strategy. Our guest remained standing at the blackboard for most of the time (the rest of us were sitting in easy chairs). He was extremely articulate, pleasant in demeanor, rarely effusive, and very penetrating in his comments. He was most buoyant when we asked him to talk about his and his company's successes, and most serious and brief when asked to discuss kinds of jobs that had not worked out well. All of the failures, moreover, were attributed to the inability of clients to use his services appropriately. Most of us were quite impressed, some of us awestruck, by the time the session was over. It was as if we had just attended a presentation to a group of important executives.

Our guest for the following week was a senior partner from a major firm that had made its mark in high-technology consulting. He was wearing a brown worsted two-piece suit (not exactly casual, but not overly formal either), sat down immediately next to me, and invited others to move their chairs closer so that we were soon all sitting in a tightly knit circle. Upon being introduced, he hunched over slightly, smiled quietly, and said, "Well, fellows, what kinds of problems would you like to discuss?"

We spent the afternoon talking about all sorts of inventions and engineering problems. Our guest was highly involved throughout, seemed to love controversy, and talked about successes and failures with equal interest so long as they involved interesting insights. By the time he left, we were highly impressed by his knowledge but equally intrigued with some of the technical issues he had raised. It was as if we had attended an interesting seminar at an engineering school.

Week 3 brought us a senior partner from a consulting firm that specialized in government lobbying. Our guest was a tall, handsome character, dressed in a sporty suit. He arrived with a broad welcoming smile on his face and had us in stitches with a series of clean but very funny jokes almost before we sat down. We spent the afternoon listening to him relate a wide variety of stories, mostly about interesting people and events in government circles. While he never named names or betrayed a confidence, he left us with the impression that he was someone who really knew what was going on in Washington. Equally important, he portrayed a sense of dynamism, sometimes sitting, sometimes standing, always in motion or just on the verge of it. He was the essence of a government lobbyist who knew his trade and could get something done. The atmosphere he had created was that of a Washington cocktail party.

Within the rather loose confines we had set for them, all three of these individuals managed content, process, and context in ways that were mutually reinforcing and that comprised a consistent message about who they were and what they could do for someone. In terms of content, one man focused attention on a specialized set of management concepts, another on technology, the third on people and relationships. Regarding process, the business strategist reinforced his message by choosing his words strategically, carefully, politely, and with an eye on maximum impact, treating us indeed as if we were members of a top management team. The high-technology consultant, by contrast, modeled a problem-solving process—analyzing, questioning, probing, discovering. He helped us become for the moment a group of sophisticated engineers and scientists. Likewise, the lobbying consultant behaved in ways that would put us at ease and made us willing to listen to him, thus suggesting to us that he was capable of doing this with anyone. What more could one ask for in a lobbyist?

Finally, each consultant made use of the little control he had over the context of our meeting to reinforce content and process. None of them could change the fact that this was a class, that it was to be held in a lounge at a certain time and place, that 27 people would attend the meeting, and so forth. These aspects of the context were indeed the things I had chosen to control and had presented them as requirements for our encounters.

Within these confines, however, the strategist affected the underlying tone of his meeting through his conservative dress, his ramrod posture, his choice to stand most of the time at the symbolic center of the action (the blackboard), and his quiet but punctuating voice. Anyone entering the room could see that something important was going on and that he was in charge.

The technologist managed his context by dressing a bit like an academic or an engineer. Even his attaché case reeked of functionality; the large, brown, bulky, rectangular type as opposed to the strategist's shiny, gray, slim model. He got us into a circle, making the lounge into a seminar room, and hunched over a little, thus making himself less visible and focusing attention on what was said rather than on who was saying it. It was clear that he made his money through the world of ideas, not imagery. And yet the imagery he created was none other than that associated with the world of ideas.

Last, our lobbyist created a Washington cocktail party as if that was what the lounge had been built for; no attaché case, no concern over whether one was sitting or standing, no overt distinction between work and play. Friendliness and conviviality pervaded his countenance and the room, and yet from time to time serious issues were discussed.

Interestingly, I found out later in my personal conversations with these three people that none of them made deliberate use of behavioral science concepts to guide their behavior. The first two even admitted that they were surprised that this course was being run by the Organizational Behavior Department, as opposed, say, to a policy group, and that they had felt a little anxious about how personal the conversation might get.

Instead, it was clear to me that all three had learned to behave the way they did because of the work cultures they had each spent the past 20 or more years in. As senior partners in their firms, they had come to embody those cultures, implicitly shaping and being shaped by them. Thus their seemingly careful orchestration of content, process, and context was from their viewpoint simply behaving in a professional manner, one that they had developed through experience and that they knew led to success.

Such success, moreover, could be attributed at least in part to the fact that these ways of behaving (of managing content, process, and context) were consistent with the cultures surrounding the functional specialties for which they consulted. Put broadly, effective strategy consultants learn to behave verbally and nonverbally, physically and intellectually, as top-level managers do, engineering consultants as do engineers, and so on. This congruence or fit in ways of behaving opens the door to comfortable relationships between client and consultant, especially if the consultant embodies what others value in his or her functional culture. Thus, a maximum amount of energy can be spent in addressing technical problems and a minimum on relationship building.

All of this is fine for the management consultant who has a technical body of expertise to offer once he or she gets a foot in the door, but what about the OD consultant? This person's mission is ultimately to change an organization's culture itself so that it is more consistent with OD values. Hopefully, this will help all technical functions perform more effectively. One is not in the business of adapting totally to a culture that is already there, and this is where conscious management of culturally impactful behaviors becomes relevant. For only by living in both worlds simultaneously, that of OD values and that of the organization, and by knowing where the line is between the two, can one accomplish one's objective.

The OD consultant gains entry to the culture of the organization by adopting its basic values around project management. Thus, upon learning that South City Chemical coordinated its work around fairly detailed contracts, we decided to make a fairly detailed contract ourselves. We made it our business to learn how the power system worked and used it to our advantage in selling the project to the rest of the management group. Whenever we wrote a memo to the membership at large, we first showed a draft to key managers and asked them to edit it so that it would look and read like a legitimate South City memo; we also made sure that it had the right signatures on it so that it would be read, and that it was sent to the right people in the right sequence to fit the prevailing hierarchy.

We dressed formally when working with management and more casually when we were with the hourly personnel. At least in the beginning, we met people on their own turf, where they felt most comfortable, and talked in casual moments about whatever they were interested in. We met our deadlines meticulously and prepared well for any presentations we made because we knew the organization valued these behaviors.

This, however, was only part of what we did, and in terms of what was important, probably only a small part. For just as the management consultants in the example above used the freedom they had to model the cultures of their organizations, we used the freedom we had within these constraints to mold content, process, and context in ways that portrayed OD values. The difference was that, to a very large extent, we did this deliberately and monitored our impact in doing so. In essence, we made use of the fact that South City Chemical, like most organizations, was not rigidly organized against the pursuit of values related to OD. While our data revealed that, in general, it was pyramidal in management philosophy, dependence oriented in its face-to-face groups, and developmentally oriented in its interpersonal relationships, there was plenty of variety in orientations at all three levels. Depending upon the function and the task at hand, all three of the other forms of organization, face-to-face orientation, and relationships were permissible and often supported. This made it possible to make a case for OD-oriented values by orienting as much of our behavior as we could along these lines. Our project thus represented a test case, with us as guinea pigs, of the OD approach.

MANAGING CONTENT, PROCESS, AND CONTEXT AT THE ORGANIZATIONAL, GROUP, AND INDIVIDUAL LEVEL

In Chapter One, I discussed OD values at three system levels—organizational, group, and individual relationships. An OD consultant needs to manage content, process, and context on all of these levels in order to enhance the chances for success. In the following sections, I want to show how the conceptual maps presented in Chapter One can be elaborated to indicate what needs to be done at each system level to foster OD values and to show some of the ways in which we did these things at South City. The conceptual maps also indicate what someone who chooses to pursue values that contrast directly with the OD stance might do to achieve his or her objectives. As noted earlier, awareness of these alternative stances is important, because it clarifies what OD does not represent and, therefore, allows one to make more informed choices and to recognize when others are doing likewise.

The Organizational Level

Figure 3–1 articulates the directions for managing content, process, and context at the organizational level in ways that are consistent with OD values (the upper right-hand quadrant) and the three other value sets that contrast directly with them.

Context.　　Much of what we did at South City in terms of the way we contracted for and managed the project as an organizational activity was consistent with the tenets of a collaborative organization. In terms of managing *context*, we had an important ally in the division manager (a major context setter), and, in fact, his own philosophy did most of the work for us. He promoted and publicized the project as a division-wide need. He sanctioned the time and space for everyone to participate. He made sure that there were no serious reservations from other key managers and opinion leaders before giving the final go-ahead. He made sure that we did not become aligned with the small subgroup that had brought us in originally. He bent over backward to facilitate union participation once the concept of the project was accepted by his management team. He provided access to the feedback data for all organization members. And when it came to action planning, his bottom-line mandate to each of the task forces was that they "consult widely" with all those concerned before formulating their proposals. All of these actions helped to create an underlying atmosphere within the division for pursuing shared goals with respect to the project under the assumption of a shared interest in the organization's welfare and for recognizing many members' control over important resources for the task.

We enhanced this context, moreover, in a number of less significant but still useful ways. These included: contracting for and thereby helping to sanction an analysis procedure that highlighted broad participation and the identification of common goals, arranging meeting spaces in ways that minimized hierarchy (sitting around square tables or seats in circles), setting up group discussion procedures that encour-

FIGURE 3-1
Managing Content, Process,
and Context at
the Organizational Level

Assume That Many Members Are
Committed to the Organization's Welfare

Pyramidal Organization

Content: Brings attention to:
- Issues of concern to many members
- Importance of a few members' resources for dealing with these issues

Process: Consultants' behavior models:
- Commitment to shared goals
- Recognition and use of a few members' resources

Context: Creates incentives for:
- Pursuing shared goals
- Recognizing and using a few members' resources

Collaborative Organization

Content: Brings attention to:
- Issues of concern to many members
- Importance of many members' resources for dealing with these issues

Process: Consultants' behavior models:
- Commitment to shared goals
- Recognition and use of many members' resources

Context: Creates incentives for:
- Pursuing shared goals
- Recognizing and using many members' resources

Assume That Only
a Few Members Have
Important Resources
to Offer

Assume That Most
Members Have
Important Resources
to Offer

Passive Organization

Content: Brings attention to:
- Issues shared by a few members
- Importance of a few members' resources for dealing with these issues

Process: Consultants' behavior models:
- Commitment to individual or subgroup goals
- Recognition and use of a few members' resources

Context: Creates incentives for:
- Pursuing individual or subgroup goals
- Recognizing and using a few members' resources

Competitive Organization

Content: Brings attention to:
- Issues shared by a few members
- Importance of many members' resources for dealing with these issues

Process: Consultants' behavior models:
- Commitment to individual or subgroup goals
- Recognition and use of many members' resources

Context: Creates incentives for:
- Pursuing individual or subgroup goals
- Recognizing and using many members' resources

Assume That Few Members Are
Committed to the Organization's Welfare

aged inputs from all present and established the identification of common concerns as a critical goal, dressing in ways that did not highlight our own status beyond those we worked with, sitting among other managers at meetings rather than in a tightly knit group around the most senior person present, and moving frequently around the entire facility, thereby making ourselves accessible to the membership at large rather than staying close to the top management offices.

There were, of course, some clear limits to the extent to which the project context followed the OD ideal. First, we were obliged to work through the hierarchy at every step of the way. It was their choice to initiate the project and to limit collaboration at any time they desired. For instance, it was not the membership at large that sanctioned the project but the relatively small management team. Participation among the professional staff was basically mandatory. Union participation was avoided until after the project had been sanctioned by management. This was probably the cause of the union's eventual lack of wholehearted support for the analysis, which, in turn, led to limited participation by hourlies in the interviews.

It would be hard to conceive of defying any of these constraints in an organization such as South City. They represent the culture of the pyramidal organization (upper left-hand quadrant in Figure 3–1) that pervades much of modern society. We simply wish to point out that this culture places boundaries around the collaborative model and needs to be dealt with realistically on this basis.

Content.   While the people at the top of the pyramid played the key roles in sanctioning the project and creating a largely collaborative context, we as consultants were a lot more active in reinforcing this context through our management of content and process. In terms of *content*, such documents as the description of our approach, the project contract letter, the format we used for the feedback documents, the reports we made of various meetings, and the presentations we made of the total study results all highlighted the identification of shared goals and concerns and the importance of the resources every member had to offer in making the project a success. With these documents as the jumping-off point for most of the meetings we attended, the content of what we said also tended to bring attention to these values.

Process.   Finally, at the level of *process* (of human interaction itself) we continuously tried to focus our discussions with all members, both individually and in groups, to division-wide problems and opportunities, and to how one might contribute one's resources and the influence one derived from them to division-wide objectives. Of course, we did not do this all of the time since the tasks of personal relationship building and the creation of effective group process required our attention as well. More often than not, however, and especially in the group feedback meetings and in the workshops, we would find ourselves shifting the focus of conversation from individual or subgroup concerns to the division-wide perspective and from discussion of what can/ should the division do for me to what can/should I be doing for the division.

The Group Level

Managing content, process, and context at the group level deals in particular with how the consultant prepares for, sets up, and actually behaves in small group problem-solving sessions. Ideal behavior at this level reinforces OD values at the organizational level but is intended in particular to encourage an effective interpersonal learning process. Figure 3–2 articulates the values paradigm in terms of content, process, and context for group activity. Once again, the upper right-hand quadrant of the figure represents the ideals of Organization Development. What follows are some of the ways in which we attempted to manage context, content, and process to fit these ideals.

FIGURE 3-2
Managing Content, Process and
Context at the Group Level

Being Candid about One's
Organizational Experience

Dependent Orientation

Content: Brings attention to:
- What is the problem
- What an expert can infer

Process: Consultants' behavior models:
- A rational problem-solving cycle
- Dependence in decision making

Context: Creates incentives for:
- Recognizing others' feelings, assumptions, perceptions
- A few people making choices for others

Consensus Orientation

Content: Brings attention to:
- What is the problem
- What has actually been said or written

Process: Consultants' behavior models:
- A rational problem-solving cycle
- Consensus decision making

Context: Creates incentives for:
- Recognizing others' feelings, assumptions, perceptions
- All members making choices for themselves

Give Responsibility for One's Behavior to Others

Take Responsibility for One's Own Behavior

Apathetic Orientation

Content: Brings attention to:
- Who is the problem
- What an expert can infer

Process: Consultants' behavior models:
- Attempts to problem-solve without shared data analysis
- Apathy in decision making

Context: Creates incentives for:
- Ignoring other people's feelings, assumptions, perceptions
- A few people making choices for others

Gamesmanship Orientation

Content: Brings attention to:
- Who is the problem
- What has actually been said or written

Process: Consultants' behavior models:
- Attempts to problem-solve without shared data analysis
- Gamesmanship in decision making

Context: Creates incentives for:
- Ignoring other people's feelings, assumptions, perceptions
- All members making choices for themselves

Being Closed about One's
Organizational Experience

Context. An important part of the context in which our meetings took place at South City was, of course, the project itself. This helped create an atmosphere in which candidness was important and expected at meetings, because the major initial task of the project was to surface members' personal perspectives regarding what it was like to work at South City. Our presence in any meeting was likely to evoke memories of sharing personal data with us in the interviews. Thus, we had a private connection with each person who had been interviewed as well as a public purpose for being at a particular meeting. Because of the interviews, we were also in a position to refer to personal positions people might take on various issues. By doing this without betraying confidences, we set the stage for discussing sensitive issues in a safe way.

For instance, one of us might observe that project leaders in general were frustrated with the lack of authority to make others comply to their needs. This would make it unnecessary for a particular manager to introduce the subject. But, once introduced, any attendee could elaborate on the issue for others' understanding without being tagged as an instigator. Often, when a manager found that an issue was being discussed with a minimum of tension, this person would take the next step of revealing his or her personal position on the subject.

The project as a context for group meetings also encouraged members to make choices for themselves, at least at the level of saying what was important in the data and what was not. For the total design stressed the need for the members themselves to identify their priorities and not to rely on us or on any particular manager to do this. Note, for example, that we did not even weight the relative support for various positions in data we fed back. We suggested instead that each group of managers do this for itself. Other OD specialists, especially those who use a written survey feedback approach, do provide quantitative weighting of results, but they also pretest their questionnaires and design them collaboratively with their clients to make sure that the statistics they compile deal with issues their clients are clearly interested in. Thus, they provide for personal choice in a somewhat different manner.[2]

Creating a context in which personal candidness and self-responsibility were encouraged was also accomplished through planning for each meeting with the senior manager who would chair it and encouraging him to introduce the session with open requests for these kinds of behaviors. The fact that these values already represented legitimate ways of behaving within the division was also important. This is not to say, however, that these were the only acceptable ways of behaving. There was some legitimacy for behaving in ways consistent with all four styles in Figure 3–2. Nonetheless, setting the stage in this way enhanced the chances for people to pick the ideal style for interacting around the project.

Content. When it came to the management of content in our meetings, the feedback documents themselves did much of the work for us. We had designed them specifically to bring people's attention to what were the problems and opportunities facing the division, not who were problem people or potential heroes. And we used a format that highlighted what the clients themselves said rather than what we as experts could infer from the data. Thus, the documents consisted mostly of verbatim quotes organized around the problem areas that many respondents had mentioned. The quotes, in turn, had been modified where necessary to disguise individual authorship or a particular individual as the target of a comment. Finally, we kept our written analysis to a minimum and did little more than summarize what was said and suggest ways of analyzing the data.

We thought it important to focus on what were the problems rather than who were the problems for two reasons, both of which are related to the development of can-

[2]David A. Nadler, *Feedback in Organization Development: Using Data-Based Methods* (Reading, Mass.: Addison-Wesley Publishing Co., 1977), pp. 94–99.

didness. First, it has been our experience and that of others,[3] that when groups attempt to search for the source of a problem in a particular person, members refrain from being candid for fear of revealing reasons that would make them the individual to be blamed. By contrast, when people search for the source of a problem in the ways of thinking and behaving that they are all parties to, they experience less of a need to be self-protective and more of a need for candidness. Everyone has had a share in creating the problem. Therefore, there is logically no particular individual to blame. Moreover, because everyone contributed to the problem, everyone's experience might help in resolving it.

Second, we have found that focusing attention on the problem as a separate entity (a "what") encourages systemic thinking and the search for multiple causes. This again encourages candidness, since the shared assumption that there are multiple causes stimulates inquiry in many directions and makes each person's experience potentially relevant.

Limiting what we fed back to the data the respondents themselves created was intended more directly to enhance self-responsibility. By the time we had finished collecting and analyzing the interviews, we had a great many theories about the division. We chose quite purposely not to present these interpretations formally in the initial feedback sessions in order to allow our clients to work with the same data we had. They were in a much better position to identify which data were relevant to themselves and their particular subgroups, to identify where their own energy was for change, and to develop ways of interpreting the data that made sense to them. This was critical since they were the ones who would have to act on the data and deal with other managers' proposals as well.

While one aspect of the content in these meetings was the feedback materials, another comprised the words that were actually spoken. We influenced this aspect by curbing what we ourselves said to fit the desired pattern. For example, more often than not, the interpretations we did offer were systemically oriented and not focused on a particular individual. We also were careful to share our own experiences in gathering the data and to own our interpretations as products of our unique experience, which might differ from others' in the group.

These actions comprised a relatively small part of our behavior at the meetings, however. For once the discussion started, we were much more concerned with how people attended to the data (process) than to what they were discussing.

Process.   Ideal process under the consensus orientation in group activity involves the treatment of subject matter in a rational, problem-solving manner and the development of decisions where participants feel that others understand their position, where they have had a chance to persuade them to follow it, and where they are willing to accept a course of action that may not be their first preference but that they sense is what the group wants. Such a process dovetails nicely with attention to what is the

[3]Herbert A. Thelen, *Dynamics of Groups at Work* (Chicago: The University of Chicago Press, 1954). Part II of this book (pp. 219-332) represents an in-depth treatment of this issue.

problem and to what has actually been said or written, because this facilitates collaborative effort at problem definition based on shared data. The latter, in turn, is the first step in the rational problem-solving cycle.

The notion of a rational problem-solving process may mean different things to different people. Thus, a brief conceptual digression at this point seems appropriate. In the field of OD, Edgar Schein's formulation is probably the most well accepted and represents how we will use the term in this book.[4] According to Schein, problem solving in its ideal form involves a six-step iterative procedure, as shown in Figure 3–3.

A group begins with a felt need—for example, evidence of controversy around a particular issue as revealed in a feedback document—and proceeds to work at formulating a definition of the problem that clearly speaks to the data and is also consistent

FIGURE 3·3
A Model of the Stages
of Problem Solving

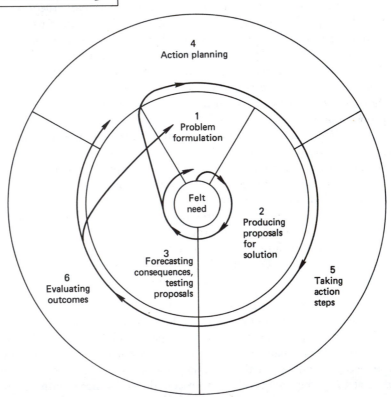

Source: Edgar H. Schein, *Process Consultation: Its Role in Organization Development* (Reading, Mass.: Addison-Wesley Publishing Co., 1969), p. 47. ©1969. Reprinted with permission.

[4]Edgar H. Schein, *Process Consultation: Its Role in Organization Development* (Reading, Mass.: Addison-Wesley Publishing Co., 1969).

with the experience of the problem solvers themselves. This is followed by the creation of proposals for solving the problem as defined. Schein suggests that this stage is accomplished most effectively when no single proposal is evaluated until all proposals that members wish to consider have been shared and understood. Once all proposals are on the table, the next step is to evaluate their relative merits in terms of the logical consequences of attempting to implement them. Analysis of each proposal may lead to the conclusion that none of them will solve the problem, or at least not do so without creating even more difficult problems to solve. In this case, the group needs to redefine the problem and repeat the previous steps.

If an attractive solution is discovered, however, the ensuing steps involve action planning, implementation, and evaluation of the outcomes. Schein notes that these later steps are best accomplished when those who enact them have also been included in the earlier stages of the process. Otherwise, the implementers are likely to develop their own conceptions of the logic behind the proposed solution and depart from the proposed plan as a result.

Referring back to Chapter Two, one can see that we designed the entire project at South City Chemical to be consistent with Schein's model. However, different meetings focused on different stages in the problem-solving process. In particular, the feedback sessions around the interview data dealt with the assessment of felt needs, problem formulation, and some very tentative steps at proposing solutions. One of our major tasks as process consultants in these meetings was to ensure that these steps were followed thoroughly.

To this end, we spent a great deal of time engaging in behaviors such as: helping people articulate what the quotations were implying and checking this against their own experience, helping people to contribute additional data that were relevant to their group and discounting comments that did not seem relevant in their experience, trying out different ways of stating the underlying issues (with particular emphasis on stating problems and opportunities in systemic terms), brainstorming about possible solutions with a minimum of premature evaluation, and preparing the group leader to be able to present the group ideas to the planning committee in succinct terms. In other meetings, we focused on different stages, though always making sure that all present were aware of how the earlier stages had been completed. Thus, these initial sessions were critical in getting the process off to a good start.

Besides facilitating the problem-solving process, we also paid considerable attention to developing decisions based on consensus. Our clients were not unfamiliar with this practice, but they displayed a much stronger tendency to defer to the authority of the senior manager present. In fact, when it came to *acting* on the data, it was clear that the prerogatives of hierarchy would be followed. Nonetheless, top management concurred with us in wanting the analysis to be achieved through consensus, so that the interpretations they were eventually to act on would be as close to representing the views of the division as possible. They were quite candid about this, and thus set the stage for modeling on our part.

What we did in this direction was to clarify the distinction between analysis and action itself. For once this was done, many of the participants would air their disagreements openly and work hard at reaching a shared picture they were willing to live with. The greatest resistance came from those who were pessimistic that management would act, for if there was no action, why bother to put the effort into taking a clear stand and putting one's neck on the line?

The most difficult meetings for gaining consensus were those attended by the union personnel who had not chosen to be interviewed. In these cases, we had to go through a testing process. Typically, the history of relations between union and management would be raised by a highly vocal union member, and inputs by other union members would not be forthcoming until the managers present admitted that this kind of collaboration had not been encouraged in the past. Thus, all agreed that this was only a first step. Basic support for the overall effort would not be forthcoming until further action had been taken by management.

The Individual Relationship Level

Managing content, context, and process at the level of individual relationships is central to a consultant's dealings with particular clients. The consultant needs to work toward creating situations in which the client feels comfortable in treating him or her as an equal and in relating with the person holistically, and thus where the boundaries of conversation are not closely defined by official roles. Under these conditions, a sense of colleagueship is established that maximizes mutual contribution to the project and represents a way of relating that is consistent with OD values. Figure 3–4 delineates the appropriate forms of content, context, and process for fostering a collegial relationship (the upper right-hand quadrant) and shows the contrasts between this and the other logical types. Let us now look at some of the tactics we used to foster collegial relationships at South City Chemical.

Context.   One aspect of context that can have an impact on relationship development is the physical settings in which conversations take place. Meeting in a client's office, with the client behind his or her desk and you, the consultant, on the other side in the "guest" chair heightens formality and thus both role playing and hierarchy. Meeting side by side in two guest chairs on the other side of the office helps to diminish this atmosphere a little. Meeting in a conference room around a circular table is even better. Meeting in a restaurant or cocktail lounge is probably the best one can do. While never making an issue of it, we did as much of our interpersonal business as we could at South City in the latter settings. After reading a draft of Chapter Two, one of our colleagues even went so far as to remark that it looked as if we got most of our work done when either eating or drinking.

Perhaps the most poignant example of this dealt with the events surrounding the beginning of the project. Having been mailed a schedule of activities before making my first visit, I saw that I might have a choice of introducing my ideas either in a conference room on the morning of my first full day at the site (where this activity was officially to take place) or over cocktails and dinner with the same people on the night before. I preferred the latter and prepared a casual but thorough presentation for this setting as well as a more formal one for the conference room.

After our first drink in the bar before dinner, the division manager asked me

FIGURE 3-4
Managing Content, Process, and
Context at the Individual Level

Relating Holistically

Developmental Relationship		Collegial Relationship	
Content:	Brings attention to; • Holistic experience of organization life • One of the party's issues	Content:	Brings attention to: • Holistic experience of organization life • Both parties' issues
Process:	Consultant's behavior models: • Exploration of whatever is relevant to the topic being discussed • Explorations of one party's needs, etc.	Process:	Consultant's behavior models: • Exploration of whatever is relevant to the topic being discussed • Mutual exploration of interests, needs, etc.
Context:	Creates incentives for: • Engaging the other as an individual • Treating the other as more or less important than oneself	Context:	Creates incentives for: • Engaging the other as an individual • Treating the other as an equal

Relating as
Unequals

Relating as
Equals

Service Relationship		Political Relationship	
Content:	Brings attention to: • Expectations and results of role performance • One of the party's issues	Content:	Brings attention to: • Expectations and results of role performance • Both parties' issues
Process:	Consultants' behavior models: • Exploration of role-related issues only • Exploration of one party's needs, etc.	Process:	Consultants' behavior models: • Exploration of role-related issues only • Mutual exploration of interests, needs, etc.
Context:	Creates incentives for: • Engaging the other as a role player only • Treating the other as more or less important than oneself	Context:	Creates incentives for: • Engaging the other as a role player only • Treating the other as an equal

Relating Strictly
in Formal Role

to say a little about myself and my background. I used it as a springboard to relate my experience to what I had heard so far about the proposed project. After about 20 minutes, one of the managers noted that I was really getting into the following day's agenda. I asked if this bothered him, and he said no. We spent the rest of the evening talking about the project and ourselves. This made it easy to discuss people's personal concerns about Organization Development, to trade war stories about good and bad consultations from both sides, and to discuss major concerns people had about the proposed analysis in a very nonthreatening atmosphere.

We met at the appointed hour the following morning in a spartanly furnished room. I sat on one side of a table with a blackboard to my back. The selection team sat on the other side. I was given a typed sheet of questions to address. The atmosphere was formal. But, given the previous evening's events, I had already gotten to know each person present as an individual, and vice versa. Equally important, almost anyone in the room could already answer most of the questions on the list. Also, I had spent the last part of the previous evening before retiring composing my responses to the issues I thought might be raised again. Given my knowledge of these people as individuals, I had a much better sense of what to say than if I had come in cold. As a result, rather than be an examination of a sort, our meeting turned into a problem-solving session with all of us working together on how to deal with issues such as confidentiality, raised expectations, and time demands. Even if I had not been chosen to do the project, I think we would have parted company with some useful learnings and a sense of camaraderie.

Readers familiar with the world of marketing might react to the foregoing with the comment that I was simply using good sales tactics. I would heartily agree. My point is that this kind of relationship building is also part and parcel of OD, and that the use of informal settings to create the context for doing so is equally important.

The initial meetings just discussed suggest another aspect of context management for relationship building. This is the sequencing of types of interpersonal activities. It may not always be possible to set the tone of an interaction so that formality is minimized and basic equality is highlighted. But one's chances of doing this can be enhanced in any setting if one's interactions in the recent past have embodied this tone. Prior interaction creates contexts for current interactions. This can be taken advantage of by sequencing one's meetings with clients so that more formal interactions are interspersed with informal ones. Thus, in the example above, the formal atmosphere of a morning meeting was strongly affected by what had happened in a more informal context the evening before.

We used this principle throughout our work at South City. There, as in other organizational cultures where certain physical settings tend to dictate the level of formality, this amounted to maintaining contact with at least some of our clients throughout the day. And, indeed, the critical relationship building did seem to occur during meals, car rides, walks in the hallways, plant tours, and coffee breaks.

Content.   The key principles for managing content so that it reinforces collegiality are to bring attention to one's own and the other's total experience of organization life and to distribute this attention to both parties' issues and not just to the client's or one's own. Some readers may find the latter tenet illogical. The client is paying the consultant to help him or her. Therefore, why not focus more attention on this person? But unless the client/consultant relationship is experienced by the client as a shared one, the client cannot use it as a model for relating collegially with more permanent workmates. Clearly, there are times when either party needs more attention and should be given it, just as there are in any work relationship. In the long run, however, the distribution needs to be fairly equal to foster an OD approach to work. If this does not make sense in a given relationship, the OD approach in general may not either, for this relationship or for the pattern of activities surrounding it.

As in other projects, we usually found that we could get our clients at South City Chemical to relate to us on a more holistic level by asking them, as soon as it seemed appropriate, to tell us how they liked playing their roles. It was rather difficult for most of our clients to sustain a conversation along these lines and still remain in role. To the extent that we could get any conversation going in this direction, we looked for interests, perspectives, and frustrations we had in common and let our clients know this by disclosing our own thinking and philosophy about the roles we played, and then openly appreciating and highlighting our commonalities. We refrained from talking about major differences we saw between us until we had gotten some mutual appreciation going.

We did this also with respect to nonbusiness activities by inquiring about family life, hobbies, politics, and so on. Our intent was to develop some ongoing topics for conversation that transcended the role relationship of client and consultant, to which we could turn for mutual appreciation, support, inquiry, debate, or whatever throughout our relationships. In the process, we also tended to steer away from topics where we had clear status differences. These were likely to invite more general attributions of inequality that could reduce the desire to share on a personal level.

Paying attention to the things we had in common, of course, was only one side of managing content to foster collegiality. Eventually, we had to recognize the ways in which we differed in our interests and values. Mutual knowledge of the latter, however, came more slowly. We learned gradually that some managers simply valued a more authoritarian posture toward organizations than we did, that some were uncomfortable with discussing emotional issues, and that some had very little in common with us as individuals or with our work at this point in their lives. We were by no means a homogeneous mutual admiration society, nor were our clients in their relations without us. Recognizing this, even if in many cases only tacitly, led us to relate more closely to some clients than to others, but it also made our relations in general more authentic. Those who interacted with us only when asked to buy their colleagues or as part of a specific task, seemed more relaxed and willing to engage once they realized that we did not intend to pursue the many personal topics we had discussed in our initial interviews.

Even with clients we were close to, moreover, it was occasionally important to focus our attention on areas where we did disagree. Without confronting these issues squarely, our own integrity would have been jeopardized. Happily, there were only two issues during the first year of the project around which confrontation was necessary. Since even the most minor tiffs with clients are underreported in the consulting literature, it seems worthwhile to review these incidents here.

The first concerned Alan Jensen's sudden departure, noted in a footnote to Figure 2-6, and Gervase Bushe's subsequent limited participation. Alan's departure was unforeseen and a blow to all of us, but we the consultants agreed that it was necessary for him to complete his Ph.D. work and that the time demands of the project would be too great for him to cope with simultaneously. We were also convinced that we had access to other consultants, such as Gervase, who would carry competently the work load of a fourth person when necessary.

Our primary client, the division manager, was upset because we had listed Alan's name on the contract letter, and he had assumed that Alan would be with us throughout the project. After sharing his annoyance with us and listening to our reasoning, he was willing to accept our position. Later, when we found that Gervase, Alan's replacement, could not be present for the feedback sessions, the division manager made it clear that he did not want any more additions to our staff. Clearly, as senior consultant, I had not managed the manning issue very well, but I personally felt much better from gaining closure on these issues, and I think all of us benefited from clearing the air. The relationship we had developed with the division manager made dealing with this issue rather straightforward, with little lasting tension on either side.

The second incident occurred 11 months into the project. It had been almost three months since the all-day planning session that had served as a capstone to the feedback process. We were visiting the site to present our ideas for a workshop that would officially begin the activities of the administrative management team. The reader will remember that this was one of two teams that the top management group was being reorganized into, so that it could respond separately to administrative and innovative issues.

A secondary purpose for the visit was to assess the progress of the various task forces and to provide help when invited. We soon learned that the various teams were still in the organizing stages and that little further analysis or action had been taken thus far. This made me anxious. I began to envision considerable dissatisfaction by the rest of the division for having engaged in a massive analysis with few results. I voiced my concerns at the planning meeting attended by the newly formed administrative management group.

The division manager responded by saying that my comments were unduly harsh. Steps were being taken at an appropriate rate and commitment to the total project had not died down. I elaborated on my position, noting that the problem of taking action after analysis was endemic to OD projects in general, and that I saw my role in this stage of the project as one of maintaining momentum in order to avoid this. We dropped the matter at this point and turned to other issues that were dealt with quite smoothly.

Cocktails and a dinner to celebrate the promotion of one of the product group managers to a position on the corporate staff followed. The division manager and I rehashed our positions over a drink and agreed that we simply were disagreeing at the moment. Aside from this, several of the other managers, in separate conversations through the evening, raised the subject of our disagreement. None of them agreed with my position on the matter, but they did say that they could empathize with my concern. They said that this was just the way the division operated. People moved deliberately and carefully on important matters, and this could seem like foot-dragging to an outsider.

Interestingly, I felt emotionally closer to several of the managers during the evening than I had throughout the project to date. They seemed to include me in more of their private jokes, laughed with me more, and in general behaved more spontaneously. One might interpret the dynamics behind this in a variety of ways that I will not deal with here. In retrospect, however, the most important lesson for me was that my confrontational behavior had strengthened my relationships with them. The division manager and I never raised the matter explicitly with each other again. He turned out to be right in the sense that many useful things did happen in the months to follow. I never will know what my impact was on this, but I remain convinced that the act of confrontation itself was a healthy one.

Process.   Ideal process in a collegial relationship involves continuous inquiry into the present state of mind of each party and the collaborative pursuit of activities that are both mutually rewarding and responsive to the situation at hand. It involves being playful when both parties are in the mood and when the conditions under which they are meeting do not require task behavior to meet either party's broader commitments. It involves working hard together when either party needs to. It involves confrontation when either party feels uncomfortable with the behavior of the other. It involves focused attention on one or the other party's problems when this person is the more needy at the moment and the other is willing and able to help. But perhaps most important, it involves mutual exploration of oneself, the other, and the situation to ensure that whatever is happening is what both parties see as in their best interests.

The general posture we took to manage process with our clients at South City Chemical should be apparent from the preceding discussion. We tried to follow the guidelines of the paragraph above as these made sense from situation to situation. In doing this, however, we relied on two techniques in particular that draw on basic counseling skills at the interpersonal level. We will devote considerable space to these techniques (and two others) in Chapter Eight. It seems appropriate here, however, to describe them briefly in order to give you some idea of the behaviors we modeled for our clients.

One technique that we used continuously was active listening.[5] This involved behaviors such as: (1) trying to restate what the client was saying in our own words until the other agreed that he or she had been understood; (2) asking nonevaluative, open-ended questions about the client's experience that helped this person further articulate the latter; (3) making empathic statements that indicated our appreciation on an emotional level of what the client was experiencing; and (4) disclosing our own feelings, assumptions, and perceptions in ways that showed the client we were on board with him or her, while not putting our own issues in the forefront. It also involved not engaging in behaviors such as: (1) asking leading questions that guide the client to our own conclusions and prevent the other from revealing the unique quality of his or her own experience; (2) making evaluative statements around an issue before both of us understand our respective positions; (3) offering advice without a careful exploration of the situation; and (4) making light of the client's experience when it is stated seriously.

We were not always successful in living up to these guidelines. Doing so takes a great deal of self-discipline, to say the least. But this was the path we tried to follow. It was especially important to do so during interviews and whenever important issues were being discussed. It was often rewarding, moreover, to see our clients adopt the same behaviors in their dealings with us and, at meetings, with each other. In this sense, active listening is one of the easiest techniques for teaching others through example.

---

[5]Carl R. Rogers and Richard E. Farson, *Active Listening* (Chicago: Industrial Relations Center, The University of Chicago, 1957).

The second technique we followed was an adaptation of the problem-solving model that builds closely on active listening. It involves following a three-stage process in discussing any particular issue. Each party starts with sharing data descriptively about his or her understanding of the situation and helping the other do the same. This is followed by an exchange of opinions about the issue. The trick here is to respond to the other's opinion with one's own opinion, rather than to return to more description. The exchange of opinions may reveal that more descriptive data need to be shared for one of the parties to feel satisfied that he has stated his or her case, but one does this only after an interchange has been completed between opinions.

The third step, once a set of opinions has been agreed to, is to exchange action suggestions. Once again, every action suggestion needs to be responded to with an action suggestion. (I think that should be done too, or my alternative would be _____.) This, in turn, can lead to more exchanges of opinion and possibly then to more description. Thus, one moves from completed exchanges of descriptions to opinions to action suggestions and back as the topic requires.

Researchers in the field of communication have found that matching these different kinds of statements enhances rational dialogue.[6] The participants have a better sense of what they have accomplished at any point in time and find their exchanges more satisfying. We used this approach in important meetings and dropped it during casual conversation. Like active listening, it was easy for our clients to pick up.

We used a number of other techniques as well to enhance our relationship building not only through effective communication, but through bringing our attention to each other's interpersonal needs and defenses. These will be covered in later chapters. The point I wish to convey here is that much of our interaction process was deliberate and conceptually guided. As with the other levels, building collegial relationships requires both a viewpoint and a method.

CONCLUSION

Influencing the members of an organization to pursue OD values is a complex and subtle process. OD consultants arrive on the scene presumably with a reputation for helping organizations function more effectively through interventions into the behavioral side of management. But, unlike other management consultants, they tend not to have a specific subculture to welcome them and support their efforts to make a useful impact on the organization. Instead, they enter at the bidding of important managers who have a general sense that they the consultants might be helpful around issues that do not fit easily into the ongoing distribution of labor. Clients may share with their consultants a humanistically oriented management philosophy but they are also likely to have little knowledge of how the consultants accomplish their objectives or the concepts they use to guide their behavior.

It is up to the OD consultants to develop their own support system and to endow it with the qualities that will make it a model of OD in action for the rest of the organization to observe, interact with, and try out on its own. They do this by using

[6] William R. Banaka, *Training in Depth Interviewing* (New York: Harper and Row, 1971).

themselves as instruments and by managing the little control they are given over people's attention (content), the way they deal with what they attend to (process), and the conditions under which they do this (context) to convey the basic principles of OD in everything they do.

They write project proposals and reports that respond logically to their clients' felt needs. And they write them in a way that encourages a sharing of commitment by everyone involved to the project's objectives and that recognizes the potential resources that many organization members have to offer. They organize and execute their work in ways that their clients consider professional, and they encourage and portray candidness and self-responsibility in their public behavior while doing this. They develop and maintain cordial relationships with their clients that make them trustworthy and valuable contributors, and they enhance these relationships by using their skills to broaden their scope beyond traditional role definitions and to establish a basic sense of equality.

In the end, if all goes well, the initial problems and opportunities the clients brought the OD consultants' attention to are dealt with effectively, and the clients are left with something more—a working model of the OD process that they can use without the consultants' help in the future. The OD consultants, in turn, are left with a group of new colleagues who now know much more about their approach and can act as consultants to them in the future, and who have helped them the consultants grow and develop as professionals.

CHAPTER FOUR

THE SKILLS
OF
THE OD PRACTITIONER

It is one thing to review the goals of Organization Development and to see how they are pursued in the context of a particular OD project. It is quite another to establish a client/consultant relationship and to design and implement an OD project on one's own. I have begun with the former in order to give you as rich a descriptive picture as space will permit of what OD is all about. I think our project at South City Chemical was a good example, but only an example, of the OD process. However, I have never done nor will I probably ever do a project just like it. The nature of my initial contacts, the client needs to be addressed, the size and complexity of the client system, the personalities of influential managers to be worked with, and the general culture of the client organization continuously differ from project to project. Consequently, while my goals for OD and my theory of influencing clients to pursue these goals remain essentially the same, I am obliged to alter the way I introduce, design, sell, and implement any OD project.

I believe this is true for any OD practitioner. It is, indeed, what makes OD an interesting field of endeavor. Unfortunately, this also makes it difficult for anyone new in the field to start off with an accurate picture of its breadth and depth. Let us assume, however, that for the purposes of getting started, I have given you enough of a sampling of OD for you to have developed a general idea of its goals and activities. Now the real work begins.

The real work of becoming an OD practitioner lies in developing a series of basic skills. These skills are applicable to any OD project. Mastering them allows one continuously to be innovative in designing all aspects of an OD project to meet a client's particular needs without losing sight of OD's underlying goals. The greater one's mastery of them, the less one has to rely on any particular technique or bag of tricks and the more one can use any technique, old or new, in a deliberate and timely manner.

These skills fall into four basic categories: conceptual, interpersonal, technical, and integrative. Conceptual skills are critical for managing content, interpersonal skills for managing process, technical skills for managing context, and integrative skills for managing a total project. Each kind of skill has a public and private side to it. The public side is what your clients see and experience through your behavior in their presence. The private side is what enables you to choose what to say to and do with particular clients at particular points in time. The public side enables you not only to fulfill your commitments but also to teach your clients new ways of thinking and behaving. The private side helps you both to prepare for your interactions with your clients and to remain centered as a professional. Continuously employing both sides helps you learn and grow as a professional.

In subsequent parts of this book, we will consider how each of these kinds of skills can be developed for work at the organizational, group, and interpersonal levels. The rest of this chapter will be devoted to an elaboration of each kind of skill and what it entails, regardless of the level at which one is working.

CONCEPTUAL SKILLS

Conceptual skills comprise, on the public side, the capacity to guide the client's attention to problems, opportunities, and ways of thinking about organization life that are consistent with OD values. On the private side, they involve the capacity to theorize about what one is trying to accomplish and to accumulate new knowledge continuously to do this. Let us deal first with the public side.

The public side of conceptual skills is essential for defining OD projects in collaboration with one's client. Every client has a particular set of needs and a relatively unique language for stating them. The task of getting started together requires considerable skill on the consultant's part in building a project definition that responds to those needs from the client's viewpoint, and yet simultaneously frames the issues in ways that ensure a commitment to an OD style of inquiry.

Initial conversations are not only mutual tests of compatibility in terms of needs and interests, but also implicit negotiations over the conceptualization of the work to be done. The same activity—for instance, an attempt to improve a division's functioning—can be conceived in different ways—for example, an assessment by an expert outsider, a top-down reorganization, a renegotiation of roles and responsibilities, or a collaborative analysis and action program. The more an OD specialist can emphasize collaborative principles in the way he or she defines the project with the client, the easier it is for the client to embrace this particular orientation. Every report, memo, or conversation can thereafter be used to reinforce the same. While the words themselves may rarely include OD theory, they need to be consistent with it if the consultant is to succeed in getting his or her basic message across.

A client is also exposed to an OD consultant's conceptual skills throughout a project in terms of the ideas the latter offers for planning each component event, making it understandable as it progresses, and studying its implications once it is over. Organizations maintain their direction in large part through the conceptual maps their members share—goals, roles, decision-making logic, and procedures. It is up to the OD consultant to continuously integrate the logic of a project into these maps. Broad theoretical positions and their action implications need to be distilled into pithy, easily understood statements that make sense in terms of the client's frame of reference. At the same time, one of the major objectives of the OD consultant is to broaden his or her client's thinking so that it includes attention to OD-related issues.

For instance, during the individual feedback sessions at South City Chemical, we put considerable effort into restating issues for our clients in ways that heightened awareness of their behavioral implications. In the course of doing this, we left many a manager's office with a brief conceptual scheme on his blackboard—for example, a model of the communication process or group development or leadership style or organization design principles. More often than not, these schemes did not spring spontaneously from our minds as we talked with the client. We had planned to present them if the opportunity became available as part of our preparation for these meetings.

Both the capacity to select or conceive such schemes and to determine when it is appropriate to use them in conversations with a client are important components of the private side of the OD consultant's conceptual skills.

We presented, in Chapter One, a brief overview of the goals of OD for work at each system level. Developing effective conceptual skills on the private side involves one's mastery of the logic behind each set of goals and of the relevant literature in the applied behavioral sciences that supports them. This requires, as do all the other skills, a commitment to an ongoing learning process.

Knowledge in the applied behavioral sciences is expanding rapidly. Much of what is useful to an OD practitioner does not appear in practitioner oriented journals. Sometimes even the most turgid academic texts contain the germ of an idea that can enhance a consultant's thinking. Effective OD consultants are avid readers of anything that deals with people and society. The trick, of course, is to discover the relevant connections in whatever one reads that will lead to new insights for one's own theorizing. This is where the basic concepts of OD enter in. They provide a focus for organizing one's inquiry so that one can juxtapose new ideas against old ones and expand one's theorizing rather than merely accumulate interesting facts.

The next step is to distinguish between those ideas that can be used to guide one's own thinking and behavior but need not be shared with a client and those that the client would find useful. Different ideas may be useful to a particular client at a particular point in time, and this points ultimately to the need to use one's theorizing in concert with one's observations to decide when and what to share.

When one is working with a client, it becomes obvious that no one intellectual paradigm, including any of those presented in this book, is likely to capture all of reality at any given point in time. And what any single scheme does capture may not be relevant to the participant's concerns at the moment. For instance, I may enter a meeting preoccupied with developing people's skills at effective communication and have a number of concepts relevant to this activity in my awareness. I may find, however, that the participants are actually doing quite well on this level relative to their inability to cope with an especially powerful and antagonistic member. Unless I can shift my focus to problems of inclusion and control, and theories related to them, I may be unable to understand the importance of what is going on and, therefore, will not help the group to deal with this more important concern.

In summary, every OD practitioner needs a theory to guide his or her behavior, one that he or she is continuously testing and elaborating both for professional development and for understanding the situations one encounters. And this person also needs a repertoire of conceptual inputs and ways of deciding when to use them that allows one to share one's perspective with others, so that they can join in this endeavor according to their own needs and interests. This is what is involved in developing conceptual skills.

INTERPERSONAL SKILLS

The *interpersonal skills* of the OD practitioner involve the ability to connect emotionally with clients in ways that make it comfortable for them to accept the consultant as a role model for dealing with the issues raised during a project. Thus, just as conceptual skills form the resource for managing content, interpersonal skills form the resource for managing process.

On the public side, this entails the capacity to invoke in clients and in oneself a number of important feelings and attributions. These include, first, a mutual feeling of acceptance and positive regard for each other as individuals, regardless of the particular problems being faced at the moment. In reviewing the literature on the results of various techniques for individual therapy, Rogers found that the patient's experience of unconditional positive regard by the therapist was an important criterion for success, regardless of the technique used.[1] My own experience in OD suggests that this basic criterion is also important, with the caveat that it needs to be mutually experienced. I have been most successful when, from very early on in a project, I liked my clients as individuals and found that the feeling was mutual. While interpersonal differences and project difficulties were inevitable, bonds of this sort made it much easier to overcome them. Equally important, I have found that, to a considerable extent, one can learn to like one's clients. It is a skill rather than an unalterable predilection.

Second, a consultant needs to behave in ways that provide both himself/herself and clients with a sense of security when trying out new behaviors that are scary or unfamiliar. Some of this can come from mutual positive regard, but much of it derives from two other sources; first, the consultant's experience in doing these things elsewhere and, second, successful past experiences in trying out new behaviors with the same clients. Since OD projects are collaborative in nature, this last factor is especially important. I have found that both my clients and I take the most risks in almost all areas (confrontation, self-disclosure, commitments to change structure and policy) only after we have worked together for several months and have a series of successes around less important issues.

A third important feeling state that a consultant needs to induce is that of mutual empathy. This comes primarily from training in active listening and general interviewing skills. Presumably, this is an area in which the consultant has had

---

[1]Carl R. Rogers, *On Becoming a Person* (Boston: Houghton Mifflin Co., 1962), pp. 39-49, 243-73.

considerable practice before engaging with a client, and we will devote a major section to it later in this book. But equally important, as we noted in Chapter Three, it is a skill that a consultant can teach clients by using it in interactions with them.

Fourth, an effective OD consultant has the capacity to generate a spirit of playfulness into much of his or her dealings with clients. This is not to say that the many situations calling for serious dialogue should not be responded to with an appropriately sober demeanor, but that playfulness—Freud called it regression in the service of the ego—is often a very helpful ingredient in dealing with sensitive issues.

Sobriety is closely associated with adulthood, and behaving as an adult in most cultures involves injunctions such as being totally in control of one's feelings, behaviors, and cognitions. One's self-concept as an adult member of the community must be maintained at all costs. And this can get in the way of expressing one's anxieties, responding to events spontaneously, and trying out new behaviors.

Playfulness, on the other hand, is associated with childhood, and in most cultures it is legitimate for children to express their emotions, to behave spontaneously, and to experiment continuously with their behavior. When adults give themselves permission, if only temporarily, to be playful, they often surprise themselves by discovering how much of their concerns they share with others, how instructive spontaneity can be, and how effective new ways of working together can be if they only give themselves a chance to learn them. There is a child in all of us, and effective OD consultants learn to show this side of themselves and to provide others with the opportunity to do the same in the service of very adult objectives.

Finally, effective OD consultants succeed in generating feelings of mutual respect for personal boundaries and cherished values. This comes from training one's senses to be immediately aware of changes in one's own and others' anxiety levels and to respond in thoughtful ways to these changes. Skill needs to be developed in recognizing changes in tone of voice, body language, and spoken language patterns and in interpreting these appropriately. A further requirement is to know when to test boundaries and confront differences because this is critical for a project's success. The failure to confront may often be more damaging than the consequences of confrontation. When confrontation is handled well, moreover, mutual respect tends to increase.

The capacity to induce these states—of mutual positive regard, security, empathy, playfulness, and mutual respect—is what makes an effective OD consultant a different kind of individual in most clients' lives. These are scarce phenomena in the day-to-day organizational world. Consultants who can create them gain the potency necessary for clients to treat them as role models even though they, the consultants, are outsiders and only temporary visitors to the organization.

Developing and maintaining this capacity represents the private side of the OD consultant's interpersonal skills. This involves first and foremost the continuous pursuit of self-knowledge. It is extremely difficult to help other people on an emotional level without being able to manage one's own emotional world. OD practitioners, like everyone else, have their own emotional needs. They grow up learning to satisfy them in many ways, including some that are destructive to other people's interests. They are susceptible to the same emotional forces in relationships, groups, and organizations that everyone else is. They become upset, unstuck, and uncentered under particular conditions that their unique life experiences have made them susceptible to, just as all people do.

Much of what makes them effective with others is their capacity to deal with these issues with respect to their own lives. Some practitioners are natural at this, just as there are naturally interpersonally skillful people in all walks of life. In fact, my own experience in training OD consultants has been that the most effective people, at least initially, are already seen by their colleagues as interpersonally skillful and self-knowledgeable and, indeed, that this was one of the reasons why they are either encouraged or allowed to pursue OD training in the first place.

For the bulk of us, however, the alternative has been to develop these skills more systematically. A number of avenues are open for doing this. Individual and group therapy is perhaps ideal but also very expensive. A more typical route is through participation in T-groups and human interaction and personal growth labs. These are available throughout the country at modest cost, and they are often included as elements in professional OD training programs. Their emphasis is not on dealing with major personal problems, but on expanding the self-awareness and the capacity to deal with the emotional problems of everyday life. Such training then sets the stage for learning to be helpful to others, and in most cases the two go hand in hand.

This book does not devote a great deal of attention to personal growth activities per se, although many of the topics included in it are likely to be helpful to those interested in this area. Readers who wish to become OD consultants, however, should seriously consider enrolling in one or more of the aforementioned programs early in their training. OD requires a commitment to deal continuously and deliberately with this aspect of one's life.

The private side of an OD specialist's interpersonal skills includes two other components: (1) the capacity to use colleagues as resources, and (2) skill in finding ways to rejuvenate oneself in times of stress and/or low energy. Both are important because of the nature of the OD consultant's role. It should be apparent by now that doing OD requires one to approach organization life from a markedly different perspective from other participants. The very fact that the task requires one to model new kinds of behaviors for others and to take risks in raising sensitive issues that others are afraid to deal with, makes the OD practitioner a marginal figure. At times it can be a very lonely, frustrating, and tension-filled job. The way to cope with this is to find colleagues who can act as both technical and emotional sources of support.

This is not as easy as one might think. Revealing one's problems to a fellow professional can threaten one's ego. Skill at giving and receiving feedback with colleagues comes only with practice and a commitment to collaboration in one's own life as well as with one's clients. Using colleagues for emotional support can be even more difficult, especially if one is working alone on a particular project and essentially has to intrude on their lives in order to do this.

Both skills, once again, are learned most easily in personal growth labs. Here relationships can be developed with trainers and fellow participants in an atmosphere where constructive critique and mutual support are primary objectives. Particularly rewarding relationships can then be maintained and rejuvenated through help on a *quid pro quo* basis when everyone is out on his or her own.

In summary, interpersonally skillful OD consultants consult widely with each other and practice what they preach with each other as well as with clients. They learn how to create conditions of mutual regard, security, empathy, playfulness, and respect for each other, and use these experiences and the relationships evolving out of them as reference points for maintaining their capacity to do so with clients on the job.

TECHNICAL SKILLS

The *technical skills* of the OD practitioner involve, on the public side, the ability to conduct the wide variety of programmed procedures available for implementing many aspects of the OD process. These can involve work at all system levels (individual, group, organizational) and all phases of a project, from conducting an initial meeting with a prospective client to ending a relationship. The bulk of OD technology, however, deals with methods for responding to specific client needs — for example, organizational analysis, team building, and intergroup conflict. For instance, the basic form of the interview/feedback activity we engaged in at South City Chemical would fall under the rubric of an OD procedure and so would some of our follow-up interventions such as the step-by-step role negotiations between superiors and subordinates that we did with the pilot plant. Today there are dozens of clearly distinguishable technical procedures that practitioners use at one time or another, although I suspect that any one OD specialist uses at most 15 to 20 with any frequency. In the following chapters, we will probably address about a dozen basic techniques, covering all system levels. This should give you a core to start with. Broadening this repertoire is up to you.

The private side of the practitioner's technical skills involves the capacity to select and modify already established procedures and to develop new ones that meet the needs of a particular client at a particular point in time. Only the most basic techniques are applicable to most situations with little modification. Clients can often sense when they are being asked to engage in a programmed activity that is not meeting their needs. Because any technique involves the deliberate investment of time and energy by the client, this can reduce the consultant's credibility and cause people to lose interest in the project as a whole. Commitment to and skill at custom-designing any procedure is critical for an OD consultant.

Technical skills are relevant most directly to the management of context. Any OD procedure guides the participants' attention to particular kinds of content and prescribes particular processes for responding to that content. Thus, it represents context in the same way that such factors as the physical setting, project definition, ongoing relationships, organizational climate, and formal structure and policies do. The OD consultant as author/selector and interpreter of a given procedure is thus acting as a manager of organizational context while he or she is conducting it. This requires that he or she develop certain general skills on both the public and private sides that are germane to the use of any techniques. While we consider particular techniques in detail later on, these general skills are worth noting here.

Three capabilities are especially germane on the public side: (1) polish in presentation, (2) manual dexterity, and (3) the ability to respond to unforeseen contingencies. Many practitioners who are excellent conceptually and interpersonally are poor presenters. Excellence at presentation involves the ability to describe clearly and distinctly what a given procedure will involve and to give the impression that one knows what one is doing and can be relied on for guidance as the activity unfolds. This takes practice and the self-discipline of careful preparation, regardless of the number of times one has used a particular technique.

Many procedures involve some form of manual dexterity. These can range from the almost trivial—penmanship, correct use of flipcharts, on-the-spot mathematical calculations, creating appropriate seating patterns—to fairly complex skills such as questionnaire design, statistical analysis of survey data, qualitative data analysis, and creating provocative presentation formats. These too require practice and often considerable training. They are typically skills that are important for professionals in general. They need to be mastered by the OD practitioner and tailored to the needs of his or her procedures because problems in these areas both reduce credibility and get in the way of the real business at hand. When the issues being addressed create tension for the people involved, the last thing one wants are technical *faux pas*.

Finally, the implementation of any technique requires the capacity to modify it on the spot in light of unforeseen events. For example, in conducting the feedback sessions on the interview data at South City Chemical, we had envisioned a situation in which most of those attending each group meeting would have taken part in the interviews. Accordingly, we had designed a procedure in which the meeting would begin with each person present offering three to five minutes of comment about the feedback document. We would put each person's comments on flipcharts and then use these data to design an agenda for the ensuing discussion.

We had not foreseen that almost all of the union personnel would attend along with their respective managers and professionals. As noted earlier, the first time this happened, we found that the most important issue to address was not in the interview data fed back, but in what the union people had to say about being invited into the activity, why they had resisted earlier, why they were attending now, and what this did or did not imply. Rather than proceed as intended, we opened the floor to a general discussion of these issues and put the union members' comments on flipcharts before attending to the feedback documents. In the first meeting, this required us to rush the rest of the procedure we had laid out. Subsequently, we found a way to abbreviate the original agenda and include the treatment of new issues brought up on the spot. Had we not done this, we would have lost an important opportunity to get the union personnel on board and probably would have lost their participation thereafter.

My experience is that a great many well-planned procedures suffer a similar fate. A crisis has occurred that requires immediate attention, a particular method of generating data proves annoying to several participants or unexpectedly makes one person especially vulnerable to attack, some prospective participants whose inputs are critical are absent, a relationship has to be cleared up before full energy can be devoted to the planned agenda, and so on. There are times when it is better to proceed with what was planned. Nonetheless, the more the consultant can respond thoughtfully and rapidly to such events, the more he or she gets done what he or she sets out to do.

General technical skills on the private side involve a slightly different form of preparedness. A great many OD techniques are effective because they cause participants to reexamine their assumptions about how they are seen by others, about what their colleagues think and feel about various issues, and about how their organizations operate. As a result, participants occasionally become unstuck, emotional, and frequently defensive. Unless the consultant has been through similar activities as a participant in the past, the same procedures can unfreeze himself or herself emotionally and cause one to behave ineffectively in helping others to deal with them. It is very easy, for instance, to become emotionally involved in defending an interpretation of some data one has spent many hours analyzing, even when one has asked everyone to state his or her views candidly before evaluating any position; or to want to come to the aid of a particular client being given negative feedback even when one has suggested that each person's views be explored, understood, and appreciated before entertaining responses to them. In short, an OD consultant needs to know through experience what to expect from a particular technique and to learn how to deal with this, just as one needs to do this when dealing with more spontaneous interpersonal issues.

A second requirement closely related to this is for the consultant to be able to choose interventions that get the most work done with the least emotional stress. Roger Harrison has called this the art of choosing an intervention with the appropriate depth.[2] There are often many ways to get the same objective accomplished. For instance, one can provide opportunities for people to give each other feedback through procedures that focus on (1) ideal roles, (2) actual behavior in role, (3) behavior regardless of role, or (4) personal feelings about and perceptions of another, regardless of the latter's specific behaviors. The latter procedures in this list typically provide data relevant to the earlier ones but, when handled well, they also generate more emotions and make the consultant a more prominent figure. A consultant needs to decide just how much emotionality to risk in order to accomplish a given objective and forego the ego rewards of deeper interventions when the latter are unnecessary.

Two colleagues, for instance, who work with each other night and day may need to confront each other on a very personal level in order to resolve an issue, while a pair who see each other rarely and in the context of programmed routines may be able to resolve all they need to through the exchange of guarded statements about their ideal roles. A well-accepted consultant may be given permission to conduct either procedure. If this person chooses the emotionally more potent intervention, he or she may gain the lasting admiration of both parties because of the intensity of the experience, but may also create unnecessary risks or loss of energy. This could hinder the successful treatment of subsequent situations where deeper interventions are more critical.

In summary, OD specialists need technical skills to select, design, and implement the field's programmatic techniques. This is a major tool in the management of the little amount of context they are given direct control over by their clients. To do this

[2]Roger Harrison, "Choosing the Depth of Organizational Intervention," in *The Journal of Applied Behavioral Science*, Vol. 2, No. 6, pp. 182-202.

well they need to be familiar with what the field has to offer, to plan innovatively on their own, and to assess client needs accurately. This, in turn, requires sound general skills in presentation, execution, and spontaneous adjustment, plus enough experience to transcend their own emotions in the act of execution, and a willingness to intervene only as deeply as necessary.

INTEGRATIVE SKILLS

Conceptual, interpersonal, and technical skills comprise what it takes to manage content, process, and context, respectively. To make all three skills blend into the management of a total project requires yet another kind of capability, which I will call integrative skills. *Integrative skills* on the public side involve the ability to conceive, sell, and manage a total OD project in a way that both responds to the client's needs and enhances the pursuit of OD values. On the private side, integrative skills involve the capacity to coordinate any given project's activities with the rest of one's professional life.

We mentioned in Chapter Two that OD projects are a blend of the usual with the unusual from the clients' perspective. The details of specific activities are often unusual, but the basic concept of an OD project is the same as it is for most other kinds of consulting or staff projects. There are certain predictable stages—entry, contracting, analysis, actions to respond to the analysis, evaluation, and termination. Certain phases may lead to the repetition of others; thus, evaluation may lead to more analysis or a new contract. Project activities have to be buffered from and/or kept in synchronization with other organizational activities to prevent undesired interference in either direction. Official approval and financial resources have to be maintained to support project activities.

On the public side, one very important aspect of an OD consultant's integrative skills is that of managing these issues in ways that are consistent with the project's philosophy and objectives. It involves the melding of two worlds, that of OD project activities, on the one hand, and day-to-day management, on the other. The contract has to make sense in economic terms and yet not make promises that are unrealistic. Evidence of hard work and expert contribution by the consultants needs to be provided without sacrificing the project's basically collaborative nature. Specific interventions need to speak to the problems identified without sapping the organization's resources for day-to-day work. Evaluations need to be hard-nosed without ignoring the many qualitative and subtle changes that OD projects create. Even though ideally the senior managers who invite the consultant in also share the burden of integration at this level, the focus is usually on the consultant at the beginning and tends ultimately to remain this person's responsibility throughout the project.

A second integrative skill that impacts directly on clients is the consultant's ability to orchestrate various kinds of activities in ways that reinforce one another. Any phase of a project cycle can take place on several levels (individual, group, organizational) and with different individuals, groups, and major organizational subunits. Careful planning is required to make sure that each member of the client organization experiences the project in a logical sequence. For instance, at South City Chemical we spent many hours planning both alone and with senior managers. Topics included

devising a sequence of activities so that everyone knew about the project before participating, making sure that influential people would have their say before activities affecting their concerns were undertaken, making sure that data were fed back more or less
simultaneously to people who worked closely together, and sequencing action steps to
match the division's priorities.

Finally, on the public side, OD consultants need to be able to manage their
own teamwork so that it maximizes use of each team member's skills, provides opportunities for personal development, and makes up for particular personal weaknesses.
Much of this depends on team members' use of their interpersonal skills in working
with each other, but it also has an integrative component in that dealing with these
issues has to take place at times and places that make sense for the project as a whole.
One cannot work on important issues with colleagues and clients simultaneously without one side getting short shrift. At South City we made sure that each day's activities
were interspersed with clinic sessions with each other. Since the client came first when
we were onsite, this often meant meeting very late at night, a typical situation for most
team-based OD projects.

The private side of the OD practitioner's integrative skills involves, once
again, some basic issues in self-management. OD projects tend to be long-term, intermittent activities. They have major peaks and valleys in work loads and emotional intensity for the consultants as well as for the clients. Over the course of a project, it is
just as true to say that the consultants let the organization enter their lives, altering
their attention patterns, their ways of doing things, and their contexts as it is to say that
the organization lets the consultants in with similar effects. Consequently, yet another
quality a consultant needs to possess is the capacity to deal with this intrusion in all its
manifestations.

Cognitively, this means separating the reality of the organization from that of
one's own professional life. Sometimes when I become intensely involved in a project, I
find myself using words, phrases, concepts, and whole sets of assumptions that I pick
up on the job, in settings where they make much less sense. For instance, after working
with a group of surgeons for several months, I found myself talking about OD techniques as if they were medical operations and fantasizing a whole complex of procedures that translated OD into a medical framework. Some of this was useful and stimulating, but it was only after I had been away from this group for awhile that I could see
the effect it had had on me and appraise it realistically.

Emotionally, one needs to put the relationships one develops during a project
into perspective. It is easy for your clients' problems to become your problems. When
onsite, this can be quite functional, but more effective OD consultants have the capacity to refrain from taking their emotional involvements home with them. The same
principle, of course, holds for work in general. It is an especially difficult problem for
OD consultants, however, because of the emotional intensity in their work. Working
on an OD project in a large organization and dealing with many people's emotional
worlds simultaneously can be taxing. Because one's role is to attend to emotional
issues, the intensity of the experience is likely to be considerably greater than one's

everyday life. Very active consultants, especially those who work alone, without colleagues to keep things in perspective, frequently complain of becoming emotionally burned out as a result.

On a technical level, there is an endless amount of innovation and fine-tuning to make every procedure meet the needs of a particular client. All efforts in this direction require time and energy, however, and one needs to set clear priorities in order to run a well-organized professional life. The opposite problem also needs to be avoided. Too little custom designing can seduce one into using a set of canned techniques that save time and energy but also impoverish one's learning and eventually leave clients unhappy. The first error can be tied to excessive emotional involvement, the second to one's defense against it.

Finally, effective OD consultants make sure that no single project becomes so important to them for either financial or status reasons that they lose sight of their professional identities and responsibilities. Once again, strong ties with colleagues both on the job and elsewhere help one to deal most effectively with these hangups.

In summary, integrative skills involve the capacity to coordinate the requirements of modern management with the logic of an OD project, to orchestrate component activities so that they reinforce and complement one another, and to deal with colleagues on the job in ways that maximize the effectiveness of the consulting team as a total unit while fostering individual growth from within. Underlying these abilities is the capacity to run one's own life effectively by recognizing the impact of OD project work on oneself, and learning to use it for one's own development without being dominated by it.

CONCLUSION

The skills requirements I have posited above for an effective OD consultant may seem excessive. In one sense, this is intentional. I do not want to give the impression that any single book can give someone all the tools necessary to be successful in this field. Personal competence in OD, I believe, requires a multiyear commitment and a willingness to pursue learning along several dimensions on one's own. The requirements are holistic, dealing with intellect and emotion and relating to self-management as well as one's interaction with others. This is consistent with the goals of the field, which promote responsible self-management in every organization member and a commitment to deal holistically with colleagues.

At the same time, I have tried to paint a picture that helps to reveal the varieties of relevant skills already present in almost every reader. The same categories I have presented are applicable to any profession. OD has its own particular emphasis but it draws on a universal set of human resources. In this sense, the only thing that is particularly unique about it is its emphasis on the whole person. Thus, the task for the beginner is to start off thinking holistically, to appreciate all the skills he or she already has, and to use a book such as this to integrate and continue to develop these skills in a particular direction.

CHAPTER FIVE

THREE APPROACHES TO BUILDING A COLLABORATIVE ORGANIZATION

In the next several chapters we will explore the conceptual, technical, and interpersonal details of doing the kind of OD portrayed in chapters Two and Three. This chapter, however, is devoted to the important prior task of putting our approach into context. The kind of OD I have discussed thus far represents only one of three basic approaches that OD consultants have used over the past two decades. While each approach has its merits, the focal one for this book is particularly suited for new consultants and internal practitioners. It requires the least amount of external credibility to initiate. It provides the most opportunities for gaining credibility, and it allows one to meld in elements of the other two as a project unfolds. After examining all three approaches, we will explore how and why it does this.

COLLABORATIVE ORGANIZATION

Let us begin by reviewing the objectives of doing OD at the organizational level and the major forces affecting such an effort. The primary objective at this level is to build or at least encourage a client to experiment with what we have termed a collaborative form of organization. This type of organization in the ideal can be characterized by qualities such as the following:

- Structures and policies that facilitate broad-based understanding of and commitment to organization goals and that maximize the coalignment of authority, expertise, and relevant information in the roles created for achieving these goals.
- Reward systems that, without dismissing the importance of individual contributions, acknowledge the interdependent nature of organization life by placing considerable emphasis on group performance.
- Measurement systems that are used by both those who are doing the measuring

and those who are being measured as imperfect yardsticks for indicating progress toward particular objectives, rather than as rigid performance criteria that become ends in themselves.

- Staffing and personal development procedures that involve the actors in question, as well as the people responsible for these activities, in a shared analysis of individual career needs and aspirations in the context of the organization's long-term interests, and of the current and potential resources the individual can offer the organization.

As noted earlier, the collaborative form is also an ideal context for fostering people's pursuit of OD values and practices in groups and relationships. Specifically, this form facilitates candidness, self-responsibility, consensus decision making, relating to others holistically, an underlying sense of egalitarianism, and collegial relationships.

Collaborative organization, according to our model, flows most naturally from the day-to-day activities of leaders who assume (1) that their followers are basically committed to the welfare of the organization, and (2) that every member is a potential source of valuable resources for promoting the organization's welfare. The assumption of shared commitment induces leaders to err on the side of trust rather than mistrust in sharing and exploring important issues with the membership. While some damage may be done because of this, the general effect, I believe, is to induce greater trust and commitment in return. Trust breeds trust. Commitment breeds commitment. Likewise, the assumption that every member is a potential holder of valuable resources encourages leaders to inquire continuously into their followers' thinking in a respectful manner and to help them grow and develop. In this way, they enhance the resources each member has to offer and maximize the chances of discovering ways in which these resources can be used to benefit both the individual and the organization.

According to our model, a leading group's choice to operate under these assumptions is itself determined largely by two underlying conditions: the leading group's management ideology and their perceptions of the current distribution among the membership of the resources (potential and immediately available) necessary for the organization's survival.

A basically humanistic orientation (one that asserts the essential dignity of every individual and his or her capacity for self-realization through reason) justifies the characterization of each member as worthy of being courted, listened to, and supported. By contrast, other orientations, such as those that attribute different levels of basic value to different economic classes, status, and power groups, justify more selective patterns of attention and support.

Likewise, perceptions of a highly skewed distribution among the membership of the particular resources necessary for the organization's survival, are likely to drive even the most humanistic managers to sacrifice balanced attention and support in favor of more selective patterns, at least in the near term.

Figure 5–1 identifies the relevant forces that determine the organizational form a leading group is attempting to implement. Note that, while we have been discussing these forces above in reference to the collaborative form, different forms can be explained in terms of different ideologies, experiences, assumptions, and so on, in the context of this model.

FIGURE 5-1
Forces Determining
a Leadership Group's Pursuit
of a Particular
Organizational Form

MANAGEMENT IDEOLOGY AND
PERCEPTIONS OF THE DISTRIBUTION
OF RESOURCES CRITICAL FOR
THE ORGANIZATION'S SURVIVAL

↓

ASSUMPTIONS REGARDING THE
TOTAL MEMBERS' COMMITMENT
TO THE ORGANIZATION'S WELFARE

AND

MEMBERS' CONTROL OVER RESOURCES THAT
MIGHT BENEFIT THE ORGANIZATION

↓

THE PARTICULAR
FORM OF ORGANIZATION
CURRENTLY USED

Doing OD at the organizational level involves the consultant in an attempt to provide a series of experiences for the leadership group that represent both a convincing case for pursuing the collaborative form and some clear guidelines for doing so. Three basic strategies are currently used. Their most important distinguishing features can be characterized by referring back to the central concepts of Chapter Three.

CONTENT, PROCESS, AND CONTEXT REVISITED

Chapter 3 talked about three ways of influencing a client: (1) molding content, that is, bringing the client's attention systematically to particular subject matter; (2) molding process, that is, interacting deliberately in a particular way with the client; and (3) molding context, that is, attempting to structure the conditions under which one interacts with a client. The power of the consultant's message comes from its consistency across these three ways rather than from its intensity within any one of them.

The same concepts can be used when conceiving a large-scale project. Here, however, they are applied to the total organization, as opposed to the consultant/client relationship, and the emphasis in their use changes from internal consistency to the highlighting of a particular dimension. Specifically, the content, process, and context, respectively, of a particular organization's operations represent three distinct areas to which one might bring a client's attention. Each can be treated by organization members from different value orientations, and each interacts with the other two. Therefore, working with the client explicitly to change one of them — for example, the content of organization members' daily concerns, or the processes through which members interact, or the context in which the organization operates — can serve as a starting point for changing all three.

The three basic approaches to OD at the organizational level all involve the consultant in managing content, process, and context in his or her relationship with the client group. But they differ in the extent to which they explicitly emphasize the *organization's* content, process, and context, respectively, as the primary arena for change and experimentation. One approach focuses explicitly on changing the processes or ways in which organization members interact with each other. Thus, the focus of the project is the organization's social processes, and the consultants use whatever control they have over their clients' attention to this topic, the processes through which they discuss it, and the contexts in which they do so to convince them to change these processes to be more consistent with OD values. The second approach focuses explicitly on changing the ways in which managers interpret and set policy in response to the context in which the organization operates, again with the consultants using the process and context of the client/consultant relationship to do this as well. Likewise, the third approach focuses explicitly on changing the ways in which managers interpret and set policy in response to the content of the organization — that is, the day-to-day task and social concerns of each other and the rest of the membership. Figure 5–2 represents the foregoing argument in schematic form and provides some tentative labels for the three approaches.

In the following sections we will review each of these approaches briefly, saving the one we will elaborate on in subsequent chapters for last.

FIGURE 5–2
Approaches to OD
on the Larger System Level

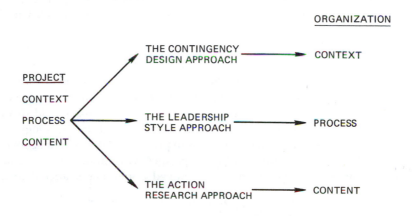

DEVELOPING EFFECTIVE
LEADERSHIP STYLES
THROUGH
LABORATORY TRAINING
AND INTERPERSONAL
ANALYSIS

One of the important precursors of OD in the applied behavioral sciences was the T-group movement. Beginning in the late 1940s, managers, consultants, academicians, and practitioners in the helping professions began to experiment with the use of unstructured groups as vehicles for helping individuals develop greater self-insight, interpersonal skills, and the capacity to improve the functioning of the groups with which they worked. The quotation below from one of the classics in this field summarizes the nature of these kinds of activities:

> A T-Group is a relatively unstructured group in which individuals participate as learners. The data for learning are not outside these individuals or remote from their immediate experience within the T-Group. The data are the transactions among the members, their own behavior within the group as they struggle to create a productive and viable organization, a miniature society; and as they work to stimulate and support one another's learning within the society. Involving experiences are a necessary, but not the only condition of learning. T-Group members must establish a process of inquiry in which data about their own behaviors are collected and analyzed simultaneously with the experience which generates these behaviors. Learnings thus achieved are tested and generalized for continuing use. Each individual may learn about his own motives, feelings, and strategies in dealing with other persons. He learns also of the other and seeks help from others in converting potentialities into actualities.
>
> Each individual may learn also about groups in the process of helping to build one. He may develop skills of membership and skills for changing and improving his social environment as well as himself. The staff who work with T-Groups do not see any necessary opposition between participation in groups and autonomous individual functioning, though they are well aware that opposition does occur in many associations of our lives and that group forces may be used to inhibit personal development. In the T-Group, on the contrary, the objective is to mobilize group forces to support the growth of members as unique individuals simultaneously with their growth as collaborators. Influences among peers are paramount in this learning process. In the T-Group, members develop their own skills in giving and receiving help. They learn to help the trainer (or teacher) as he assists in the development of individual and group learnings.[1]

As one can see from the description above, T-group training or laboratory training, as it is more often called today, embodies essentially all of the values we have identified in this book as underlying OD, and in fact much of the underlying philosophy of OD was originally developed by leaders in the T-group field. It was a natural step for early practitioners of this art to attempt to use this methodology to develop organizations as well. The initial thrust was to provide groups of managers in an organization with new interpersonal skills and perspectives through the laboratory training process. The assumption was that those trained would then change their work-related

---

[1]Leland P. Bradford, Jack R. Gibb, and Kenneth D. Benne, *T-Group Theory and Laboratory Method* (New York: John Wiley and Sons, Inc., 1964), pp. 1-2.

interpersonal behavior and organizational decision-making practices to fit the underlying values of this methodology.

Weaknesses of the Approach.   Major problems were encountered almost immediately, however. To begin with, managers returning from T-group experiences faced major difficulties in reentry. The first groups attempted were comprised of managers who did not work with each other on a day-to-day basis, the assumption being that working in "stranger" groups would facilitate personal learning by removing historical influences and important ongoing status differences. This resulted, however, in situations where managers who were basking in the euphoria of a successful group experience, full of new insights about themselves and group life, and energy to behave differently in the future, would return to a social setting in which their colleagues neither had been through a similar experience nor had been prepared to welcome new behavior on the part of their returning colleague.

The returnee would quickly experience the force of group norms operating in a different direction, his or her enthusiasm would falter, and the net effect of the T-group experience would at best be one of a very private transformation in understanding and self-insight and, at worst, bitter disillusionment.

A second major problem dealt with differences in ideology. Efforts to introduce T-group-oriented OD began in the late 1950s, a time when the basic concept of participative management was still in its infancy, far from being integrated with more traditional notions of authoritarian management. In some cases senior managers would sanction a training program for others but refuse to become involved themselves, thus missing the critical experiences that might help them to make sense out of the perspectives derived from these efforts.

At the lower levels, ideological conflict was evident around the issue of psychological safety. T-groups as management training programs were far more intrusive psychologically than traditional methods of manager development. Stories spread rapidly of managers being psychologically undressed, of being forced to change personal behaviors that were traditionally matters of personal choice and not open to public analysis, of people having breakdowns due to the emotional stress of unstructured group activities.

This led to major concerns about whether it was legitimate to introduce such activities in the first place. While most efforts were identified officially as strictly voluntary, managers complained that the realities of their day-to-day worlds made them obligatory. Those who refused to attend when given the opportunity might be seen as uncooperative or uninterested in moving ahead with the organization.

A third major problem with this initial strategy was that, while T-group work per se did provide people with a new and potentially useful way of approaching the management process on the interpersonal and intragroup levels, it offered few specifics regarding how to deal with behavioral issues at the intergroup and larger system levels. Thus, particular teams might become more effective internally only to find that they did not have the wherewithal to encounter other groups productively and promote changes in the formal organization that would be consistent with their personal learnings.

Later Developments.   In varying degrees, all three of these problems remain today. However, consultants who have continued to practice this approach have come a long way toward resolving them. Problems in reentry have been reduced significantly by training whole teams of managers who work together on a daily basis and by training line managers to be trainers. Ideological conflict at the top of the organization has been ameliorated both by the gradual acceptance of participative management into our administrative culture, a reflection of changing societal values, and by the refusal of practitioners to undertake the training approach without strong top management support and participation.

The same shift in societal values has helped to legitimize T-group kinds of activities as normal components of management and personal development, and many managers are introduced to such activities in their early schooling, church, and community programs, undergraduate courses, and MBA programs. Beyond this, numerous organizations are becoming publicly more clear regarding their philosophies with

FIGURE 5-3
The Managerial Grid

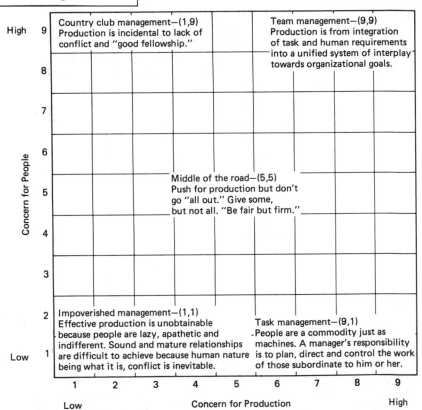

Source: Robert R. Blake and Jane Syrgley Mouton, *The Managerial Grid Laboratory Seminar Materials* (Austin, Tex.: Scientific Methods, 1962).

respect to laboratory group work, so that those who are considering employment with them can take this into account in their own choices.

Yet another way in which ideological differences have been dealt with is through the use by consultants of conceptual schemes that translate T-group values (often seen as abstract and academic) into more easily understood and (by modern management standards) culturally attractive concerns. For example, two of the originators and still very active proponents of the manager-run, laboratory training approach are Robert R. Blake and Jane Syrgley Mouton.[2] The well-known trademark of these consultants is the Managerial Grid, a typology that characterizes leadership styles as byproducts of combinations of concerns for two dimensions: production and people (see Figure 5–3).

The ideal style to pursue, according to Blake and Mouton, is the (9,9) Team Management approach. When translated into concrete behaviors, this style is very similar to both the underlying values of the T-group movement and the upper-right hand quadrants of the value paradigms used in this book.

Finally, the problem of translating the underlying values of the laboratory training approach into perspectives and procedures for dealing with larger scale (intergroup and organization design) issues has been dealt with through the creation of multistage programs that follow up group training efforts with explicit attention to these other issues. For example, Blake and Mouton offer a multiphase program that begins with training, and proceeds through efforts at intergroup development, the creation of an ideal organizational blueprint, and, ultimately, the implementation of this blueprint.

Blake and Mouton's program is probably the best-known example of the leadership style approach, but it is by no means the only one. Hersey and Blanchard offer an interesting variation on the same model, and numerous less well published consultants have developed their own variations on the same themes as well.[3]

In summary, the basic elements of this approach today are:

1.   The use of some conceptual model that brings the client's attention to the process of managing the organization (usually in terms of a leadership or personal style paradigm) and that provides a vehicle for highlighting the merits of behaving in ways that are consistent with OD values.

2.   Group training activities that facilitate the assimilation of the model, skill building in the identification and enactment of particular styles, and exploration of the problems and opportunities associated with each of them.

3.   Follow-up activities that provide guidelines for and practice in using particular styles and the values underlying them for dealing with larger system issues.

[2]Robert R. Blake and Jane Syrgley Mouton, "An Overview of the Grid," in *Training and Development Journal* (The American Society for Training and Development, Inc., May 1975), pp. 29-37.

[3]Paul Hersey and Kenneth H. Blanchard, *Management of Organizational Behavior: Utilizing Human Resources*, 4th ed. (Englewood Cliffs, N.J.: Prentice-Hall, Inc., 1982).

CONTINGENCY DESIGN APPROACH TO ENHANCE FIT BETWEEN ORGANIZATION'S STRATEGY FOR DEALING WITH ENVIRONMENT AND INTERNAL STRUCTURE AND POLICIES

Something else besides the T-group movement was happening in management circles between the end of World War II and the 1960s. Large organizations and business firms in particular were facing the task of integrating their organizational learnings from their participation in the war effort. The demand to produce both old and totally new products under emergency conditions had forced them to break many of the traditional tenets regarding how to organize effectively.

Up until this time, the predominant focus in the management sciences had been on the pursuit of greater efficiency through task specialization, standardization of roles facing similar tasks, and routinization of rules and regulations. These strategies for organizing were intended to achieve ends such as minimizing skill requirements, thereby reducing training costs, increasing the predictability of and control over people's behavior, and increasing the extent to which day-to-day operations could be handled by lower level managers, while those in the upper ranks attended to broader policy issues.

It was an ideology that emerged out of the experience of running large organizations such as foot soldier–dominated armies, railroads, steel mills, and assembly line–dominated manufacturing organizations. It had been bolstered by the birth of "scientific management" and the discovery that human behavior could be measured and made more efficient through the application of hard science techniques. And it provided a stable conceptual underpinning for the rapid emergence of more and more large organizations in the first half of the century that other developments, such as better communication and transportation systems, were allowing.

World War II, however, generated massive demands for new products and technologies, more rapid production rates, and extremely complex patterns of integration and coordination both within and across organizations. Scarce resources simultaneously made efficiency even more critical. The result was the emergence of a whole new array of systems-oriented management techniques and innovative organizational designs created on the spot to achieve results, regardless of prevailing organization theory.

The postwar period presented a time when organization theorists caught up with these events. As managers began to apply their learnings to business in general, administrative scientists began to hail the benefits of decentralization and participative management, and to justify conceptually the need to manage scientists and other professionals in more flexible ways. This led ultimately to what has come to be known today as the contingency approach to organizational design.

Lawrence and Lorsch's Contingency Theory

While a number of behavioral scientists made important contributions to the development of the contingency approach, Paul Lawrence and Jay Lorsch were the first to develop something of a unified theory in this area and to apply it programmatically in OD efforts.[4] Other writers with their own variations on this theme have

[4]Paul R. Lawrence and Jay W. Lorsch, *Organization and Environment: Managing Differentiation and Integration* (Boston: Division of Research, Graduate School of Business Administration, Harvard University, 1967).

since followed—for example, Jay Galbraith, and David Nadler and Michael Tushman.[5] But for purposes of this overview, we will confine our attention to Lawrence and Lorsch's concepts.

As one can imagine from the foregoing, a critical problem organization theorists faced in the early 1960s was how to reconcile the tenets of traditional organization theory, which was continuing to provide an important focus for designing and managing many organizational tasks, with more recent ideas that stressed flexible job design, short hierarchies, minimization of rigid rules and regulations, lateral communication, and decentralized decision making. Lawrence and Lorsch proposed a method of reconciling the two approaches by tying them to contrasting environmental demands and, in particular, to the concept of task certainty.

These authors advanced a conception of the modern business firm as a network of interdependent groups each performing a different task—for example, marketing, research, and production—whose successful execution was necessary for implementing the firm's overall strategy. Building on the work of Burns and Stalker, and Woodward,[6] they argued that a work group must vary the degree of formality and structure in its organization in direct proportion to the certainty of its task. Specifically, the less certain the task a group faces, the more it can benefit from minimal structure and informality in achieving its goals.

In an early phase of their own research, Lawrence and Lorsch used this idea to explain a finding that ran counter to the classical notion that effective firms must organize their major functional departments in similar ways, according to the tenets of maximum specialization, standardization, and routinization. The data they gathered on six firms in the plastics industry indicated that research departments consistently displayed less structure and formality than marketing departments, which, in turn, displayed fewer of these qualities than production departments. Moreover, these differences were accentuated in the more effective firms in their sample. This finding made sense in terms of the certainty principle when further research revealed that, in the segment of the plastics industry they were studying, research tasks tended to be considerably less certain than marketing tasks, which were themselves less certain than the production tasks.

While these findings represent Lawrence and Lorsch's initial break with classical theory, a follow-up study they made of interindustry differences was probably more important. Here they compared pairs of more and less effective firms in each of three different industries (containers, food processing, and plastics). They were able to show that, while the basic kinds of differences they had already documented remained the same, regardless of industry, these differences were smaller in some industries than in others. Moreover, the variation in these differences could also be explained in terms of task certainty. For the firms displaying smaller differences in the formality of their departmental organizations operated in industries where levels of certainty in the major functional tasks were also less different.

[5]Jay R. Galbraith, "Organization Design: An Information Processing View," in *Interfaces*, Vol. 4, No. 3 (May 1974), pp. 28-36; and David A. Nadler and Michael T. Tushman, "A Model for Diagnosing Organizational Behavior," in *Organizational Dynamics* (New York: AMACOM, Autumn 1980), pp. 35-51.

[6]Tom Burns and G. M. Stalker, *The Management of Innovation* (London: Tavistock Publications, 1961); and Joan Woodward, *Management and Technology* (London: Her Majesty's Printing Office, 1958).

Lawrence and Lorsch used the term "differentiation" to mean the "difference in cognitive and emotional orientations of the managers in different functional departments."[7] They operationalized their concepts of cognitive and emotional orientations through measures of time orientation (long versus short), interpersonal orientation (task versus social), and structure (many versus few rules and procedures, levels in the hierarchy, performance criteria, etc.). Their results supported the proposition that, in order to be more effective, the level of differentiation in an organization must vary directly with the degree of diversity in the certainty of its functional tasks.

Besides the foregoing proposition, Lawrence and Lorsch's findings also offered support for three other hypotheses dealing with closely related issues. First, data from the plastics industry suggested that the quality of relations between pairs of interdependent departments in an organization varies inversely with the degree of differentiation between them—that is, the more the members of two departments that have to work together differ in terms of their cognitive and emotional orientations, the worse they are likely to get along with each other. Second, they were able to show that, while this relationship held across all six plastics firms they studied, the more effective units in this industry were able to achieve higher average levels of integration.[8]

They went on to show that this finding could be attributed to the more frequent presence in these units of a number of conditions that seemed logically to contribute to effective conflict resolution. Specifically, individual personnel assigned integrating tasks in the more effective firms were found more often:

- to have time orientations which fell between those of the departments they coordinated, and to have socially oriented interpersonal styles that were effective for dealing with interpersonal differences;

- to have integrating team structures whose elaborateness was similarly intermediate;

- to have more balanced personal concerns with the goals of the departments they were integrating;

- to identify the main source of their rewards in the total performance of their project groups rather than in other sources such as individual performance; and

- to have not only high levels of perceived influence around the critical integrating tasks but also influence based on perceived expertise rather than positional power.

Other conditions were also identified that referred to the character of the firm as a whole:

- Better integrated units were reported by their managers as using problem solving or confrontation techniques to resolve conflict (a component of Blake and Mouton's 9,9 style), as opposed to tactics such as forcing decisions through positional power or avoiding tension creating issues.

[7]Lawrence and Lorsch, *Organization and Environment*, p. 11.

[8]*Ibid.*, p. 11. Lawrence and Lorsch define the term *integration* to mean the "quality of the state of collaboration that exists among departments that are required to achieve unity of effort by the demands of the environment." They operationalized this variable by having managers rate the quality of relations among pairs of departments on a 1–poor to 7–excellent scale.

- More of their managers thought they had high influence over major decisions, a fact which corresponded nicely to the complexity of their industrial environment.

- The distribution of influence within particular departments more often coincided with where the knowledge to make important decisions was located.

Subsequent findings on the food and container industries added more support for these last three observations. The more effective firms in these industries also used confrontation tactics more often, and the level of influence and its distribution among managers made sense in terms of their particular environments. For instance, fewer managers in the more effective container firm reported having high influence over product development decisions (a key integrating task) and the distribution of influence was skewed toward the top of the hierarchy. This made sense in terms of the particular requirements of this industry, since most of the necessary knowledge for making these decisions rested only at the top of the three basic departments.

Third, comparisons between more and less effective firms within each of the three industries revealed that the more effective firms displayed simultaneously:

- a pattern of differentiation which fit environmental demands more closely, and
- a higher average level of integration.

Lawrence and Lorsch concluded that both appropriate levels of differentiation and high levels of integration are necessary for any organization's effective operation. Moreover, they went on to argue that, in order for these states to occur, structures and policies that respond to the demands of the environment are not the only things that have to be created. Equally important, a human resource system has to be established that promotes the selection, development, and assignment of individuals to tasks whose demands, as determined by the environment, call for talents they can and are willing to offer, and a work environment that fits their interpersonal and cognitive styles. The critical fit is not just between the organization and the environment but also between the individual and these two elements, with environmental demands as the driving force. Later work by Morse and Lorsch provided research support for these arguments as well.[9]

Putting the Theory to Work.   These findings and the basic questionnaire instruments that helped to generate them, subsequently became the conceptual and research base for a normative model of organization design. As they describe in their book, *Developing Organizations; Diagnosis and Action*, Lawrence and Lorsch's basic approach to OD involves using these tools in two ways:

(1) . . . to make an analysis of the environmental or task demands facing the organization and/or to analyze the needs of individual contributors with whom we are concerned. From these sorts of analyses we can make a *normative prescription* as to what organizational characteristics would provide the best fit with task requirements and individual needs.

[9]Jay W. Lorsch and John Morse, *Organizations and Their Members: A Contingency Approach* (New York: Harper and Row, 1974).

(2)   . . . to make a *descriptive diagnosis* of the current state of the organization. How differentiated is the organization? Where are problems occurring in achieving integration? How are members managing conflict? What are the sources of individual satisfaction and dissatisfaction? Where do members feel the individual contribution contract is inadequate, etc.? This description of the organization's state along with the normative prescription can then be utilized to determine the desired direction for change.

In essence, the *diagnosis* provides a snapshot of where the organization is currently, while the *prescriptive analysis* sets the targets for change. By using these concepts in this manner, we attempt to determine in any particular situation the directions of change which will develop the organization to fit the needs of its members and the demands of its environment.[10]

The design principles advanced by Lawrence and Lorsch are excellent guidelines for client/consultant teams to follow in their attempts to enlist the commitment of and to provide important developmental opportunities for the membership. The contingency approach provides an easily understood logic for making sense out of the organization as a whole. This, in turn, enables every member to see where he or she fits into the larger picture, to understand how one's personal commitment to a particular role ultimately contributes to the organization's welfare, and to collaborate with others in honing one's role so that it is even better suited to task demands. Likewise, the matching of individual needs, styles, and psychological orientations to roles where such qualities are responsive to task demands, facilitates personal development as well as technological effectiveness.

Weaknesses of the Approach.   However, the approach also has certain drawbacks that warrant consideration. First, careful attention needs to be paid to both the content of the total membership's concerns and the process through which the design principles are applied, if the use of the contingency model is to be seen as an authentic OD effort. Paying attention to the content of the membership's concerns is important because the relevant parts of an organization's environment are not givens. Rather, they are byproducts of the organization's overall strategy. When numerous strategic choices are available, as they frequently are, different parts of the membership may be committed to different strategies. Consequently, the pursuit of any one strategy in terms of the contingency approach, no matter how well articulated, can lead to alienation and conflict for some members rather than the cementing of broad-based commitment.

For instance, in the not-too-distant past, firms manufacturing equipment for the paper-making industry had the choice of either staying with a 100-year old craft technology, in which case the research function was fairly certain and of relatively little importance to corporate success, or shifting to a higher technology that required a much greater investment in research, higher levels of uncertainty in the research function, and more complex integrating demands to coordinate new designs with production and marketing. In a firm I worked with that faced this choice, there was consider-

---

[10]Paul R. Lawrence and Jay W. Lorsch, *Developing Organizations: Diagnosis and Action* (Reading, Mass.: Addison-Wesley Publishing Co., 1969), p. 19. ©1969. Reprinted with permission.

ably more conflict over which strategy to pursue rather than what needed to be done once the strategy was chosen.

Second, since the primary focus of the contingency approach is on the relationship between the environment and the organization's overall structure and operating policies, the consultant's initial contacts are almost invariably with members of the organization who are officially in charge of defining the environment and who have control over structure and policy for either the organization as a whole or a major and moderately autonomous subunit of it—for example, a division or product group. This is responsive to the need of any OD project to have top-down involvement, but it also makes it very easy to limit client involvement to this particular group. While this group may indeed be very powerful, failure to include other powerful individuals and subgroups—for example, the corporate group or certain classes of professionals within a division—in the prior task of clarifying the basic corporate strategy to be pursued can lead to major problems.

Moreover, there are organizations in which by their nature several powerful groups have an important say over strategy, structure, and policy—for example, physicians, administrators, and boards of directors in a health care system or faculty, administrators, and government officials in a state-run university. In situations such as these, the respective traditions and orientations of each power group may be so different that the development of a shared strategy may be next to impossible. Pursuit of the contingency approach under these conditions may have major limitations, and a consultant's work with any one group may be severely curtailed by the boundaries set by the others.

Finally, paying attention to the process through which the principles of the contingency approach are applied is equally important. For just as the nature of the approach can seduce the consultant into limiting his or her attention to a small power group when setting up the basic parameters of the project, implementing a design, once created, can lead one into becoming preoccupied with the design per se rather than the membership's understanding of it or their capacity or desire to play their appointed roles in it.

It is quite possible, given enough management control, to implement a design by fiat. This may be a preferred choice in situations where the top management foresees the development of a great deal of resistance were the change made gradually and its logic shared. For instance, the more rational pursuit of the organization's strategy through use of the contingency approach might create major shifts in the relative influence of key groups or break important traditions and habits. The organization may change for the better several years down the road when the members have discovered the benefits of their new roles through the gradual impact of the new structure on them, and those who have not been able to do this have left. Such a strategy is likely to reap havoc in the short run, however, and is inconsistent with the underlying OD values of candidness and self-responsibility.

Educational Enhancement.   A more prudent change strategy and one that is more consistent with OD values involves a major effort at educating the membership in the logic of the new design and enlisting their assistance in making the transition. Besides the human courtesies involved, this has the added benefit of access to a much wider distribution of resources. The membership as a whole can be asked to think through the logic of the changes required as they affect their particular roles, to identify problem areas where task logic runs up against important traditions and prerogatives that may not be worth changing, to identify new skills they may have to develop in order to respond to new task demands, to share their anxieties about the change, and to develop timetables and action plans that will facilitate a smooth transition from old to new practices.

All this is likely to require the assistance of the consultants, other human resource personnel, and other organization members who are already on board with the change effort. It may take from several months to several years, but the outcome is likely to be a shift in values that are more consistent with the contingency approach as well as a shift in the structure and policies themselves.

A particular benefit of educating the membership in the logic of the approach as part of a contingency design effort, is the further surfacing of important data on the fit between the individual and the organization. Major redesign tasks, by their nature, require their designers to make very broad and occasionally tenuous assumptions about the interplay of these two forces. For instance, it may hold on a general level that production personnel, because of the certainty of the tasks they face through their careers, are most comfortable when working in a highly routinized structure with clear performance criteria, frequent appraisals, and short time frames for assessing performance.

This may indeed be the case for most of the production units in the particular organization one is working with, but perhaps not for all of them; for instance, a team in charge of a pilot plant operation that requires continuous innovation and experimentation to meet task demands. A systematic assessment of the task requirements and personnel preferences of every department to be affected by a design project maximizes the chances of spotting such exceptions.

Perhaps even more important is the ability of the educational process to uncover situations in which the proposed change requires individuals to develop interpersonal skills that relatively few members of the organization possess. For instance, new integrating roles may be allocated to individuals who are known to have the requisite mix of technical skills, or the capacity to develop them rapidly, to manage the interfaces between several different groups. In situations where prior integrating activities have been managed by a relatively small number of skillful senior managers, there may be few role models for helping the new incumbents to develop the critical interpersonal skills that their roles also require. An educational, participative approach that allows members to explore the requirements of their new jobs before diving in increases the likelihood of spotting this deficiency and providing the necessary training early on.

The emphasis in the preceding paragraphs on the pitfalls of the contingency approach is not intended to warn one away from using the latter, but to indicate what needs to be done in order to use it successfully as a vehicle for OD. Organization designs based on contingency principles are probably the best the field has to offer today. The specificity of these ideas and their close relationship to organizational strategy and technological effectiveness make them extremely attractive to managers and administrators, and they are currently taught in many MBA programs.

The major message I want to get across is that an organization design by itself, not even an ideal one that logically facilitates the pursuit of all the values stressed in this book, is not the sum and substance of OD. Lawrence and Lorsch, in their own book on using the approach as an OD tool, are careful to point out the importance of pursuing their principles in the context of a collaborative effort. Michael Beer's case on the Corning Glass Works, which is to my knowledge the most well-documented study of the use of this approach in the context of an OD project, does likewise.[11]

The ultimate objective of an OD effort at the large system level is the creation and continued enhancement of an organization design that facilitates the pursuit of OD values. But to make this happen, the consultant has to work with his or her clients to bring both parties' attention to the primary professional concerns of the membership as a whole, and to create a process through which these concerns can be addressed that both models OD values and leads to their continued use. Providing a client with an ideal design is not enough.

ACTION RESEARCH OF A COLLABORATIVE NATURE TO ENHANCE COMMITMENT AND INDIVIDUAL DEVELOPMENT

A third approach to OD at the large-system level centers around the development of action research programs aimed at responding to important organizational problems and opportunities through collaborative analysis and experimentation. Chapter Two represents an example of this approach, and the next several chapters will discuss its implementation in considerable detail. In this section I want to present a general overview of the approach so that we can compare it with the two discussed above, and then set the stage for a step-by-step analysis.[12]

Action research is a term coined by John Collier while he was commissioner of Indian affairs in the United States from 1933 to 1945. Collier used the term to characterize the nature of the activities he and his colleagues engaged in with behavioral scientists in their attempts to improve race relations between whites and American Indians. It refers to a kind of research in which researchers/consultants and the people who govern the systems they are attempting to help, work collaboratively as both students of and interveners into the vital concerns of the latter's social system. Its focus is

[11]John P. Kotter, Leonard A. Schlesinger, and Vijay Sathe, *Organization: Text, Cases, and Readings on the Management of Organizational Design and Change* (Homewood, Ill.: Richard D. Irwin, Co., 1979), pp. 607-30.

The Kotter book contains the A case only, with the B and C cases in the instructor's manual. See also:

Michael Beer, *Corning Glass Works (A)* (Boston: HBS Case Services, Harvard Business School, 1978), 9-477-024.

Michael Beer, *Corning Glass Works (B)* (Boston: HBS Case Services, Harvard Business School, 1977), revised 7/78, 9-477-073.

Michael Beer, *Corning Glass Works (C)* (Boston: HBS Case Services, Harvard Business School, 1977), 9-477-074.

[12]French and Bell provide an excellent review of the conceptual and historical underpinnings of the action research paradigm. Since my own biases are similar to theirs, I will only review the highlights here. Wendell L. French and Cecil H. Bell, Jr., *Organization Development: Behavioral Science Interventions for Organization Improvement*, 2nd ed. (Englewood Cliffs, N.J.: Prentice-Hall, Inc., 1978), pp. 80–100.

on problems and opportunities that key members of a system, be it an organization, a community, a social class, or a small group, have defined for themselves as important and as requiring action. Its dynamics involve a sequence of activities in which research aimed at understanding a problem alternates with planning and action to resolve the latter, the results of which, in turn, become new data to be understood for planning further action.

As it is used today in OD projects, action research tends to follow a specific sequence of steps:

1. systematically collecting research data about an ongoing system relative to some objective, goal or need of that system;

2. feeding these data back into the system;

3. taking actions by altering selected variables within the system based on both data and on hypotheses; and

4. evaluating the results of actions by collecting more data. [13]

This cycle, moreover, can be repeated with the same or different parts of a system as the results of evaluating the initial actions (step 4) provide new perspectives on the problems and opportunities being studied.

A wide variety of projects that could be characterized as action research were conducted in the 1940s and 1950s. Many of them addressed the management problems of large organizations—for example, hotels, oil refineries, and factories. Likewise, many of the researchers who conducted these projects were either participants in or the mentors of those who conducted the earliest OD projects, and many of the same group also participated in the birth of the laboratory training movement.

Action research was part and parcel of the integration of the T-group movement into OD, and vice versa. Action research provided an organizational focus for the application of interpersonal skills once learned in the laboratory. The T-group movement helped to expand the collaborative relationship in action research between researcher and organization leader, to relationships between organization leaders and their subordinates. While contingency theory had somewhat different intellectual roots, its practitioners also embraced the action research paradigm as a general model for applying their design tenets in consulting relationships.

Despite this blending of historical sources, OD-oriented action research can be distinguished today from the other approaches we have discussed by its explicit attention to the immediate content of a client's organizational concerns and, in particular, to the interplay between the concerns of the leaders who ask a consultant to help them and the concerns of the rest of the organization's membership. Rather than lead with positions that place either interpersonal skills or environmental demands in the forefront, practitioners who use the action research paradigm as their primary focus, begin their

---

[13] *Ibid.*, p. 92.

relationships with clients by encouraging them to engage in a study of the internal workings of their systems. Particular emphasis is put on studying how the larger body of organization members currently experience their roles, on how they interpret the problems and opportunities the organization is currently facing, and on how this total array of viewpoints can be used as a tool for placing particular members' concerns in perspective.

The underlying assumption is that the bulk of an organization's problems are systemic in nature. Consequently, no one individual is likely to have a complete understanding of the dynamics surrounding a given issue. Collaborative analysis involving inputs from many members and collaborative experimentation involving the careful reworking of whole sets of technical and social relationships are usually necessary for enhancing the organization's effectiveness.

With neither an explicit approach to building OD-oriented interpersonal skills nor a set of design tenets for creating structures and policies that encourage collaborative behavior, one might wonder how an action research approach can effect change in organization members' values. The answer, quite simply, is that the primary message is in the medium.

We argued at the beginning of this chapter that collaborative organization flows most naturally from the actions of organization leaders who assume commitment of the total membership to the organization's welfare and who think about all members as possessors of potentially important resources. Action research programs that tap into and attempt to respond to the current concerns of an organization's membership are consistent with both of these assumptions. A leading group's sanctioning of a project that invites input from the membership around important personal and organizational issues, can be interpreted as a significant gesture of concern for the development of each member. Follow-up action programs that both utilize members' ideas for organizational improvement and provide opportunities for their personal development in the process, provide significant evidence of trust in the membership's commitment to the organization's welfare.

Consequently, both leaders and followers obtain important outcomes. Leaders gain access to new data and critical problem-solving resources from the membership. Followers gain evidence that their commitment is wanted, and that at least some of their concerns will be responded to if they voice them. Both groups gain a better understanding of the benefits of collaboration. The project itself, in essence, represents an experiment in working with the collaborative form. Thus, it sets the stage for still more analysis and experimentation that is likely to move the organization as a whole toward more thorough use of the collaborative form.

Equally important, the action research approach rules out neither interpersonal skill building nor efforts at contingency design. Both of these strategies are frequently identified as appropriate action steps to be taken, based on an initial analysis.

Weaknesses of the Approach.   The action research approach has its pitfalls just as do the other ones we have discussed. While we will address many of them in greater detail later on, three are especially important to mention here. First, careful attention needs to be paid to the kinds of data collected. By starting with a leading client's definition of a system's problems, it is easy for a consultant to develop a data gathering strategy that fails to surface the variety of concerns other members of the system may have. Other members' concerns are likely to be important, even if the primary client does not recognize this initially, because they interact with those this person does have and often in unforeseen ways.

For instance, initial contacts with an organization leader might reveal that he or she was especially worried about middle management's apparent lack of concern with opportunities for cost savings in a variety of areas. Starting with this premise, it might seem logical to try to find out whether this group was actually aware of these opportunities, or how to take advantage of them, or of top leadership's concern about them. If the consultant were to buy into this premise, he or she might create an excellent inquiry program for answering these specific questions, but fail to discover that a more direct cause for the unwanted behaviors was a broad pattern of resentment toward certain senior management practices—building new facilities, redecorating offices, or buying new equipment during an economic downturn. All of the latter activities might be ultimately justifiable in terms that middle management would accept, but the need for such justification might not reach either the senior client's or the consultant's awareness.

Moreover, an inquiry process that failed to surface these underlying concerns might alienate middle management even further and be seen as an additional waste of money. Avoiding this trap requires careful emphasis in the initial contracting stages on legitimizing a broad-based inquiry process, one that allows each person who participates in the process to express his or her own views of the organization's problems and opportunities.

A second major pitfall concerns the use of data once collected. Broad-based inquiry strategies tend to require a high degree of candidness on the part of the participants. As one can see from Chapter Two, respondents may find it important to express their concerns about their own performance, how they have been treated by others, their views of other organization members, and so on, in the course of portraying their organizational experience. While all of these data may be useful in resolving important problems, they may also be misused. Breaches of confidence, however inadvertent, can destroy a project's credibility. Likewise, failure to use the data as promised can be equally damaging in other ways. For instance, it is often tempting for leading groups to delay or subvert feedback activities when the data to be fed back may damage their own credibility or oblige them to respond to issues they find difficult or time consuming to handle. All this emphasizes the need to contract very carefully around the process through which data will be collected and how they will be used.

Finally, it is almost imperative for leading clients to commit themselves to following through on the action research cycle once they have begun it. The initial data gathering process *can* be seen as a bid for commitment and a sign of concern for others' individual development. But this is not the only interpretation possible. The same activity can also be interpreted as everything from window dressing, designed to make management "look good," to an outright attempt to obtain damaging information. The proof of the desired interpretation is in the actions of powerful figures that follow the analysis.

Contrary to the fear that numerous managers have shared with me when considering an action research program, this does not mean that all of the concerns of a particular group have to be responded to as the latter desire. What it does imply, however, is that these concerns need to be acknowledged and reasons given when action is not taken. It is also true, however, that for a project to be a success, at least some of the concerns surfaced by the membership need to be explored in considerable detail and solutions reached that most of the membership see as valid. To do otherwise is to acknowledge that leadership really is not concerned with the rest of the membership's commitment and development. In short, commitment comes at a price, the most basic form of which is the collaborative process itself. The underlying premise of this approach to OD is that the price is worth the results in terms of increased long-run organizational effectiveness.

WHY START WITH THE ACTION RESEARCH APPROACH?

Before setting the stage for the next several chapters, which will take us through a more thorough and systematic application of the action research approach, it is important to say why I have chosen to focus on this approach as opposed to the others. To begin with, let me stress that all three approaches are being used with considerable success today. When executed in a thoughtful and competent manner, no one approach, in my view, is better than any other. This is particularly true when a consultant pays careful attention to the context, process, and content of a project and aligns his or her management of each aspect with the pursuit of OD values.

Moreover, in large-scale projects, elements of all three approaches tend to be employed. The differences between them lie respectively in their differing initial emphases on interpersonal processes, responsiveness to the environment, and the immediate concerns of the membership. But initial emphasis on interpersonal skills leads almost invariably to the application of these skills to members' immediate organizational concerns, and frequently to contingency oriented design projects. Initial emphasis on the demands of the environment leads to new structures and policies for dealing with immediate concerns, and frequently to interpersonal skill building for helping people perform new roles. And action research on immediate concerns rarely goes very far without identifying the need for skill building to enhance the collaborative process, and frequently the need for contingency oriented design efforts that are intended to provide more lasting solutions to recurrent problems.

The value of starting one's career in OD with the action research approach, I believe, lies primarily in two related factors: (1) its relative accessibility to the typical middle manager or beginning consultant in terms of the credibility required to get something going; and (2) the relative accessibility of the necessary skills and techniques for providing important payoffs to an organization. This is most easily seen by first looking at what it takes to gain entry with the other two approaches.

Factors Working Against the Interpersonal Skills Approach

Convincing a client to engage in interpersonal or leadership skill building as an opening agenda for a large-scale OD effort tends to require two kinds of credibility. First, one usually needs a high level of professional credentialing in the interpersonal area in order to justify investment of time and money in didactic and workshop activities. Second, one needs a high degree of organizational credibility as someone who understands the system being worked with well enough to facilitate the application of interpersonal skills to concrete organizational problems. The original users of this approach had both kinds of credibility, and their successors have come most typically from the ranks of Ph.D.s who have been trained in both areas.

However, I have encountered a number of very skillful internal training and development personnel who are allowed to ply their trade in management workshops and training programs in their organizations, but who sadly have had great difficulties in getting opportunities to expand their roles into the management of larger OD efforts. The history of the field, I believe, has created an unfortunate prejudice in this regard. When top management wants a major skill-building effort, they tend to hire external consultants with major credentials. Internal training personnel are relegated to assistant status and less credentialed external consultants are not invited in.

Factors Working Against the Contingency Design Approach

Convincing a client to engage in a major design project using the contingency approach involves similar roadblocks. Since potential changes in major aspects of structure and policy are to be considered, entry needs to be gained at the top. Were the organization relatively small, this might not be a major difficulty for newer managers and consultants. But the contingency design approach was developed primarily for application to large organizations, where structure and policy replace hands-on management as critical sources of control for top leadership. It can be used to good effect in smaller systems, but there the need to begin from a design perspective tends to be less apparent. Leading off with one of the other approaches is likely to become more potent. Thus the less consequential a consultant's age and experience are for gaining entry, the less useful this approach may be.

Furthermore, this particular approach is heavily based in academic research. The chances of justifying its use to a client are enhanced greatly when the consultant is seen as a specialist on organization theory. Once again, a Ph.D. in organizational behavior or management is often critical, both for gaining entry and for developing the actual knowledge base for applying it competently.

The Strengths of Action Research

By contrast with these other approaches, action research does not rely as heavily on prior professional training and credentials, nor does it require entry with top management personnel to the same degree. While the latter helps, especially in highly centralized organizations, major work can be done with relatively autonomous sub-units of an organization without major sanctioning from the top. What counts here perhaps even to a greater degree, moreover, is not the consultant's professional credentials but this person's actual skills.

The consultant's opening bid is to assist the client in working on important organizational problems by analyzing these problems in greater depth, with more unusual techniques, and with inputs from more people than the client might initially think necessary. This requires skillful dialogue and a realignment of the client's thinking through competence in presenting a new and interesting research strategy, and the development of the client's confidence in the consultant's ability to carry out his or her role in the project.

Professional credentials and a successful record in conducting similar projects are clearly helpful. However, to a far smaller degree than with the other approaches, the client is not put in the position of having to trust the consultant's external credentials and status when making the decision about whether to proceed. It is much easier for this person to see himself or herself as an expert on the problem-solving process as well. This, after all, is what he or she gets paid for, that is, getting things done through people. Thus, the client is in a much better position to trust his or her own experience in considering the potential strengths and weaknesses of each element of the consultant's proposal, and to balance judgments about the consultant's credentials with judgments about the quality of the ideas this person is presenting in the here-and-now.

Of course, many executives, by the time they have reached a position in their organizations where they are able to hire a consultant, have been exposed to interpersonal skills programs and courses, and workshops or readings on contingency design. Many of these experiences may indeed have been helpful to them, and they may have integrated important parts of them into their day-to-day thinking and behavior. In fact, one might argue that not only through training but through day-to-day experience, senior executives as a group are probably equally adept at managing their interpersonal behavior and designing organizations as they are at solving problems through people. But, in the last analysis, they are not likely to see themselves as professional experts in these other areas. Our culture puts these skills in the provinces of other experts.

For the client, then, the consultant using the action research approach is more readily seen as a fellow expert in the general field of human problem solving. His or her proposals may be judged in terms of one's own experience. This gives the new external consultant or middle manager who wants to experiment with OD a much better chance at both initiating a project successfully and getting the help he or she needs from the client to grow and develop as a professional as the project progresses.

THE OD CYCLE

Regardless of the approach one uses, any OD project can be conceived as being imbedded in a somewhat larger cycle of activities than those that distinguish the approach itself. In particular, attention needs to be paid to getting into and out of the relationship as well as to

FIGURE 5-4
Phases in an OD Project

Scouting	Arriving at a decision of whether or not to enter.
Entry	Establishing a collaborative relationship, initial problem exploration, and selecting data gathering/feedback methods.
Data Gathering	Developing measures of organization variables and processes.
Data Analysis and Feedback	Interpreting and organizing the data, feeding them back to the system, developing a shared understanding of the system and its problems in collaboration with the client.
Action Planning	Developing specific action plans, including who will implement the plans and how their effects will be evaluated.
Action Implementation	Implementing specific action plans.
Evaluation	Determining effects and effectiveness of action implementation, leading to further efforts or to termination.

Source: Adapted from Mark A. Frohman, Marshall Sashkin, and Michael J. Kavanagh, "Action-Research as Applied to Organization Development," in *Organization and Administrative Sciences*, Vol. 7, Nos. 1–2 (Spring/Summer 1976), p. 134.

implementing a project itself. Figure 5–4 describes the basic elements in this larger cycle as they relate specifically to action research oriented OD.[14]

These phases, while distinguishable analytically, continuously overlap in terms of the actual activities they point to and can be seen as involving iterations among each other in various combinations—for example, data gathering difficulties can lead to further contracting, data analysis activities can lead to further data gathering. The entire cycle can be enacted in as short a time frame as a single meeting or involve a major multiyear project. The model is useful, nonetheless, as a way of conceiving the major issues to be attended to in a rational sequence. When undertaken on a sufficiently large scale, the model may help to identify behaviorally distinct activities.

Each of the phases will be covered in considerable detail in the next few chapters as they apply to a fairly large-scale OD project such as the South City example. Bear in mind, however, that they are equally applicable to much smaller projects, in-

[14]In subsequent chapters we will also include the additional phase of contracting, which occurs after entry and before data gathering. It involves exchanging expectations and coming to an agreement about specific objectives, procedures, rules of conduct, costs, and time tables. In terms of the general cycle, however, it can be viewed as part of the entry phase.

cluding specific interventions within a larger one. The model describes both a process and a useful way of thinking about the history of any client/consultant relationship.

CONCLUSION

This completes our review of the three current approaches to OD, the relative merits of each, and my rationale for focusing on the action research approach. One last point, it is important to note that I will be discussing only one major variant of large-scale, action research oriented OD. We will focus on the implementation of an interview/feedback program where the primary research tool is a series of face-to-face interviews with a large sample of the client group. Two other variants are popular in the field today, and both have already been treated extensively in the literature. One of these involves the use of structured questionnaires as the primary research tool. This particular form was developed at the Massachusetts Institute of Technology and later at the University of Michigan in the 1940s and forms the backbone of most of the survey research done today. David Nadler's *Feedback and Organization Development* is an excellent treatment of this methodology, and while I will discuss questionnaire design as it relates to the interview method, the interested reader should refer to Nadler's text for a more detailed treatment.[15]

The third major variant emphasizes data gathering through workshop designs and group problem solving sessions. Again, while our treatment will overlap in some degree, a more detailed analysis can be found in Richard Beckhard and Ruben Harris' *Organizational Transitions*.[16]

In contrast to these two variants, the interview/feedback method highlights the face-to-face interaction between client and consultant, and it relies heavily on the capacity of the consultant to use the totality of himself or herself both as a research tool and as a helper to the client. It is this particular dynamic that we will stress throughout the rest of this book.

[15]David A. Nadler, *Feedback and Organization Development: Using Data-Based Methods* (Reading, Mass.: Addison-Wesley Publishing Co., 1977).

[16]Richard Beckhard and Reuben T. Harris, *Organizational Transitions: Managing Complex Change* (Reading, Mass.: Addison-Wesley Publishing Co., 1979).

CHAPTER SIX

A MODEL
FOR
ACTION RESEARCH ANALYSIS

The primary focus of the action research approach to OD consulting is the on-going array of concrete problems an organization's members face. Ultimately the concerns of the entire membership are germane. One begins on a much smaller scale, however, by forming a relationship with the individual or individuals who have invited one in, usually important leaders of the system and known in the vernacular as one's primary client(s). The stated purpose of this relationship is to explore the problems of major concern to the primary client(s) and to develop innovative ways of discovering and implementing long-term solutions to them.

The expansion of one's concerns to the entire membership, or hopefully at least a major proportion of it, is achieved by viewing the particular concerns and perspectives of the primary client as symptoms of larger problems that are imbedded in the way the system as a whole is operating. The consultant's challenge is to convince the primary client that this is the most useful perspective to take and to gain this party's cooperation in examining the organization from a broad-based systemic perspective.

To do this it is important to have a conceptual roadmap for conceiving and analyzing the organization in systemic terms. While the action research approach is problem oriented, it is by no means devoid of theory. In fact, it represents a style of consulting that requires theorizing on many levels, thus making it critical for the consultant to have a sound conceptual framework to guide his or her behavior.

A wide variety of systems models of organization dynamics are available in the literature. The one I will present in this chapter is based in part on the work of one of the major systems thinkers in modern sociology, Talcott Parsons. Parsons' work is little discussed in the field of OD but I have found it helpful, especially in providing simple ways to organize very complex bodies of data.[1]

---

[1]Talcott Parsons, "General Theory in Sociology," in Robert K. Merton, Leonard Broom, Leonard S. Cottrell, Jr., eds., *Sociology Today: Problems and Prospects* (New York: Harper and Row, 1959), Volume I, pp. 3-38.

The other concepts I will draw on come largely from the work of James D. Thompson, whose book *Organizations in Action* is one of the seminal works in the field.[2] Because this is intended to be a practitioner's handbook rather than a theoretical treatise, I will not cite the intellectual sources of each of the model's concepts. Suffice it to say that most of the ideas to be presented are not new. My own contribution, hopefully, has been to synthesize them in ways that make them immediately useful to the practitioner.

Readers who are already familiar with various systems models in the behavioral sciences will find the one presented here somewhat more elaborate than most of those currently used. This elaborateness is intended to give the user a broad range of choices about what to attend to in the context of a particular problem. In essence, it enables the user to build his or her own working model from a fairly comprehensive menu of choices. All the elements of the model need not be applied in their entirety for any given project.

DIMENSIONS OF THE MODEL

The model contains sixteen elements as outlined in Figure 6-1. Before reading further, look over this figure and familiarize yourself with the labels to the right of the first column and beneath the first row. These labels identify the specific elements of the model and they span a great many topics, and any one or a particular combination of which might be of concern to one's clients. At the broadest level, the model is simply a menu of potential project topics or the building blocks for one. It is useful in this respect as a reminder of just how wide-ranging the concerns of one's clients might be.

Beyond this, the elements themselves are organized in terms of two dimensions: function—as indicated in the top row of Figure 6-1; and system—as indicated in the first column. With respect to the first of these dimensions, the model is based on the assumption that any organization has to perform, or get performed for it, four basic functions in order to survive.

First, it has to adapt to its environment in ways sufficient to obtain the resources and knowhow necessary for producing its goods and services and for rewarding its members for their contributions. For the typical modern enterprise, this can be referred to as the *technoeconomic function*.

Second, no organization can survive without continuously identifying and pursuing particular sets of goals that are acceptable both to its surrounding community (for a business enterprise this might be the government, shareholders, and customers) and to its members. While organizations can exist with many and often competing goals, they are unlikely to do so for long without any goals whatsoever. Likewise, the continued pursuit of goals that are not consistent with the demands of important internal and external constituencies is likely to lead to the organization's dissolution. Identifying goals and mobilizing support for them is referred to as the *goal-setting function*.

Third, every organization has to find ways to integrate its members into some level of harmonious and relatively stable participation. While conflict and change are inescapable facts of life, individuals join organizations in order to achieve goals they

[2]James D. Thompson, *Organizations in Action* (New York: McGraw-Hill Book Company, 1967).

FIGURE 6-1
A Roadmap for Analyzing
An Organization

	TECHNO-ECONOMIC FUNCTION	GOAL-SETTING FUNCTION	REGULATORY FUNCTION	HUMAN RESOURCE FUNCTION
COMMUNITY AND OTHER GROUPS	Relevant sciences & economic conditions	Constituency demands Strategic constraints & opportunities	Government regulations Contracts with other organizations	Labor force size, availability, characteristics
FORMAL ORGANIZATION	Technology Work systems Equipment Facilities Property Finances	Formal mission & strategy	Formal structure & integrating mechanisms	Membership size & characteristics Formal policies for human resource management (recruiting, staffing, etc.)
INFORMAL ORGANIZATION	Access to organization resources Team skills & knowhow	Interest group goals & strategies	Informal structure, roles, norms	Informal groups & networks Membership size & criteria Internal HR management
INDIVIDUAL ORGANIZATION	Individual access to organization resources Individual technical & interpersonal skills	Personal aspirations & preferences for organization	Individual's formal & informal roles & relationships Individual's management style	Individual's upbringing & career Personal characteristics Psychological contract

could not achieve alone. This requires the development of mechanisms for defining and maintaining legitimate patterns of cooperation, both internally and in the organization's relationships with other social systems. The creation and maintenance of these mechanisms comprises the *regulatory function*.

Finally, organizations in the behavioral sense of the term, as opposed to corporate fiction, need people in order to exist. In most large modern organizations, the people who are willing, able, and needed to contribute to the organization's operation come from many walks of life, possess diverse social and demographic characteristics, and place many different demands on the organization in return for their services. Consequently, organizations need to develop mechanisms for finding, hiring, training, measuring, rewarding, and promoting their members. The pursuit of these objectives represents the *human resource function*.

While it is easy for us to think about all of these functions as being performed solely by an organization and as being manifested primarily in formal structures, policies, rules, regulations, and work systems, a more realistic way of conceiving their pursuit is to think of them as involving several different systems, of which the organization, or more specifically the *formal organization*, is only one. The formal organization never does all the work of ensuring its survival by itself. It exists alongside of (in some cases within and in other cases surrounding) other social systems, and the latter help it to survive because they, in turn, depend for their survival on the formal organization.

The second dimension of our scheme takes this into account by identifying three other kinds of systems that operate interdependently with a given formal organization in the course of ensuring their own welfare. These are the surrounding community (including other formal organizations), informal organizations or face-to-face groups, and individuals.

Each of these other systems also needs to perform all four of the functions noted above to survive. A *community*, in which many organizations are embedded, needs a stable economy and the capacity to produce a vast array of goods and services in order to meet the survival needs of its population. Shared goals for the community have to be continuously established in order to fight stagnation and entropy. Stable patterns of cooperation are necessary for keeping the peace. And opportunities for the pursuit of wide varieties of careers and life styles are needed to provide the population with sufficiently meaningful lives for them to choose to remain within the system and to continue to contribute to it.

The fate of an organization is bound up in the fate of the community or communities within which it exists. The surrounding economy affects the availability of money and the need for goods and services. Community goals serve as important constraints and opportunities in strategy formulation. Community legal systems and regulatory activities affect the internal regulation of the organization, and labor force availability and values determine the potential pool of organization members and their needs. Depending on the size of the organization in comparison to the larger community, the community in turn can experience important economic effects, strategic constraints, and opportunities, and so on in response to the organization's dynamics.

Likewise, the fate of many other formal organizations is usually interdependent with one under study. For instance, organizations such as competitors, consumer groups, unions, professional associations, creditors, and vendors all rely on a typical manufacturing organization in some degree for their survival, and vice versa. The same would be even more true of a parent company if the system being analyzed were a division of a larger enterprise. And, in turn, how each one of these other organizations tries to perform its own survival functions can often affect the ways in which the others do this.

Formal organizations also have their informal counterparts, that is, systems of personal relationships based on ongoing, face-to-face interaction, shared experience, and personal ties. *Informal organizations* tend to involve subsets of a single formal organization's membership. They develop out of their members' needs to achieve ends that are either not being met or are not being met as well as they could be by the formal organization. For example, informal groups of blue collar workers who are rewarded through piece-rate incentive schemes often cooperate to limit their production to a single, agreed-upon level. Among other things, this responds to the need for predictable and noncompetitive interpersonal relationships and, at least from the workers' viewpoint, enhances job security by masking the actual capabilities of the group's members. While senior managers may not appreciate restriction of output, such groups in turn often help the formal organization to survive by training their members informally, reducing absenteeism, and maintaining harmony. At management levels, informal groups develop to enhance communication and personal support beyond levels currently provided by the formal organization. This can help group members' careers and simultaneously enhance formal operating efficiency.

These informal systems however also have to satisfy needs for resources, goals, internal regulation, and human resource management in order to survive. They draw heavily on the formal organization to help them do this and, in turn, the formal organization relies on them to do much of its work.

Finally, the primary motive power of all organizations comes from their *individual members*, the only systems that have any chance of surviving without the other three. A sufficiently socialized individual can live alone in the wilderness and perform all four survival functions in isolation, although this option is vanishing rapidly, while the other systems need interdependence with individuals in order to survive. The individuals one finds in an organization, moreover, have by definition given up the escape option and have chosen to be interdependent with the formal organization, and all the other systems.

Thus, each type of system exists interdependently with the other three. Relations between the systems need to be neither completely harmonious nor long lasting to ensure the survival of all. For instance, individuals continuously come and go without affecting the stability of the larger organization; informal groups can go through periods of intense conflict with the formal organization only to follow this with just as intense periods of cooperation with it. Whole organizations move from one community to another, while the latter continue to survive.

Equally important, shared needs for survival provide opportunities for cooperation, but there is no guarantee that these opportunities will either be recognized or exploited. For example, an individual may leave an organization, fully believing that there is no job available in it that would satisfy his or her needs, when the opposite is the case. Likewise, asymmetrical patterns of interdependence encourage compliance by the more dependent systems to the demands and needs of the more independent ones, but such compliance is never guaranteed. Informal groups of middle managers, for instance, may insist on maintaining guerilla-like warfare with certain senior managers regardless of the career risks involved.

An important implication of all this for the practice of OD is that any aspect of the formal organization, or any other aspect of organization life that a client attends to, is embedded in a complex set of interdependencies. These interdependencies are ultimately so complex and changing that it is impossible for any given problem to be understood in its entirety. Thus, any way in which a client frames a problem stands a good chance of ignoring relevant variables.

The same is also true, ultimately, for any interpretation a consultant arrives at, whether it be alone or in close collaboration with the client. But there is a difference. By using a roadmap for guiding analysis that recognizes the breadth of these interdependencies, the consultant stands a better chance than the client of identifying relevant conditions that might be changed to resolve a problem or to redefine it so as to make it easier to cope with.

This is only one of the advantages a consultant has in the problem-solving process. His or her relative lack of emotional involvement in particular aspects of the organization and the fact that this person is at least initially not part of the problem also help. For the meantime, however, let us focus on the advantages of using a more comprehensive map.

In the following sections, we will first provide a series of questions that can be used to guide exploration of each topic in the roadmap, (refer again to Figure 6-1), and then discuss some principles for analyzing the answers in the context of the client's problem. Bear in mind that the questions are designed to be comprehensive, to point to a wide variety of phenomena that might be relevant, rather than to issues that need to be covered in depth in every instance. As we will suggest in Chapter Seven, it may even turn out that if some of the elements are especially relevant to a client's concerns, then other kinds of consulting rather than OD might be more appropriate.

Technoeconomic Factors in the Organization's Environment

1. What is the general state of the economy in which the organization is operating?
2. What areas of scientific knowledge does the organization draw on in order to produce its products and services?
3. How, if at all, has each of these factors changed over the past several years, and what trends, if any, are apparent in the ways each is changing today?

Goal-Setting Factors in the Organization's Environment

1. What are the major organizations and groups in this organization's environment that have a major interest in the goals and strategies it is currently pursuing and/or might pursue?
2. How much and what kind of power does each of these systems have to block or facilitate the pursuit of the organization's potential and current goals?
3. How much and what kind of countervailing power does the organization have to control the goal-setting activities of each of these groups?
4. What is the nature and quality of the relationship between the organization and each of these groups?

5. How, if at all, has each of these factors changed over the past several years, and what trends, if any, are apparent in the ways they are changing today?

Regulatory Factors in the Organization's Environment

1. What kinds of government regulation does the organization have to conform to?

2. What other organizations (unions, professional and community associations) does the organization have agreements with? What is their nature and duration?

3. What other organizations is it feasible for the organization to make agreements with in the foreseeable future? What might be the nature and duration of such agreements?

4. How, if at all, has each of these factors changed over the past several years, and what trends, if any, are apparent in the ways they are changing today?

Human Resource Factors in the Organization's Environment

1. What categories of people does the organization employ — for example, unskilled, semiskilled, blue collar, white collar, professional?

2. What is the size and age distribution of the available labor pool in each category?

3. What is the nature of the values of people in the different categories as they relate to work, authority, and career?

4. What are the typical wage rates for the people in these categories, and what other rewards do they typically expect from an employer?

5. How, if at all, has each of these factors changed over the past several years, and what trends, if any, are apparent in the ways they are changing today?

Technoeconomic Factors in the Formal Organization

1. What is the nature of the organization's technology, facilities, equipment, and real estate?

2. How are the organization's facilities, equipment, and technology distributed geographically?

3. What is the current monetary value of the organization's plant, equipment, and technology?

4. What is the financial status of the organization?

5. How, if at all, has each of these factors changed over the past several years, and what trends, if any, are apparent in the ways they are changing today?

Goal-Setting Factors in the Formal Organization

1. What are the organization's current objectives and operating strategies?

2. What formal procedures are used to determine objectives and strategies?

3. What formal procedures are used to measure progress toward the achievement of the organization's objectives?

4.   How, if at all, has each of these factors changed over the past several years, and what trends, if any, are apparent in the ways they are changing today?

Regulatory Factors in the Formal Organization

1.   How is the organization formally organized in terms of functions, products, service groups, departments, divisions, operating units, and so on?

2.   What is the nature of the formal hierarchy in terms of rank, prerogatives, and responsibilities?

3.   What other mechanisms does the organization use to integrate the activities of its subunits (integrating roles, teams, task forces, meetings, rules, and policies)?

4.   What is the organization's management philosophy (general expectations with respect to its members, the physical environment, customers, suppliers, shareholders, unions, communities, and governments)?

5.   How, if at all, has each of these factors changed over the past several years, and what trends, if any, are apparent in the ways they are changing today?

Human Resource Factors in the Formal Organization

1.   How many people does the organization employ?

2.   What is their distribution across job categories (blue collar, clerical, professional, managerial, etc.)?

3.   What formal policies and procedures does the organization have for recruiting, developing, and placing its personnel?

4.   What formal policies does the organization have for assessing, rewarding, punishing, and terminating its personnel?

5.   How, if at all, has each of these factors changed over the past several years, and what trends, if any, are apparent in the ways they are changing today?

Technoeconomic Factors in the Informal Organization

1.   What organizational technologies, equipment, facilities, and moneys does each group work with or within?

2.   What kinds of technical knowhow and interpersonal skills has each group developed as a team?

3.   How well does each group work as a team in comparison to other groups in the organization, especially those whose interests are directly intertwined with its own?

4.   How, if at all, has each of these factors changed over the past several years, and what trends, if any, are apparent in the ways they are changing today?

Goal-Setting Factors in the Informal Organization

1.   What is the nature of each group's view of the larger organization, how it operates, and how the group fits into it?

2.   What specific organizational goals, strategies, operating conditions, and management philosophies does each group want to maintain and enhance, and why?

3.   What specific changes, if any, would each group like to have happen in the larger organization's goals, strategies, operating conditions, and management philosophies, and why?

4.   How does each group make decisions about its position on the above issues?

5.   How, if at all, has each of these factors changed over the past several years, and what trends, if any, are apparent in the ways they are changing today?

Regulatory Factors in the Informal Organization

1.   What is the nature of the status hierarchy among the informal groups in the system in terms of their total influence over the organization's operations and their capacity to influence each other's behavior?

2.   What is the quality of the relations among these informal groups?

3.   What norms or informal rules of conduct do all or most of these groups share with respect to the functioning of the organization?

4.   For each group, what is the nature of its internal hierarchy, criteria for leadership, for being seen as a regular member, a deviant, or an isolate?

5.   How is labor divided within each group with respect to those tasks that are performed as a group?

6.   For each group, what are the norms or informal rules of conduct and thinking that all members are expected to abide by?

7.   How, if at all, has each of these factors changed over the past several years, and what trends, if any, are apparent in the ways they are changing today?

Human Resource Factors in the Informal Organization

1.   Within the segment of the organization being studied most directly, what are the major cliques and influence networks—for example, the informal relationships that have emerged apart from formal ties in the various departments, functions, and face-to-face work groups?

2.   How many people are in each of these groups, and how, if at all, do their memberships overlap?

3.   For each group, what social and organizational characteristics do its members have in common—for example, age, sex, race, ethnicity, type and extent of education and training, socioeconomic status, seniority, rank, type of jobs and specialties, shared work experiences, physical location of offices, and most typical work areas?

4.   For each group, which of the characteristics listed in question 3 appear to represent necessary (if not sufficient) criteria for membership?

5.   How, if at all, does each group recruit, develop, assess, reward, punish, and expel its members?

6.   How, if at all, has each of these factors changed over the past several years, and what trends, if any, are apparent in the ways they are changing today?

Technoeconomic Factors as They Relate to Individual Members

1.   What specific organizational technologies, equipment, facilities, and moneys does each member work with or within?

2. What kinds of technical and interpersonal skills does each member possess?

3. How skillful is each member of the organization in comparison to his or her immediate colleagues and other members of the organization in general?

4. How, if at all, has each of these factors changed over the past several years, and what trends, if any, are apparent in the ways they are changing today?

Goal-Setting Factors as They Relate to Individual Members

1. How, if at all, would each member like to change the organization or any aspect of its operations, and why?

2. What features of the organization would each member like to maintain or enhance, and why?

3. What, if anything, would each member personally like to do more of, keep doing, or do less of, with respect to activities related to his or her life in the organization, and why?

4. What are each member's career aspirations and time frames for achieving career goals?

5. How, if at all, has each of these factors changed over the past several years, and what trends, if any, are apparent in the ways they are changing today?

Regulatory Factors as They Relate to Individual Members

1. What is each member's formal and actual role in the organization's division of labor?

2. What is each member's formal position in the organization's hierarchy?

3. What is each member's informal role and influence within the various face-to-face groups of which he or she is a member?

4. How well does each member get along with his or her immediate colleagues?

5. What is each member's management or leadership style?

6. What are each member's formal and informal roles and status in the community surrounding the organization and in other organizations with which it deals?

7. How, if at all, has each of these factors changed over the past several years, and what trends, if any, are apparent in the ways they are changing today?

Human Resource Factors as They Relate to Individual Members

1. What is the nature of each member's education and career, both prior to coming to the organization and during his or her history to date within it?

2. What are each member's salient demographic characteristics?

3. What does each member want from the organization in return for his or her services?

4. How does each individual feel about the way his or her career has been managed within the organization to date?

5. How, if at all, have each of these factors changed over the past several years, and what trends, if any, are apparent in the ways they are changing today?

ANALYZING THE ORGANIZATION

Using this scheme to direct one's inquiry into an organization sets the stage for exploring the client's presenting problems from several different perspectives. The essential conceptual ingredient for doing this is Thompson's concept of coalignment.[3] *Coalignment* refers to the situation in which two or more conditions or aspects of a social system are in harmony with each other, so that their actions reinforce rather than conflict with or disrupt each other. The same idea is also referred to today as simply alignment, congruence, or even more simply "fit."

Specifically, it is possible to think about each element in Figure 6–1 as a subsystem that may or may not exist in a state of coalignment with each of the other elements or subsystems. The manager's job is to attend to coalignments across both functions and levels and within aspects of particular subsystems, when such conditions are relevant to the organization's success. In the management literature, for instance, it is common today to assert that effective organizations are those whose missions and strategies are consistent with their structures, operating policies, membership characteristics, and technical and financial resources. That is, all four of the elements in the *formal organization* row of the model fit or work in harmony with each other.

Likewise, one can argue that the pursuit of a given strategy is accomplished most efficiently when there is consistency not only between the organization's strategy and the demands and opportunities presented by its external constituencies, but also between both of these factors and the goals of interest groups within the organization and, ultimately, the goals and aspirations of each of the organization's members. Here, there is a pattern of fit or coalignment between all four elements in the *goal setting function* column of the model.

In line with this reasoning, a basic way to analyze one's data is to look for patterns of coalignment, or the absence thereof, throughout the roadmap. The basic questions to ask in examining any two subsystems are first, "To what extent do these two aspects of the organization's functioning reinforce each other, and if not, what in particular seems to be getting in the way?" And second, "How might this condition be affecting the problems being experienced by the membership?"

For example, the recruiting policies of a business organization (*human resource function at the formal organization system level*) might be out of alignment or fit with the organization's formal mission and strategy (*goal setting function at the formal organization system level*) were they to attract upward oriented and aggressive managers at a time when the firm was not pursuing growth and thus was not promoting its managers rapidly. The condition might have been created by the fact that the organization had been pursuing a growth strategy until the recent past, when an economic downturn re-

[3]See Thompson, 1967, pp. 147-48. John Kotter has made similar use of the term in connection with his own models, which involve conceptualizations of somewhat different elements. John P. Kotter, *Organizational Dynamics: Diagnosis and Intervention* (Reading, Mass.: Addison-Wesley Publishing Co., 1978). Jay Lorsch uses the term "fit" for describing essentially the same phenomenon. Jay Lorsch, "A Note on Organizational Design." (Boston, Mass.: Intercollegiate Case Clearing House), 9-476-094, 1975. David Nadler and Michael Tushman use the term "congruence" to do likewise. David A. Nadler and Michael T. Tushman, "A Model for Diagnosing Organizational Behavior" in *Organizational Dynamics* (New York: AMACOM, Autumn 1980).

quired a more conservative posture, and the personnel department had yet to revise its recruiting strategy to be consistent with the new, no-growth strategy. This condition might in turn be contributing to a particular client's problems by forcing him or her to work with new and talented personnel who leave the organization as soon as they realize how constrained their career opportunities currently are.

Selecting Elements for Analysis

It is important to recognize at the outset in doing this kind of analysis that an exhaustive assessment is next to impossible. For instance, there are 120 pairings to examine even if one assumes that all community groups are identical, and that so are all informal groups and all individual members in a particular formal organization under study. Thus, in any given analysis one needs to be quite selective about which particular subsystems to examine.

Where one starts depends upon the central interests of the client. While they may not be framed initially in ways that acknowledge many of the interdependencies involved, the client's immediate concerns can be used to identify the more important aspects of his or her organizational world that require attention. For instance, if at the outset of a project my client's immediate concern is with the organization's internal operating efficiency, I can begin to truncate the model as we converse by:

1. inquiring into only the most important external groups at the community level (since the client is concerned primarily with internal issues);

2. asking for a general analysis of each of the subsystems at the formal organization level;

3. focusing on the top leadership group at the informal organizational level, attending to only the most salient features within each of the subsystems for this group;

4. focusing on the leader of the organization as the only individual to be studied initially, and paying primary attention to this person's expectations, aspirations, and leadership style.

This allows one to characterize the organization in terms of the major system levels noted in the left-hand margins of Figure 6–2. The field of possible topics that one might attend to is still huge. But they are not out of reach if one uses this initial model as a menu for further exploration in conversations with the primary client. By inviting the client to talk further about the specifics of the problem as he or she sees it, a considerably smaller set of relevent topic areas is likely to surface.

For example, further elaboration by the client might reveal that most of this person's examples of poor operating efficiency deal with the recent introduction of a new and complex technology designed to help the organization expand in a particular market. New staff have been hired to manage this technology, and my client's comments suggest that they differ markedly from other employees in terms of their more advanced education, younger age, experience in different industries, and preference for more autonomy and less structure in their dealings with their leader and other senior managers.

FIGURE 6-2
Focusing the Roadmap
for Analyzing
an Organization

	TECHNO-ECONOMIC FUNCTION	GOAL-SETTING FUNCTION	REGULATORY FUNCTION	HUMAN RESOURCE FUNCTION
COMMUNITY AND OTHER GROUPS (KEY GROUPS ONLY)	Relevant sciences and economic conditions	Constituency demands Strategic constraints and opportunities	Government regulations Contracts with other organizations	Labor force size, availability, characteristics
FORMAL ORGANIZATION (MAJOR FEATURES)	Technology Work systems Equipment Facilities Property Finances	Formal mission and strategy	Formal structure and integrating mechanisms	Membership size and characteristics Formal policies for human resource management (recruiting, staffing, etc.)
INFORMAL ORGANIZATION (TOP GROUP ONLY)	Access to organization resources Team skills and knowhow	Interest group goals and strategies	Informal structure, roles, norms	Informal groups and networks Membership size and criteria Internal HR management
INDIVIDUAL ORGANIZATION (LEADER)	Individual access to organization resources Individual technical and interpersonal skills	Personal aspirations and preferences for organization	Individual's formal and informal roles and relationships Individual's management style	Individual's upbringing and career Personal characteristics Psychological contract

At the same time, I am told that this group seems to have excellent relations with new customers and government regulators, that they seem to be solidly behind the organization's strategy, and that their credentials are excellent in terms of the available labor pool of people in their field. They also appear to have all the financial and technical resources they need and know how to use them. My client also tells me that these people seem to work extremely well as a team, but that their inefficiency seems to occur in their relations with three senior production personnel and with a particular marketing manager who had previously been in charge of the area they were now working in. My client's own problems with this group center around their failure to meet key deadlines and to make reports in the level of detail expected of other managers. My client is open to being flexible but sees no rationale for being tolerant at the present time.

These data allow me to truncate the model even further. For the purposes of a followup analysis involving other members of the organization besides my primary client, I might:

1.   ignore the community subsystems altogether;

2.   focus on the production/research, marketing/research, and top leadership/research interfaces at the formal organizational level and attend in particular to the technoeconomic and regulatory subsystems as they relate to these interfaces;

3.   explore differences and similarities in the informal cultures of the new team, as compared to production leadership, marketing leadership, and top management, especially as they relate to the regulatory and human resource functions;

4.   Explore the personalities of the leaders of each of these subsystems and the relationships of these people with each other.

This is clearly a much more manageable set of issues to work with. I have a limited number of key interfaces to explore at the organizational, informal, and individual levels, and I will give special emphasis to the regulatory and technoeconomic functions at the formal level and the regulatory and human resource functions at the informal level. At the same time, I can remain aware of the potential interactions of these subsystems with others as my analysis progresses, gather data on them (especially at the individual level since some sources of tension remain unspecified), and alert my clients to these possibilities as well.

Finally, it should be apparent from this example that there is no strict formula for deciding which subsystems to study and in what configurations. In this sense, the analysis process remains something of an art. The client's immediate concerns provide an important starting point, although one that may be highly biased, diffused, or too focussed and therefore in need of a more systemic perspective. The roadmap as a whole provides a menu of possible areas to explore. The consultant's experience, intellect, intuition, and his or her capacity to relate to the client provide the rest.

PHASES IN THE ANALYSIS PROCESS[4]

So far we have discussed a general model for analyzing an organization, the concept of fit or coalignment as a way of making sense out of the data gathered, and the possibility of truncating the model in various ways in order to make its application

[4]Some of the examples in this section were first reported in an article by the author, "The Human Side of Growth," *Organizational Dynamics*, Summer 1978, pp. 68, 69, and 75. © 1978 by AMACOM, a division of American Management Associations, New York. All rights reserved. Adapted by permission of the publisher.

manageable in the context of particular client needs. In the rest of this chapter, I want to offer some suggestions for how to interpret the patterns of coalignment and misalignment one identifies in ways that will increase one's capacity to be helpful to one's clients.

I find it useful to think about the process of interpreting one's findings in terms of four phases: (1) appreciating the organization's strengths and ethos, (2) identifying recurrent problems that invite experimentation and change in the organization, (3) understanding how the organization is evolving on its own and how it might evolve, and (4) assessing the ways in which the organization is currently addressing its problems.

As Figure 6–3 suggests, the process taken as a whole allows one to examine the organization in terms of two dichotomies; the organization as a problem-solving system versus the organization as an opportunity system, and the organization as a static set of problems and opportunities versus the organization as a mechanism for problem solving and opportunity creating. In the following sections we will discuss how the analysis process can be applied to organizations taken as single corporate entities. Note, however, that the same diagnostic process can be applied to any subset of an organization one chooses to study, or any informal group, or even a single individual.

FIGURE 6–3
Interpreting the
Organization's Dynamics
from Four Perspectives

THE ORGANIZATION
AS A PROBLEM-SOLVING SYSTEM

Identifying recurrent problems
and their sources

Assessing the organization's
problem-solving capacities and style

STATIC ASPECTS

DYNAMIC ASPECTS

Appreciating current strengths
and ethos of the organization

Understanding how the
organization is evolving and might evolve

THE ORGANIZATION AS
AN OPPORTUNITY SYSTEM

Appreciating Current Strengths and Ethos

Consultants typically are invited to help an organization when the latter is facing problems it cannot resolve by itself. The consultants are quite aware of this, and the net result is that they often dive headlong into efforts to resolve whatever problems are presented to them, plus any others they might find that fit their skills, without first coming to a thorough appreciation of what the organization is doing well already. Discovering what an organization's strengths are, and the particular ethos that provides the organization with its vitality, is for me an essential first step that needs to be accomplished before any serious problem-solving activities can be undertaken.

To begin with, if I do not do this, I do not know what my client wants to protect in the course of examining other things he or she might want to change. I stand a good chance of developing positions that are likely to be seen as dangerous if not sure signs of incompetence. Occasionally, my client may not know some of the organization's real strengths either and may only discover them, regrettably, after the fact, unless I help this person discover what makes the organization work as well as it does already.

Appreciating the organization is also useful as a first step, because it goes hand in hand with simply finding out how this system works. Moreover, despite the problems they are facing, clients also like to talk about what they think they do well. Inviting this and being able to show one's appreciation for the organization helps to build strong relationships where my clients feel that I am working with their best interests in mind.

The diagnostic roadmap helps one do this, because identifying important patterns of coalignment is a necessary counterpart to identifying their absence. Rather than start by focusing on the negative, one simply begins by searching out the critical fits among and within the elements and by thinking about how they interact with each other, and how they have done so in the past, to make the organization a viable operation in the first place.

Frequently, it is possible to discover what one might call a key pattern of ingredients that has been leading to whatever level of success is currently being experienced. For example, a metal parts stamping firm grew from its infancy largely through a close match between the needs of a small number of customers and its production capabilities, combined with a match in management styles between the leaders of the customer organizations and its leadership. Over the years, the stamping firm's willingness to grow in tune with the emerging needs of these customers became a key strength and its primary way of doing business. In working with this firm, I learned very early that people prided themselves on this posture and that the firm's unique ways of doing things, its ethos, revolved around it.

Key customers were consulted continuously about the utility of possible changes in the stamping firm's production methods. Managers who were being groomed for important positions were exposed to leading managers in these organizations, and part of the criteria for their success was determined by their ability to work well with the latter. The choice to become a supplier for a new customer was an event that involved considerations of the similarities and differences in the two organization's operating styles, as well as the financial opportunities involved.

The key pattern of ingredients, the operating ethos surrounding it, and the matches or coalignments involved, are likely to be different for every organization one encounters. For some firms, it might be a critical match between engineering and production. For others, it might be a close alignment between production and sales. For still others, it might be the fit between the president's operating expertise and style, on the one hand, and the complementary strengths and styles of other leaders, on the other, or between a particular technology and operating style and the relatively unique ongoing availability of a work force whose values and skills match these things. For a hospital, it might be a match between a particular group of physicians and the typical needs of their clientele, on the one hand, and the facilities, climate, billing procedures, and support staff of the hospital itself, on the other.

Organizations grow and prosper in the context of these patterns. They emerge initially out of an organization's efforts to survive and, over time, the organization builds itself around them. To know what these patterns are is to know the essence of the organization.

Identifying Problems

Identifying patterns of misalignment within and between elements goes hand in hand with identifying patterns of coalignment. Thus, by the time one has developed an appreciation for why the organization is successful to the extent that it is, one is also likely to have discovered a number of important weaknesses and specific problem areas. And just as some of the strengths one will have discovered will be well known to the organization's members and major sources of pride, while others may be less well known, some of these problems are likely to be well known to management already, while others may be beyond this group's awareness. At the same time, some of them are likely to represent aspects of the organization that the primary client will have immediate energy to experiment with, while others represent aspects that this person would rather leave alone without considerable persuasion from the consultant and/or other colleagues.

Whether a client is aware of a particular problem or not, and whether this person has the energy to experiment with it or not, are important factors to bear in mind when the time comes to feed back one's data and analyses. In Chapter Ten we will have a great deal to say about the implications of action planning under each of the possible combinations of these conditions. Consequently, it is also important to try to understand clients' problems from the beginning in terms of them.

Problems that the client may not be aware of and that he or she may initially resist acting on after discovering them. Once one has discovered the strengths and ethos of an organization, a natural next step is to address the client's weaknesses in the context of these factors. Sometimes, doing this leads to the identification of particular problems that the client may not be aware of, and which he or she may not want to deal with initially after discovering them. One of Karl Marx's seminal ideas (really an adaptation of the philosopher Hegel's) is especially useful for doing this task. Marx argued that every new productive system sows within it the seeds of its own destruction. Likewise, in the context of a particular firm, one can argue that a management's preoccupation with the strengths and ethos that have made their operation a success is also a major cause of the recurrent problems they encounter.

For example, in the case of the stamping firm referred to above, there came a time when the firm had grown so large that the ability to get along with key clients in terms of management philosophy and personal style was no lnger as important a criterion for promotion in the management ranks as it had been. The sales service department in particular needed managers with a broad array of technical as well as interpersonal skills, because the task of servicing the technical needs of a dozen major customers was now too large for the firm's engineers to do this job on a sporadic basis and still complete the rest of their work.

Several sales managers with excellent records in other organizations had been hired to meet expanded sales, but interpersonal skills and general management philosophy had been key criteria in the selection process, not technical expertise. Reports of their ability to help customers had been disappointing, and this was eventually traced to their lack of technical knowhow. Given a very able engineering department that had always responded to technical service needs effectively, top management had never seen any cause to think about technical competence in its marketing group as a critical criterion until it was too late. In fact, some very thorough soul searching had to be done in the process of selecting new recruits for these jobs. The introduction of the technical competence criterion complicated the process and represented the beginnings of a new hiring philosophy for this part of the organization.

Thus, a first place to look for important problems that are likely to be difficult for one's clients to deal with is in those features of the organization that are closely related to the organization's strengths and that are likely to have been overshadowed by them. If an organization prides itself on its cost effectiveness, as did South City Chemical in Chapter Two, think about what the unintended consequences of excessive cost consciousness might be. What subsystems are likely to be involved—for example, equipment and facilities, reward systems? What important mismatches might this be creating—for example, between meager reward systems and recruitment policies aimed at hiring top-rate people, and between threadbare facilities and management's characterization of the enterprise as a modern place to work?

Taking another example, suppose success has been due to an ethos of innovation. Consider whether people are trying to be too innovative and feeling frustrated because they are not living up to their own and others' expectations, or whether productivity has fallen because they are not paying enough attention to sheer craftsmanship.

The same strategy may also be important to pursue on a more subtle level. For instance, a particular management group may have developed the practice of promoting only men into its senior ranks. While this might not be a critical criterion for organizational success in any objective sense, it might be felt to be so by the group involved because it was culturally sanctioned in the past. The same might be true for a wide variety of practices—for example, the promotion of minorities in general, the recruitment of people with particular social backgrounds, the maintenance of particular management prerogatives designed to indicate status differences (special parking spots, office space, special dining areas), the involvement of top management in decisions that they no longer have the information or expertise to contribute to effectively, and the maintenance of particular stereotypes of people working in different functions. Any of these practices might no longer be relevant to the organization's success in the present. Indeed, they might be getting in the way of continued success, but they might still represent important traditions that are felt to be part of the organization's ethos.

Problems that the client is unaware of but that it would want to act on after discovering them. Problems in this category usually fall under the rubric of poor communication. They are especially germane to two types of organizations: those that are growing very rapidly and those that have been running smoothly for an extended period of time.

The managers of rapidly growing organizations are typically overworked and underinformed. Adding on new products and services, developing new divisions, and so on require attention to what is new about the organization and divert attention from ongoing practices and conditions. In the process, considerable autonomy tends to be given to personnel throughout the organization. New managers are hired and others promoted without being socialized into the normal way of doing things. Consequently, these people do what makes sense in terms of the training they do have and the demands of the situations immediately facing them. New policies and practices are adopted without a thorough analysis of their potential impact on the rest of the organization. While much of what is done may be effective in the short run, problems in many areas are likely to develop simply because no one has had the time to attend to the systemic conditions creating them.

Problems of this variety are often the easiest to cope with, since the only barrier to their resolution is ignorance. OD projects, by their very nature as information gathering and dissemination activities, are likely to surface many of them. And often this is all that a consultant needs to do. Once they are identified, the organization takes over.

Organizations that have been running smoothly for an extended period of time are apt to encounter similar problems, especially if they are highly decentralized. Continued success encourages complacency in monitoring ongoing practices. The practices seem to be working well enough, so why bother to surveil them closely and assess them for long-term effects? Problems arise because change is inevitable. Managers grow older and develop different interests. Work groups become solidified and gradually develop practices to their liking that may be inconsistent with other subsystems. Work force values change. Hiring, evaluation, and promotion practices gradually become outmoded. Incremental changes in technology gradually generate major differences in skill demands, and so on.

Much of what we did at South City Chemical was simply to surface problems of this variety, and the task forces that were appointed to respond to them needed little assistance in resolving them.

Problems the client is already aware of, has yet to find a way to resolve, and is still addressing. Many of the immediate problems a client invites a consultant to deal with fall directly into this category. Examples might include:

"We are aware that the work values of our labor force are changing, but have yet to find an effective way to deal with this."

"These two groups have had poor relations for years. Their mutual cooperation is now too vital to tolerate this."

"Our staffing practices are not in tune with the times. What new practices would fit our needs?"

"Some of our managers are getting excellent results without following the procedures laid down for everyone. How do we get them to conform without reducing their effectiveness?"

In cases such as these, the consultant's own analysis of the situation, using the diagnostic roadmap, may often be similar in some degree to the client's. At first blush, this might suggest that one's diagnostic abilities per se are of little use to the organization. What it needs is expertise in developing appropriate action programs. Sometimes this is clearly the case. Just as often, however, new insights can be achieved from *additional* systemic analysis because it opens up new perspectives on old issues.

While a client may have correctly identified a lack of fit between a particular group's informal operating style and formal organizational procedures, it may not have discovered the interplay between this condition and the relatively unique logic, compared to the rest of the organization, of the group's assigned tasks. For example, an engineering group in a manufacturing plant appeared to upper management to be doing a shoddy job in providing quarterly goals and detailed reports on their progress. Its own investigation revealed that the informal norms of this group were far less deadline-oriented than other professional groups at the plant and it was searching for a new leader to remedy this condition. However, further analysis of the situation revealed that this group's task was considerably more uncertain than those of other groups reporting to the same managers. Consequently, longer range goals and more intermittent progress reports were both more appropriate and easily justified to the rest of the organization. Thus, what was necessary was a new way of defining the problem, not a new solution to a problem poorly framed.

In a sense, the task of analyzing the organization in this situation is no different than it is in the others discussed above. Its ultimate objective remains that of developing new perspectives that provide the client with an expanded set of options to work from. The only difference is that some perspectives have already been identified as unfruitful.

Problems the client is aware of and has chosen not to address. Problems that fall into this category may seem pointless to examine, other than as guidelines for what to avoid. Trying to get a client interested in issues that have already been bounded off may seem like a fruitless task, if not a source of tension in the relationship. Careful analysis is important, however, because sometimes the client's position is based on assumptions that no longer hold.

For example, one of my clients had long since decided that trying to promote rank and file personnel into the management ranks as a way of keeping the hourly workforce company oriented was not worth the effort. It had been tried before with little success. Few people had been interested, and most of those who had applied for promotions and gotten them had left the company within a few months after being promoted. The client's immediate concern was with absenteeism and turnover in the rank and file. The option of dealing with this by offering career advancement opportunities had been considered briefly and discarded.

In the meantime, however, conditions had changed. Prospective candidates were now better educated. Several of the middle-level managers to whom the new promotees would report were more skilled at mentoring, and worker values had changed to the point where moving into the management ranks carried less of a stigma than it had in previous years. My reopening the option to promote workers into the management ranks as a way of enhancing commitment to the firm was initially rejected, but subsequent analysis highlighted the merits of this strategy, and its eventual adoption contributed to resolving the client's problem.

Understanding How the Organization Is Evolving

Organizations are in constant flux. Their day-to-day activities fold back on themselves and change the very nature of how they operate as well as what they do. Consequently, alongside of exploring current strengths and weaknesses, it is important to consider those processes in the organization whose current nature has implications for future strengths and weaknesses.

The diagnostic model provides an opportunity for doing this by inviting attention not only to patterns of fit and misfit in the present, but also to how these things are changing over time. In this section, we will briefly consider how knowledge of current patterns of change in the organization's success formula can be used to envision future strengths. The final section will deal with how current problem-solving processes can be used to envision future weaknesses.

We noted earlier that every organization displays certain patterns of coalignment within and among its subsystem elements that appear to be its key sources of success. They are discovered through trial and error, and then built on as success reinforces their importance. What is important to point out here is that the success formula itself changes over time. For even when leaders pay careful attention to the critical issues involved, they are not always in a position to influence them in the ways they want to. Changes in technology, the economy, competition, constituency demands, external regulation, labor force characteristics, the firm's control over resources to deal with these external forces, and the needs and resources of informal groups and individual members, can all change in ways that are beyond the leadership's control. When these things happen, an organization's leadership has no choice other than to search for new ways of succeeding.

Sometimes the essential ingredients of old formulas are kept while the less important ones fall by the wayside. For example, a seam binding manufacturer grew for many years through the excellent fit between its marketing tactics and the buying habits of a large and stable group of customers. When sewing technology changed and seam binding was no longer an essential ingredient for the home sewer, the company simply adopted several lines of related products (buttons, lacing, etc.) and marketed them successfully through the same channels. The predominance of the marketing department within the firm and its close relationships with top management remained the same, while more production work was contracted externally and the traditions of the firm gradually changed.

At other times, major aspects of the original success formula may be scrapped. For example, a spring manufacturer that prided itself on customer service and had slowly built up a catalog of over a thousand types of springs, each uniquely suited to a different customer, found that it could no longer continue to grow with so many lines to attend to. The stockholders brought in new leadership that made the radical decision to drop the firm's custom service orientation. In its place it capitalized on the firm's technical knowhow by combining it with systems expertise, brought in from the outside, to reduce the firm's offerings to a hundred basic springs.

In the ensuing months, many small customers were lost while larger customers were obtained. The internal workings of the organization changed as well. The spirit of informality and craftsmanship that had gone hand in hand with the custom service orientation was replaced by a more formal, efficiency oriented atmosphere and the use of more formal systems to manage many aspects of the firm's operations. The firm began to grow again, but it was now a very different organization than it had been several years before.

For the OD consultant, discovering these shifts in the organization's success formula is just as important as identifying its current ingredients. At any given point in time, an organization's strengths are likely to be a combination of both the old and the new, and being able to recognize both and to put them in perspective is essential for understanding where the concerns of different groups and individuals in the organization are.

To put it another way, OD consulting projects are not the only things that produce change in an organization. One has to become aware of the other forces of change at work in order to build on them. The more one understands them, the more one can facilitate the development of new technical and organizational strengths in the context of influencing clients to pursue OD-oriented values.

Assessing the Organization's Problem-Solving Capacities and Style

How an organization evolves over time is not only a product of the strengths it succeeds in identifying and pursuing, but also of its capacity to resolve the difficulties that arise in the course of doing these things. Recurrent problems of all sorts are likely to arise in the future, just as they exist in the present, and how an organization deals with them plays an important role in determining how well opportunities are exploited.

Assessing an organization's problem-solving style is a critical ingredient in envisioning the kinds of weaknesses the organization may continue to have, regardless of its overall success. For how decisions are made and the conditions under which they are made determine many of the things that are likely to go unnoticed and unresolved.

One way to do this is to use the value paradigms presented in Chapter One as reference points. Each of the three value paradigms provides a way of conceiving the problem-solving style, respectively, of a particular pair of individuals, a group, and the organization as a whole. Rather than repeat what I have said already, however, I invite you to review Chapter One and consider the kinds of weaknesses that the pursuit of different combinations of values, including the OD-oriented ones, are likely to engender.

My own position is that, among these various combinations, those that represent OD values are most likely to lead to effective problem solving in the long run. Candidness, relating to others holistically, and the assumption that many organization members are committed to its welfare all enhance the search for the multiple causes of any difficult problem. They represent conditions under which people are apt to discuss problems as soon as they arise, to search for their causes in as broad a context as possible, and to be willing to listen to everyone who has something to offer. Likewise, self-responsiblity, feelings of equality, and the assumption that many members have important resources to offer enhance the identification and implementation of effective solutions. Under these conditions, more people are likely to cooperate wholeheartedly in making changes, to do so with fewer fears about what they might lose in the process, and to share their skills and personal resources in ways that provide new learning opportunities for everyone involved.

The absence of behavior consistent with these values may not hurt, in the short run. It may very well represent a realistic response to current conditions and lead to effective action in response to immediate problems. OD's mission, however, is focused on the long-run improvement of the organization's problem-solving abilities. Its overriding objective is to show organizations how to identify and treat their problems in the context of these value stances. The preceding phases of the analysis process help the OD consultant to become familiar with the organization's current and emerging strengths and the problems it is having in exploiting them. But they could be used by any consultant to improve an organization's operations.

The consultant's unique contribution as an OD specialist revolves around interventions that prove the utility of OD values as guidelines for shaping the organization's problem-solving activities. Therefore, understanding the extent to which the organization and its members have adopted these values in the present, and why they have or have not done so, is the most critical phase in the analysis process. Careful execution of the preceding phases provides the necessary data for determining where the most promising interventions might be made. However, the ultimate objective is neither to resolve the current problems of the organization for their own sake nor to tamper with the organization's formula for success, but to build in better ways of solving problems and building strengths in the future.

The final phase in the analysis process, thus, involves a careful assessment of the combinations of values that organization members are following, as they deal with each other around problems, and the reasons for their pursuit of these values:

1. To what extent are organization members being candid with each other in the course of discussing particular problems?

2. To what extent are they taking responsibility for their own actions?

3. To what extent are they relating to each other as whole individuals, as opposed to treating each other strictly in the context of their formal roles?

4. To what extent are they treating each other basically as equals, as opposed to viewing each other as unequal along such criteria as basic social worth, the capacity to grow and develop, and the importance of personal fulfillment?

5. To what extent are they showing in their interaction a concern for the organization's welfare and the commitment of every member of the organization to it?

6. To what extent do they seem to recognize the resources that others have to offer and to invite their participation in the problem-solving process whenever this might be relevant?

7. What conditions are encouraging people to pursue each of these values?

In Chapter One, I offered some general hypotheses for why people pursue particular values. For instance, candidness is closely related to issues of personal safety, and self-responsibility to a sense of competence. But these hypotheses beg the question of how the prior conditions arise in the first place. They were useful for introducing the subject matter but have less potency in an actual diagnosis. The exact causal relations that determine a person's behavior in any particular situation are in large part unique. Once again, the diagnostic roadmap provides a menu of the possible elements involved. The challenge of the OD consultant is to be able to empathize with his or her clients sufficiently to come up with viable working hypotheses that can be tested through dialogue and creative experimentation.

GUIDELINES FOR THE ANALYSIS PROCESS

The following statements and questions summarize the steps to be taken in the analysis process:

1. Describe the issues with which the primary client is concerned.

2. Select those elements in the diagnostic roadmap that are likely to be closely related to these issues.

3. Answer the diagnostic questions for each of the elements you have selected.

4. Explore the relationships among the elements for important patterns of coalignment and misalignment.

5. What are the key conditions that seem to be contributing most to the organization's current success?

6. What problems are likely to be beyond the client's awareness and difficult for this person to acknowledge?

7. What problems may be unknown to the client but that this person will have an immediate interest in exploring and resolving?

8. What problems is the client already aware of and having difficulty resolving?

9. What problems is the client already aware of and has decided to put up with?

10. What conditions are emerging that represent new ingredients for the organization's success, and how do they differ from previous conditions?

11. To what extent do the members of the organization, and the primary client in particular, address the day-to-day problems they face in a spirit of candidness, self-responsibility, holism, basic equality, concern for all member's commitment to the organization's welfare, and acknowledgment of the resources each member has to offer?

Following these guidelines requires a considerable amount of data gathering and analysis. But before one is in a position to do this, one first needs to develop a relationship with one's primary client and other important members of the organization that will make pursuing such an analysis program legitimate and worthwhile. The next two chapters deal with these issues.

CHAPTER SEVEN

SCOUTING, ENTRY, AND CONTRACTING

Scouting: Arriving at a decision of whether or not to pursue a relationship.

Entry: Establishing a relationship, discussing the issues that might be addressed initially and the techniques for doing so.

Contracting: Exchanging expectations and coming to an agreement about specific objectives, procedures, rules of conduct, costs, and timetables.

Getting started on an action research oriented OD project can be conceived as involving three stages of activity—scouting, entry, and contracting. We have already discussed how these stages fit theoretically into the larger OD cycle and have seen an example of their execution in the story of the South City project. In this chapter, we will discuss some of the practical issues one has to deal with in managing these stages from a technical or "hands-on" viewpoint.

SCOUTING

Scouting refers to the activity of deciding whether one wants to work with a client in the first place. Four criteria need to be considered in making the decision: (1) Is there a match between the client's needs and what OD has to offer? (2) Do the clients who initially request the consultant's services have the influence and resources in their organization to sanction and buffer an OD project? (3) Are the values of the organization's membership sufficiently consistent with OD values to ensure broad-based support for the project? (4) Is the client system sufficiently attractive to the consultant to make the project intrinsically rewarding?

Client Needs. The practice of Organization Development is applicable to a wide variety of situations, but in general the problems and opportunities it helps to address best need to have two basic qualities. First, they have to be recognized by the client group as having a heavily behavioral component to them and, second, they need to involve the coordinated acivities of one or more groups of people. While these criteria may seem quite broad, they do rule out a considerable range of issues that are more appropriate for other kinds of consulting (see Figure 7–1).

FIGURE 7-1

Types of Consulting
by Problem Focus and
Locus of Desired Change

Problem Focus

Locus of Change		Techno-economic	Behavioral
	The way people work collec- tively	Corporate and Functional Consulting	Organization Development
	The way people work as individuals	Technical Training	Management Development

When the focus is behavioral but the basic target for change is the individual, the broad field of management development makes more sense. Burke and Schmidt have identified a number of specific differences between Organization Development and management development (see Figure 7–2).[1] These are useful for OD consultants to refer to in conversations with potential clients, because both kinds of activities tend to be conducted by people in personnel departments or consultants with behavioral science backgrounds. In fact, many internal and even some external OD consultants develop their initial client contacts in the course of running management development workshops. Thus, many potential clients see no difference initially between the two kinds of consulting, and need to be educated about this before a meaningful OD project can be formulated.

When the problem focus is more technoeconomic than behavioral, more traditional kinds of management consulting may be called for—for example, corporate strategy formulation, market analysis, operations management. On a general level, of course, any problem or opportunity involving organized activity is amenable to OD, but there are many cases when what the client system is ready to invest its resources in is a specific area of business or economic technology, rather than a learning activity that puts behavioral issues in the foreground.

Frequently, behavioral problems are identified in the course of dealing with organization-wide technoeconomic issues, and many technical consulting firms deal

---

[1] W. Warner Burke and Warren H. Schmidt, "Management and Organization Development: What Is the Target of Change?" *Personnel Administration*, March-April 1971 (Chicago: International Personnel Management Association, 1971), pp. 44-57.

FIGURE 7-2:
Relationship of Management
Development and
Organization Development

DIMENSION	MANAGEMENT DEVELOPMENT	ORGANIZATION DEVELOPMENT
GOALS	Teach manager new skills Expand manager's conceptual under-standing Change managerial attitudes Upgrade manager's present knowledge and skills in such areas as problem solving, decision making, or evaluating subordinates	Facilitate problem solving on the job Plan and implement changes more systematically Increase sense of "ownership" of organizational objectives throughout work force Create conditions so that decisions are made on the basis of competence rather than organization role Create conditions where conflict is managed creatively rather than avoided
REASONS FOR INITIATING	Something wrong with the manager Managers do not know company policy or management philosophy Managers do not have a needed skill	Something wrong with the system Problems with a merger or acquisition Technical change may call for change in mission Present organization structure and roles within it are not effective Competition hurting more than helping
DIFFICULTIES IN INITIATING	Individual resistance and feelings of threat Making training relevant	High commitment required Support from many persons, especially top management, is needed Strong need for long-term commitment to change effort
STRATEGIES FOR PRODUCING CHANGE	Send manager to some educational program Job rotation of managers Courses and/or conferences Specialized training "packages" Reading books and/or articles	Usually done on the job; learning while problem solving and solving problems while learning Team building Organizational structure changes Job enrichment Action research Training Feedback Conflict management Business logic Management science

TIME FRAME	Short, intense	Long range
STAFF REQUIREMENTS	Diagnostician	Diagnostician
	Teacher/trainer	Catalyst/facilitator
	Program manager	Consultant/helper
	Designer of training programs	Knowledge and skill in planned change
		Skill in laboratory training
PROBLEMS AND CRITICISMS	Lack of continuity, follow-up, reinforcement on the job for transfer of learning	Can become "another program"
		Top management must provide leadership and support
	Dependence on experts	Commitment on the part of top management needed
	Lip service given but little transfer	Time demanding
	Difficult to make training relevant to manager's everyday problems	

Source: W. Warner Burke and Warren H. Schmidt, "Management and Organization Development: What Is the Target of Change?" *Personnel Administration*, March–April 1971 (Chicago: International Personnel Management Association, 1971), pp. 44–57.

with this by incorporating particular behaviorally oriented techniques into their activities. Nonetheless, their primary focus is still technoeconomic, and attention to the human side of management is secondary.

Finally, consulting services are also used to provide individual managers with particular technical skills—for example, sales techniques, financial planning, and equipment use. These objectives can be achieved most effectively through in-house training programs that parallel management development seminars and via fully external education programs. They have little place in an OD project.

Client Resources.   Once a consultant has established that a potential client is interested in dealing with behavioral issues on an organizational level, the next step is to decide whether this person or group has the organizational influence and resources necessary to manage and buffer an OD project. Any OD activity requires that time and energy be diverted from the mainstream of an organization's activities, often for extended periods of time and with little promise of benefits in the short term. Consequently, any particular manager or subgroup of managers that wants to do OD needs to be either high up in the organization's hierarchy or have the concerted backing of people who are. The literature on OD abounds with examples of projects that went awry at almost every stage, because more powerful people than those who were directly involved and committed to the project chose to interfere.

Ideally, this suggests that the consultant needs to gain the support early on of either the top leadership of the organization or, at a minimum, individuals who are at least a level above the segment of the organization to be worked with. It is also important to try to sense just how powerful these people are. For instance, a client may have an officially powerful position in the organization but still be susceptible to influence from certain colleagues around activities that may threaten established territories and routines. Thus, initial conversations that address the appropriateness of OD for the organization's needs, as seen by the client, also need to include a very frank exploration of the extent to which the project can be supported and/or what it would take to get the necessary support from other powerful groups.

Client Values.   While an OD project is not likely to get off the ground without the help of especially influential people within the organization, it is not likely to proceed very far once started unless a major segment of the client system, including one's primary contacts, have values that are basically compatible with those underlying OD. The clients' values need not be highly articulated in this regard. For instance, one need not expect one's clients to openly espouse candidness, self-responsibility, holism, equality, shared commitment, and the pursuit of individual fulfillment as the cornerstones of their management philosophies. But it is useful to keep in mind during initial dialogues and to continuously question whether there are any major aspects of the organization's operations and one's potential client's behavior, that would hinder the management of the project in ways consistent with these values.

If one found, for instance, that one's key contacts were strongly authoritarian in style, closed in self-presentation, and consistently hesitant to explore sensitive issues, such as their own power in the organization and their own anxieties about the possible consequences of doing the project, one might think twice before proceeding further.

Decisions around shared values can be especially difficult when other conditions are propitious — for example, when the issues to be addressed are ideal for OD and the key clients are powerful. It is tempting to assume that one has the skills to make converts out of everyone. Nonetheless, it has been my experience that success varies directly with the extent to which one's primary contacts already hold a number of the values we have espoused for OD and have already spent a good deal of time trying to manage their organization in ways consistent with these values. Under these conditions, an OD project has an unfolding, liberating, self-actualizing quality to it. Key managers learn to shape their working environments in ways that amplify their basic sentiments. Each step provides new learnings that they can integrate into their current thinking and that enable them to create realistic tests of their own convictions.

Managers who give only lip service to the underlying philosophy of the OD process find it harder to proceed on their own and, in my experience, rarely sustain their enthusiasm without a considerable amount of group support and encouragement. This is not to say that one requires a total population of gung ho humanists to succeed, but simply that some sentiment along these lines needs to exist within the leading group at the beginning.

Attractiveness to the Consultant.   Last, but not least, every consultant needs to ask the question, *Would I really enjoy working with these people and this organization over an extended period of time?* It goes without saying that both internal and external consultants often have clients they need rather than want, but this should not justify discounting this question altogether. My experience has been that one has to train oneself to like one's clients if one is to be more than minimally successful, regardless of one's initial impressions.

At the bottom of this question is the need to confront one's own feelings about the client from the beginning, to own up to one's own prejudices and preferences and search out ways to deal with them. If one truly dislikes a particular client or organizational setting, it may be worthwhile to withdraw quickly and suffer the short-term costs of doing so.

Regardless of my own standards and self-image, I inevitably find in retrospect that I have put more time and energy into situations and people I have been intrinsically attracted to. The more I learn about my own preferences, the more I can take this into account in organizing work with my colleagues and in making choices about avenues to pursue that I will do better at, regardless of the logic of the task. Shared values around OD are simply not enough. Preference for working with people with a sense of humor, with particular kinds of educational orientations, with a sense of optimism, and so on, often prove to be just as important for me as an individual. I cannot help but believe that this is true of most consultants.

If one is at least moderately convinced that the issues a client wants to address are amenable to OD; that the individual clients who want to spearhead the project have the resources and influence to carry it through; that there are a sufficient number of individuals within the client system (including one's primary contacts) whose values are consistent with those underlying OD; and that the people and the setting are attractive to one's own personality; then the next step is to engage in more serious conversation about the scope and objectives of the work to be done. This marks the beginning of the entry process.

ENTRY

Moving through the *entry* phase, on the surface, is a matter of trying to get to know your client, and have him or her get to know you, in a way that will lead naturally to a mutually agreeable contract. Your scouting activities have convinced you that making this effort is worthwhile, but you still do not know a great deal about your client, and vice versa. It is time to move from gathering data on the potential benefits of a relationship, to declaring your interest and saying, in effect, "Let us see if we can work something out."

There are two issues of importance in managing this process with a client: (1) how much the client knows about OD, especially the way *you* want to practice it, and (2) how voluntary your meeting is on the client's part. The first issue is germane to all of your entry efforts. The second is not likely to be problematic with the specific people who invite you in, but it may well be with many others you deal with. It can be an especially important issue for internal consultants who are assigned a particular client by their organizational superiors. Figure 7–3 indicates the difficulty of the entry process as it relates to client knowledge of OD and why this person is meeting a consultant. Let us consider what needs to be done under each condition.

Easiest.   The process is easiest when your client knows a lot about OD and has decided he or she wants to work with an OD specialist (potentially you) on a given set of problems and opportunities. Even in this situation, a great deal needs to be accomplished. A typical entry meeting, where you are talking seriously with a client for the first time, tends to conform roughly to the following format:

1. Client introduces self, role in organization, states brief reason for asking you in, asks for some background on you.

2. You (consultant) talk about yourself, organizational position, your organization's nature and the role of OD consulting in it, and nature of contacts with client system thus far, and ask for elaboration on issues client is facing that you are being invited to discuss.

3. Client describes issues, you assist by helping him or her articulate the issues, covering history, specification of current concerns, what has been done to address them so far, desired end states, and client's assumptions about how you might be helpful.

4. You elaborate on your general approach, relate past experiences in dealing with similar issues, and suggest kinds of choices that might be considered in tailoring your approach to client's concerns.

5. Both of you problem-solve around the potential fit between the client's concerns and your approach; testing out various scenarios, checking them against your respective needs, capabilities, and interests, identifying potential problem areas, and envisioning solutions to them.

6. At any time during step 5, but more typically after considerable dialogue, client broaches cost and time parameters (if not, you may want to do so at this time), and you provide tentative estimates and meld these data into the discussion of what might be done.

7. Client typically asks for your ideas about next steps, may suggest formal proposal, descriptive data, or additional meetings. The two of you work together to establish a viable set of steps. The meeting may end here or flow into more sharing of personal and organizational background data.

When the client already knows about OD (especially when he or she has been involved in such efforts before) and this person has already decided tentatively that the issues he or she is facing are amenable to it, the critical tasks of a meeting such as this revolve around (1) confirming that your scouting diagnosis with regard to appropriateness of the situation, client influence, attractiveness, and values is correct, (2) establishing your own credibility as the kind of OD consultant the client is looking for, and (3)

FIGURE 7-3
Difficulty of Entry Under
Four Conditions

	Client knows much about OD	Client knows little about OD
Client is meeting consultant voluntarily	Easiest	Harder
Client has been assigned to meet with consultant	A Real Challenge	Much Harder

establishing a mutually agreeable problem definition, action program, and picture of the desired results.

Occasionally, one's scouting activities go hand in hand with this initial meeting, in which case one uses the data one gathers under the above format to determine the desirability of the relationship as well. However, I personally prefer to get as much background data as I can from my contacts before this meeting. This gives me a chance to rehearse aspects of my own experience that may be relevant to the client's concerns and to imagine the kind of problem-solving dialogue we are likely to have.

Accomplishing each of these steps effectively requires a good deal of interpersonal skill, even under these ideal conditions. We will provide a number of basic techniques on this topic in the next chapter. At this point, however, let us consider the more difficult situations and note how the task gets amplified as conditions worsen.

Harder.   When the client calls you in voluntarily but knows little about OD, the same steps need to be accomplished in the context of an important educational effort. Steps 1 and 2 may go smoothly enough, but the client's lack of knowledge is likely to become evident at step 3 when he or she describes the situation to be addressed. Frequently, a client with little knowledge of OD will begin by locating the problem within a particular person or several people and by asking you either to implement a particular solution he or she has in mind or to identify what more you need to know to solve the problem:

> We have received complaints from the rank and file that our foremen are not treating them as human beings, and we would like you to develop a course on human relations for them.
>
> I am having problems with my subordinate. Here's what's happening. . . . What do I do?
>
> My boss has told me I am not a good people manager. What do I need to do to develop in this area?

Initial statements along these lines present you the consultant with two tasks: (1) shifting the client's attention from *who* is the problem to *what* is the problem, and (2) redefining the potential relationship as collaborative rather than hierarchical. The first is necessary unless you want to do management development, which is typically what behaviorally oriented consultants and staff personnel are identified with. It is only when behavioral concerns are defined systemically, however, that OD makes sense.

Every OD consultant, I believe, develops preferred strategies for making this transition in a client's thinking. For instance, my favorite response when I am asked to do training of one sort or another is to ask the client how he or she knows that the people in question need it. Perhaps they already have the requisite skills but either do not want to use them or do not feel comfortable using them because of the situations they find themselves in. Thus, should not the situation — that is, the total system — be assessed first? I have rarely found a client who asks for training who has actually done a careful, data-based diagnosis of the situation. In any case, this sets the stage for discussing the potential benefits of a systemic analysis, which is an essential first step in any OD project.

A popular alternative strategy is to declare explicitly one's preference for an initial systemic analysis of the situation, using the contrasts between the overall goals of OD versus management development, or other descriptions of OD and its philosophical underpinnings.

Tied in with this is the need to define the relationship initially as collaborative. Just as non-OD-educated clients are likely to associate behavioral science consultants with management development, they are also in the habit of conceiving the structure of the relationship in more traditional terms. Edgar Schein, in an early OD classic on process consultation, identified two alternative models that are more typical of other kinds of consulting.

The Purchase Model

The most prevalent model of consultation is certainly the "purchase of expert information or service." The buyer, an individual manager or some group in the organization, defines a need—something he wishes to know or some activity he wishes carried out—and if he doesn't feel the organization itself has the time or capability, he will look to the consultant to fill the need.[2]

The Doctor–Patient Model

Another traditionally popular model is that of doctor–patient. One or more executives in the organization decide to bring in a consultant or team of consultants to "look them over," much as a patient might go to his doctor for an annual physical. The consultants are supposed to find out what is wrong with which part of the organization, and then, like a physician, recommend a program of therapy. Often the manager singles out some unit of the organization where he is having difficulty or when performance has fallen off, and asks the consultant to determine "what is wrong with our _____ department."[3]

In either case, client and consultant are not conceived as equal collaborators in the analysis of the organization's problems and opportunities. The *purchase model* puts the consultant in a one-down position and places the burden of defining the major parameters of the problems in the client's lap. The *doctor–patient model* does the reverse. Neither situation models the philosophy of an OD project as a joint effort where client and consultant build on each other's resources and thinking from the beginning.

Establishing a collaborative concept of the relationship goes hand in hand with creating a systemic approach to the situation to be explored, although getting this concept across may be considerably more difficult. The client may feel the need initially either to be in control or to be dependent on the consultant as a way of coping with his

---

[2]Edgar H. Schein, *Process Consultation: Its Role in Organization Development* (Reading, Mass: Addison-Wesley Publishing Co., 1969), p. 6. **©1969. Reprinted with permission.**

[3]*Ibid.*, p. 6.

or her own anxieties. Rather than talk about the structure of the relationship explicitly, I find it easiest just to act as a coequal.

For example, in the case above where someone asks me to do a training program, the same question that induces a systemic orientation (How do you know they do not have the skills already and simply have not chosen to use them?) also performs the function of setting the stage for a collaborative dialogue. The trick is to avoid cross-examining the client and, rather, to draw his or her reasoning out in full and offer my own insights and questions in the process of doing this. My aim is to legitimize more data gathering and analysis as a next step. Thus, the ideal end point of the conversation is the identification of a whole list of questions that neither of us already knows the answers to and that need to be answered for any specific action intervention to be justified.

Occasionally, a client balks at this type of dialogue and takes the position that he or she knows what needs to be done. If I cannot convince this person otherwise, I am obliged to state my position directly. The result has occasionally been a polite termination of the relationship. At this stage of the game, there a few bonds between us to overcome such a pivotal difference in philosophies.

This is not to suggest that stating one's basic philosophy will get you into trouble with the client, but simply that if the client is ready to work collaboratively, he or she will do so. Thus, testing out this person's willingness through your own behavior is a viable way to start. There is nothing wrong with stating your position at the start, but the real response will be apparent in the client's behavior and not necessarily in his or her words.

On the other hand, I am apt to take a slightly different stance when I find a client starting off with a more dependent posture toward me, perhaps because I am starting in a more influential position than I need. If the client asks me to diagnose the situation and come up with an action plan unilaterally, I will again try to draw out his or her reasoning and collaborate in discussing ideas. If the client persists in asking me to provide all the answers, however, I will launch into a discussion of the philosophy of OD and the need for collaborative analysis to make it really work. When treated as "the doctor," OD and its philosophy are my prescriptions, and I will outline a series of steps (the OD cycle) that I think will lead us to a successful collaborative analysis.

I may still leave the meeting with a sense that the client is depending on me to solve his or her problems, but I find it a lot easier to induce people to reduce their dependency on me during the course of a relationship than for me to start off in a service position and try to become more influential with a client once a project is well under way. By then it may be too late to establish a truly collaborative program.

Much Harder.   Entering with a client who has little knowledge of OD and is also not enthusiastic about engaging with you involves an even greater challenge. By definition, such a person would not be the one who made contact with you initially, but it could be any of the following people:

- your initial contact's boss, whom you are being asked to convince that an OD project would be worthwhile sanctioning;

- a colleague of your initial contact, whose approval and/or support would be necessary or helpful for getting the project off the ground;

- a subordinate of your contact whose work unit or section would be heavily involved in the project's activities.

In these cases the person is meeting you either as a favor to your contact, or as a matter of protocol, or in response to an implied or direct command. Beyond accomplishing the objectives we have already covered, the task additionally is to convince this person that you are attractive to work with. This requires that you find a way to respond to his or her needs without damaging your relationship with your initial contact.

Much of this can often be accomplished by using the same format suggested for the preceding conditions. Following the basic format as if the client really wants to see you has a number of positive advantages. First, this person may not have wanted to see you due to a lack of information or to misinformation about your proposed activities. For instance, the client may see you initially as a source of work overload, as a misuse of organizational resources, or as a political tool controlled by your contact. Playing it straight gives him or her an opportunity to ponder such issues internally without publicly acknowledging any resistance. Depending upon your behavior, he or she may choose to develop some enthusiasm as the conversation progresses. Second, the client may discover during the course of the conversation that he or she shares important values with you and that you offer interesting insights that make you valuable or at least palatable, even if the project concept is not initially to his or her liking. This opens the door to further problem definition without the need to acknowledge that there was a disagreement in the first place. Third, the choice not to search for resistance initially saves you the trouble of having to deal with it emotionally in the event that it disappears as the conversation progresses.

Occasionally, however, one finds that one's attempt to start with a positive attitude is getting nowhere—for example, the client either declares disinterest outright or refrains from talking, looks bored, and so on. Then it is necessary to inquire directly about this person's concerns and deal with them openly. The interpersonal skills we will discuss in the next chapter are the main keys to doing this; it is important to note here, however, that the basic strategy to follow is not to argue with the client's concerns, but to help this person articulate them fully, to appreciate them, and to suggest ways of dealing with them realistically.

For example, a client may see the project as just one more work item to be added to an already busy schedule. Your initial description of your approach and the tentative plans you have been discussing with others may confirm the fear that the project would take significant time. If your inquiry into this person's concerns leads him or her to share this problem, you have the opportunity to help him or her think it through and devise strategies such as renegotiating general work expectations with others in light of the new task, or reorganizing a work schedule, or even developing a good case to present to colleagues for why the project should not be done in the first place.

My own experience has been that *how* I respond to a client's reservations is often more important that what ideas come out of the conversation. Hesitant clients who discover that I am willing to appreciate their concerns and deal with them with a sense of both realism and empathy are likely to develop a respect for me that keeps our relationships cordial and productive, even if these people are not enthusiastic about my activities in their organization. As I have learned, much to my chagrin, the problems clients challenge me with in the course of working through their reluctance often turn out to be of little real concern to them. At the time, however, they are logical ways of warding me off. Thus, working through them is worth the effort.

A Real Challenge.   We come finally to the situation in which the client does not want to meet with the consultant and simultaneously knows something about OD. Almost always these are people who have had bad experiences in other OD projects. For instance, we met a good many hourly employees in the South City project who fell into this category because of a previous OD activity that was followed by the firing of many people they had talked about to the consultants.

People who have had a bad OD experience seem to remember four kinds of negative outcomes most vividly: (1) broken agreements regarding confidentiality, (2) unmet expectations regarding project results, (3) broken promises regarding the feedback of data or the completion of planned activities, and (4) failure to transfer changes in climate and working relationships that emerged in the context of the project activities (team meetings, workshops, T-groups) to day-to-day management activities. It does not matter whether these things actually occurred in the experience of the bulk of the participants in a project. The problem to be addressed is that the client you are talking to at the moment is convinced that they did.

Beyond using the behavioral strategies already discussed, the additional tactics you might employ would be to recognize that any of these things can occur, to declare an intent not to let them happen if this is within your power, to reiterate the safeguards you are using to avoid their occurrence, and to discuss with the client additional ways he or she might find credible for preventing them from happening. Unfortunately, many of the safeguards that clients suggest are not always pragmatically achievable— such as promises from top management that no one will be fired during the duration of the project and a certain period thereafter, lack of pressure to participate when one does not want to, and generous compensation for time spent on the project in lieu of other responsibilities.

Perhaps the most important thing that can be done when a significant number of clients have had bad experiences with past OD efforts is to discuss this openly throughout the entry process, so that there is public commitment by management to safeguard against them.

In any case, it is important to recognize that if these concerns do exist and are bolstered by past experience, they are not likely to be allayed in any significant degree during the entry process. The best one can do is to recognize them, set the stage for avoiding them in the future, and hope to change people's perceptions through the actual conduct of the project in the ensuing months.

Group Entry Meetings

Thus far we have discussed the entry phase in terms of the consultant(s) meetings with particular clients. It is especially useful to bolster these meetings with group sessions. The latter need to be run by individuals you have already talked to, and to be comprised of other influential organization members who would be involved in the project. I encourage my clients to use both formal and informal status as the key criteria for selecting attendees, and to be sure to include the people they think will offer the most resistance to the project.

The consultant's behavior in these meetings should be limited to the same kinds of behavior he or she displays in one-on-one sessions. For instance, as in the South City case, the consultant ought to discuss his or her background, approach, and tentative plans created thus far, and then to field questions from those present.

These meetings have a variety of functions. They represent an efficient forum for establishing relationships with significant people in the organization who have some role in your entry — for example, a veto vote, if supported by several people — but not a large enough role to warrant meeting with them individually.

They provide an important opportunity for you to see just how potent your primary contacts are, as the latter help you introduce the project and develop support for it. They give you a chance to see how the managers you may be working with interact with each other around project concepts such as yours. They provide opportunities for establishing a common language and a set of shared working assumptions with respect to the project — project objectives, procedures, time frames, and boundaries. Perhaps most important, they lend social force to any commitments made and positions taken during them. For example, when the problem of confidentiality in data collection is voiced in such a meeting and a procedure is developed for dealing with it, all those present are bound symbolically by the procedures and are held witness to the fact that this issue had indeed been raised and dealt with at the beginning of the project.

Some consultants prefer to hold group entry meetings with all of the individuals they will work with during a project, while others will only meet with the more powerful individuals. Typically, moreover, entry sessions with less powerful participants will be held after an initial contract has been agreed to, while the more powerful people will be met with earlier in the process, so that they can have a say in whether a contract should be let and what some of its details should be. My own preference is to meet with and gain the support of all relevant power groups before the contract is let, to notify other individuals of the nature of the contract once it has been let, and then to enter with them either individually or in groups as the project unfolds.

CONTRACTING

Provided one has managed the scouting and entry phases in a thorough manner, contracting is a fairly straightforward process. A *contract* can be conceived as a formal agreement between client and consultant around three areas:

1.   What each (party) expects to get from the relationship.
2.   How much time each will invest, when, and at what cost.
3.   The ground rules under which the parties will operate.[4]

All three items should have been covered in some detail during the entry meetings. Thus, the contract per se is simply a formal agreement on the outputs of these meetings. It may be written or verbal or part written, part verbal. If I am working with a client for the first time, I prefer a written contract to start, at least regarding the activities involved in the collaborative analysis. Having something on paper provides an additional check on whether we have understood each other, makes one's involvement a matter of record in the organization's legal processes, and acts as a reference point for subsequent discussions of the relationship.

Frequently, after a major entry meeting, I find it useful to write a proposal letter to the client reviewing what we have discussed and setting the stage for a more formal document, if the latter is eventually requested. If it is not, an affirmative written reply to the proposal letter, with any changes requested, plus my responses to the latter, serves nicely as a documented contract in and of itself.

Organizations differ slightly regarding how they are used to writing contracts with consultants or internal staff groups. The rule-of-thumb I follow is to find out how my client of the moment does this and use his or her format as closely as I can. Some organizations prefer a fairly formal document that has to be approved by their legal department before it is signed, while others are content with a letter such as in Figure 2–5 in the South City case.

There are a few principles that I think are critical to follow in writing such documents. First, avoid promising particular outcomes—such as reduction of turnover, absenteeism, intergroup conflict. OD is a process with many potential outcomes, and what you are contracting for is the competent execution of a series of activities. It is often useful for you and your client to agree on some specific objectives to strive for, but since this is a collaborative effort, there is no guarantee that you will be able to achieve them nor are you asking for the influence that you might think necessary to ensure their accomplishment.

Second, make your commitments flexible—"We will interview between 30–40 personnel in group X depending upon the availability of the membership during the month of _____ and the result of continuing conversations with you and your staff." As you and your client get to know each other, you may want to revise your plan to fit what both of you want to achieve.

Third, build in a commitment to review continuously what you are doing with your client, thus confirming the collaborative nature of the project. This goes hand in hand with the preceding point.

Fourth, if costs have to be accounted for, as they do with external consultants, commit to time to be spent per dollar rather than to the completion of a particular

[4]Marvin Weisbord (Senior Vice President, Block Petrella Weisbord, Ardmore, Pa.), "The Organization Development Contract," in *Organization Development Practitioner*, Vol. 5, No. 2, 1973 (Plainfield, N.J.: National OD Network, 1973), pp. 1-4.

activity. Here it might be useful to mention an outside figure for the total cost of a given activity, but indicate also that this may not be achievable and that your promise is to keep the client informed of the likelihood of achieving your target as the activity progresses. In this way, your client can discuss with you the pros and cons of staying within the proposed parameters in light of the logic of the task and the unique conditions you may be encountering.

Fifth, be as clear as you can about the ground rules of the relationship, especially around issues of confidentiality and promises to feed back data once they have been gathered. Ultimately, I have found that few clients have ever demanded that the essential messages of the data I and my colleagues have gathered should not be fed back to those who were interviewed. But the temptation has surely been present and a clear prior commitment to feedback to everyone involved, I believe, has been helpful. Likewise, agreements to review the project as it progresses, to refrain from acting as a funnel for information on individual performance, to be willing to renegotiate, even terminate, the relationship at any time, are important items to be written down, because they represent a consulting philosophy that underlies all interaction with the client.

Finally, I think it is important to write a contract in a way that is consistent with the spirit of the OD process. Regardless of the words one uses, the more it reads as if this is an agreement to collaborate in a candid and self-responsible manner, where commitment to the organization's success and to every organization member's development are stressed, and where the parties to the agreement are treating each other as whole individuals and in a spirit of basic equality, then the more the spirit of the process is conveyed. The contract represents an important component of the context in which the actual activities are conducted. Thus through the very way it reads, it can get the project off to a promising start.

Thus, once you have completed writing your agreement and have perused it for its technical details, read it once again for the general impressions it seems to create and see if you can heighten the phraseology to convey your values as well as your expectations.

CONCLUSION

In this chapter we have reviewed some of the more practical matters one encounters in starting an OD project. Scouting, entry, and contracting are not only analytical categories for distinguishing types of startup activities, but also specific technical tasks. Each task has its own parameters and contingencies. Scouting, from a technical viewpoint, is essentially a decision-making task requiring attention to four criteria: the match between client needs and what OD has to offer; the match between project demands and client influence, resources, and organizational readiness; the match between OD values and the client's management philosophy; and the match between the personalities of consultant and client.

Entry requires the management of self-presentation, a task that takes on different levels of complexity and invites the use of different approaches, depending on two conditions: the client's knowledge of OD and the conditions under which the meeting takes place. Contracting is an exchange of mutual expectations that requires the careful integration of realistic promises, ground rules consistent with OD values, and mutual commitment to collaboration in spirit as well as in words.

Going hand in hand with these technical matters is an equally important task that we have yet to consider. This is the development of a sound working relationship on an emotional level between client and consultant. Technical proficiency on the part of the consultant helps to create this, but more purely interpersonal skills are also critical. The next chapter presents some basic techniques for developing one's skills in this area as well.

CHAPTER EIGHT

TALKING
WITH CLIENTS

The success of any encounter with a client, be it around scouting, entry, contracting, or any other phase of the OD process, hinges at least in part on the consultant's interpersonal skills, that is, one's capacity to manage one's own behavior in the presence of the client in a way that enhances both task accomplishment and the feelings both parties have about their interaction. The more the client experiences the encounter as both productive and emotionally satisfying, the more likely is he or she to view the consultant as a potentially valuable contributor to his or her world and thus to take this person's ideas seriously.

In this chapter I want to introduce both a typology for thinking about what is going on in a client/consultant dialogue and a series of behavioral strategies for dealing with each of the phenomena the typology identifies. Mastering at least some of these strategies is important for effective consultation because they multiply one's choices about how to behave with a client when working on almost any issue.

The typology divides what is going on in a conversation along two dimensions — task/social and person centered/relationship centered (see Figure 8-1). *Task phenomena* are ways of feeling, thinking, and acting that derive from each party's attempts to participate in the pursuit of some agreed-upon objective. *Social phenomena* derive from each party's attempts to reap emotional rewards from the encounter that are not necessarily related to the task, and whose pursuit may either help, hinder, or be irrelevant to it. *Person centered phenomena* involve ways of feeling, thinking, and acting that derive from a person's attempts to maintain his or her identity as a competent participant with particular social qualities. *Relationship centered phenomena* involve ways of feeling, thinking, and acting that derive from a person's attempts to make interaction with the other party both instrumentally and socially rewarding. Crossing the two dimensions yields four kinds of activity in a client/consultant dialogue that may require attention.

The task, relationship centered aspect of the dialogue is the publicly shared task that you and your client have come together to work on. It involves both creating a stream of complementary contributions and combining them in ways that get the job done. It is what most people would describe if they were asked about what they did in a meeting with someone. One underlying intent of the typology is to suggest that, while this official task activity is important, it is only one stream of action that is occurring among several, all of which need to be attended to by an effective consultant.

The task, person centered aspect involves bridging experience and language. It refers to the actions each party takes to stay cognitively attuned to what is going on. One has to make sense out of the other party's language and, simultaneously, transform one's own experience into words that someone else can understand. For the language we use to conceptualize our own experience may mean something quite different to the other party. Consequently, in order to be seen and to experience oneself as an effective communicator, the additional step of tuning one's internal language to that of the other party is necessary.

The social, person centered aspect involves each party's maintenance and enhancement of his or her broader self-concept. Task activities never take place in a vacuum. They make sense to the parties involved only as means to enacting particular parts of their self-concepts or identities, as managers, administrators, scientists, consultants, and so on. Moreover, the mere act of engaging in a single task itself is rarely enough to maintain one's identity. How one engages in it, what one says and does not say, and what one acknowledges or accepts in the other's behavior or does not acknowledge or accept, may also be dictated by one's concept of who one is.

FIGURE 8-1
Four Kinds of Activity
in a Client/Consultant
Dialogue

	Person–Centered	Relationship–Centered
Task	Bridging Experience and Language Putting one's own experience into words and relating the other's words to one's own experience.	Talking the Task Sharing relevant task data, analyzing them, and developing action plans based on the shared analysis.
Social	Maintaining and Enhancing One's Self-Concept Behaving in ways that fit a particular role or image one has of one's self in the situation and avoiding behavior that would refute this role or image.	Satisfying Interpersonal Needs Interacting in ways designed to elicit responses from the other that satisfy one's needs for appreciation, influence, intimacy, etc.

For instance, a client may be quite willing to admit ignorance on an issue around which I can offer assistance, provided he or she does not think that he or she should know these things already. The latter represents a potential cause for embarrassment that would damage his or her self-concept as a competent professional, and thus is to be avoided even if it gets in the way of proceeding with the task. Thus, involvement in the task is circumscribed by a whole series of personal dos and don'ts and a consultant needs to be sensitive to behaviors in himself or herself and the client that may stem from these requirements, especially when they get in the way of logical task demands.

Finally, the social, relationship centered aspect points to each party's attempt to satisfy interpersonal needs that require the other party to behave in a certain way. For instance, on the one hand, I may want to work hard at creating a mutually agreeable project definition with a client (talk the task), but simultaneously, I may also want my client to think I am a pretty neat person whose advice is worth following, and equally important, I may want the client to acknowledge this. My client may have similar needs and our respective pursuit of such outputs from each other may have an important effect on our task behavior.

In summary, pursuit of the shared task is only one of four streams of activity to be attended to in the client/consultant dialogue. It may be helped or hindered by the multiple ways in which each party transforms experience into language, maintains and enhances his or her self-concept, and tries to get his or her interpersonal needs satisfied. Effective consulting involves being attentive to these other streams of activity, and guiding the conversation in ways that are most likely to prevent them from becoming hindrances to task performance and, when possible, that enhance the latter.

Dealing effectively with the dynamics involved in each aspect of the conversation can be enhanced by the use of a different kind of behavioral strategy. There are ways of talking the task that are more effective than others, and simultaneously, ways of handling the other three aspects that facilitate effective task performance. The rest of this chapter describes each of these strategies in some detail. Figure 8–2 indicates the particular strategies we will cover.

Logical Communication[1]

When writing a report, most people are quite aware of what it takes to communicate logically. Like scientists, we find it natural to move systematically from providing information about a problem or issue to stating our opinions about the meaning of the information and our reasoning behind these opinions to suggesting courses of action to resolve the issue that are consistent with our opinions.

Thus, we move sequentially from information to opinion to action. We may move among these logical levels several times during the course of an analysis, but it is hard not to see the necessity of making the reader aware of the opinions upon which a suggested action is based and the information upon which an opinion is based. Logical

[1]This section draws heavily on William H. Banaka's *Training in Depth Interviewing* (New York: Harper and Row, 1971). This is an excellent training guide for those interested in becoming effective interviewers.

FIGURE 8-2

Skills for Managing the
Different Dimensions of
Activity in a Client/Consultant
Dialogue

	Person–Centered	Relationship–Centered
Task	Bridging Experience and Language requires Skill in Spotting Representational Systems and Meta-modeling	Talking the Task requires Skill in Logical Communication
Social	Maintaining and Enhancing Another's Self-Concept requires Skill in Active Listening	Satisfying Interpersonal Needs requires Skill in Spotting Interpersonal Needs and Responding Choicefully to Them

communication requires attention to each level of analysis and the sequencing of inputs so that the receiver can see the natural progression of a single argument from information to opinion to action.

Unfortunately, few people attend to these necessities very rigorously when talking to each other as opposed to writing something down. Consider the following dialogue between a client and a consultant:

	INPUT	ANALYSIS
Consultant:	Do you think you have a clear enough picture to present it to George so that he'll understand what you're doing?	Consultant asks for an opinion.
Client:	Don't worry about George. He's always done what I've asked him to.	Client ignores consultant's request for an opinion and shifts the level to an action suggestion, then to information.
Consultant:	I think George will have to be very clear on the plan if he's going to convince his people that it's worth their time.	Consultant tries to reason with client by offering another opinion, without responding to client's action suggestion.

Client:	I'll tell him to check with you if he has any questions.	Client shifts the level to an action suggestion, without responding directly to consultant's opinion.
Consultant:	But I'll be leaving here by 6:00 tonight.	Consultant responds by providing further information.

The conversation moves from opinion about one topic, to action and information about another, then to opinion about a third topic, then to action and then to information. No issue is resolved before the next issue is raised. A more logical way for the consultant to have proceeded after the client's initial response above might have been the following:

	INPUT	ANALYSIS
Consultant:	It sounds to me as if you don't want to say whether you can tell George what he needs to know. Is that true?	Consultant asks client for a direct response to his initial request for an opinion.
Client:	You're right. I guess I was hedging on that one.	Client gives a direct answer apart from other issues.
Consultant:	Can you tell me why?	Consultant stays on opinion level, asking for interpretations about why the client was hesitant to respond.
Client:	Well, when you describe the procedure, it sounds really logical and it makes great sense. But then when I try to tell it to someone else, I get all bungled up. It doesn't sound nearly as logical when I'm saying it.	Client responds with information and opinions about his abilities in relation to the consultant's with respect to communicating the plan.
Consultant:	I can understand how that must be frustrating. I think it's natural to feel that way since you haven't been through the activity yourself yet and therefore can't work from your own experience.	Consultant stays at the opinion level and on the same topic, sharing his own opinions and showing he accepts client's opinions and feelings on this matter.
Client:	Yeah, that makes sense. I guess I won't get over this problem until I have been through a few rounds. Come to think of it, if I'm in this boat, George might be too. What do you think?	Client provides closure on this aspect of the problem and discovers its logical implications for a related topic. Then he asks for opinion on this next topic.

Consultant:	My hunch is that different people respond to this problem in different ways. George may be the kind of guy who does not rely as heavily on his own experience and therefore might feel comfortable with our description.	Consultant responds with his opinions on the new topic.
Client:	I guess that's possible. So what do we do?	Client provides closure on the opinion level of this topic and indicates readiness for action.
Consultant:	Let's ask George in now and see how he responds with both of us going over the plan with him.	Consultant responds with a relevant action suggestion.

The example shows how to resolve an issue by staying on the topic and by staying at a particular logical level (here it was opinion), until closure is achieved by both parties and both are ready to consider issues at the next logical level (in this case, action). Similar scenarios might be played out on any logical level. What is essential is to deal with one topic at a time and to adhere to the logic of building opinion on information and action on opinion.

A tremendous amount of potentially sloppy dialogue can be made logical and more productive by adhering to these simple guidelines. While the client may not be asking for this particular service, his experience of it is likely to strengthen his feelings about the relationship as well. William Banaka, whose formulation we are following, has proposed four earmarks to effective logical communication that recapitulate the goals of this strategy:

1. The parties involved complete their discussion of one topic before turning their attention to another.

2. Each party is willing to provide relevant information at each logical level, that is, to justify opinions with information and to justify action suggestions with logical agreements (opinions).

3. The parties involved complete their discussions of a topic on one logical level to their mutual satisfaction before proceeding to the next logical level.

4. The parties involved cooperate in shifting to logically prior issues when they cannot gain closure on the level at which they are currently discussing an issue. For instance, if agreement cannot be reached on an action suggestion, the conversation shifts to a further exploration of opinions about the issue. If opinions cannot be mutually understood, the conversation shifts to a further provision of the information upon which the opinions are based.

These earmarks, in turn, suggest four kinds of discontinuity in the communication process, each of which can be responded to with a specific intervention (see Figure 8–3).

FIGURE 8-3
Guidelines for Restoring
Logical Communication
in a Conversation

LOGICAL ISSUE	RESOLUTION
1. Client suddenly changes the topic before finishing the previous one.	Consultant returns to the unfinished topic as soon as possible. If client persists in changing the topic, consultant confronts him about that behavior.
2. Client appears unwilling to continue giving information on a topic.	Consultant asks client if he is unwilling to continue. Consultant then tries to help client deal with the reasons for his unwillingness.
3. Client shifts the logical level before enough closure is obtained.	Consultant recognizes a priority of logical issues. If action issues cannot be resolved, he next asks client about his opinions (goals, predictions, analysis of causes). If an opinion issue cannot be resolved, consultant goes to the information level to get more facts or to clarify client's definition of terms. Consultant keeps structuring the level of communication until the logically prior issue is resolved.
4. Client refuses to cooperate in shifting to logically prior issues.	Consultant asks client the reasons for his refusal to give opinions or factual information. Client's or consultant's feelings about their relationship may be a contributing factor to be discussed.

Source: William H. Banaka, *Training in Depth Interviewing* (New York: Harper and Row, 1971), p. 7.

Holding to these guidelines may be far more difficult than the reader might think upon initially reading them. To see just how difficult it is, try tape recording five minutes of any conversation you are having with someone. Type up a transcript of the recording, statement by statement, leaving the right half of the paper for comments. Then analyze your transcript carefully for each kind of discontinuity and how either party responded to it. It often takes several hours of practice to be able to follow the intervention guidelines consistently for more than a few minutes. Having a partner who intentionally creates discontinuities for you to deal with and then discussing the results with each other afterward is a good way to speed up this learning process.

What you are likely to find as you do this is that your rate of conversation will seem to slow down considerably, but, simultaneously, your sense of where you are in any problem-solving process will become clearer. Unfortunately, this strategy can also drive out one's sense of spontaneity and excitement. Learn to use it consciously for serious business. The more you use it, the more natural it will seem.

Facilitating logical communication contributes directly to accomplishing the tasks that you and your client have agreed to work on, but, as we have been arguing, this is only one stream of activity that is going on in any conversation. As a result, there are times when it simply does not work. An action suggestion cannot be agreed to, so you move back to a discussion of your views on the issue in question. Your client's reasoning seems muddled, so you invite more descriptive data. But, ultimately, no amount of description leads back to a cogent analysis. When this is happening, one can only conclude that something other than your logical reasoning processes with respect to the issue in question is getting in the way. In short, there is a still prior issue that has to be dealt with before the task can be addressed logically. The model presented in this chapter suggests that there are three other places to look for this block to logical analyses.

Facilitating the Bridging of Experience and Language

When the logical communication process begins to break down, one highly underrated area where one might look for the causes is the way in which the client transforms experience into words and simultaneously relates your words to his or her experience. It is a truism today to say that one cannot understand another person's experience directly. One must infer it through the other's behavior. Likewise, the language another uses to convey his or her experience is only partially effective. A common linguistic culture, shared life experiences, and consensual validation in the here-and-now of what particular words refer to make the sharing of experience through language practicable but by no means totally efficient. There is, inevitably, a vast amount of data that falls through the cracks in the translation process.

Until recently, applied behavioral scientists were stuck with these insights, and were without a practical theoretical model for acting on them in a systematic way. Two authors, Richard Bandler and John Grinder, have made considerable headway in the past decade, however, in building a model that seems promising for therapists and behavioral consultants in general.[2]

Bandler and Grinder begin with the notion that just as words and gestures are not meaning, language is not experience, but a representation of experience. People build models of the world with language, and they use these models to make sense out of the world and to act upon it. But one's model (or map) is not the world; it is only a working representation of it that is continuously being elaborated and modified through new experience. The role of the helper (whether a therapist or consultant) is to enable a client to discover the limitations of his or her current model and to build a better one in its place.

The possibility of building a better model always exists because, according to Bandler and Grinder, models are created through three universal, human processes that inevitably lead to imperfect results. The three processes are generalization, deletion, and distortion.

"Generalization is the process by which elements or pieces of a person's model become detached from their original experience and come to represent the entire

---

[2] Richard Bandler and John Grinder, *The Structure of Magic I* (Palo Alto, Calif.: Science and Behavior Books, Inc., 1975).

category of which the experience is an example."[3] Thus, many a child learns through experience that a particular dog can bite and *generalizes* this to other dogs and animals with teeth. How elaborate this model gets depends on the variety and frequency of experiences the child has with dogs that bite. The principle can be applied to all human experience.

Problems arise with the process of generalizing when the model thus created fails to reflect accurately a particular situation. For example, an individual who has failed on several occasions to get a superior to take his or her ideas seriously may conclude that "this person never listens to me." Consequently, he or she may refrain from presenting more ideas to the superior based on this assumption even when some of the ideas might be well received.

Deletion, the second basic modeling process, is the way in "which we selectively pay attention to certain dimensions of an experience and exclude others."[4] Such selective attention is critical to avoiding data overload as we attempt to make sense out of the world around us. We learn to focus on what is relevant and ignore the rest. The dysfunctional side of deletion is that we may selectively attend to the wrong things or to not enough of the things that are necessary to attend to in order to understand our own and others' behavior. People do this conversationally when they fail to specify who, whom, and what in their descriptions of events and conditions. Helping a client fill in the unspecified elements not only enables the listener to understand better what he or she is saying, but also helps the speaker clarify his or her own thinking.

Finally, "distortion is the process which allows us to make shifts in our experience of sensory data."[5] It involves making inferences about the world that do not follow logically from our sensing but that are often useful heuristically for planning action or creating pleasurable experiences. Thus, a painting by Dali of a watch pouring over the side of a table is not meant to be real but one may consider it aesthetically pleasing. A utility curve in a financial analysis is not meant to be an exact representation of reality but, nonetheless, it can be useful in planning a budget.

The negative side of *distortion*, as with the other processes, occurs when it prevents us from discovering relevant aspects of the conditions we face that would enable us to act with more choice or sophistication. For instance, assuming that one can tell a colleague's mood by how this person has dressed for the day may be useful some of the time but may discourage one from checking one's predictions at crucial moments, for instance, by simply asking.

Bandler and Grinder have developed a set of specific linguistic tools, which they call the Meta-model, for helping clients deal with the dysfunctional aspects of these basic modeling processes. Leslie Cameron-Bandler has compiled an excellent summary of these tools that we have included below. These conversational guidelines were originally created for use in therapeutic relationships. I think they are largely applicable to client/consultant relationships in an OD project as well.

[3]*Ibid*, p. 14.

[4]*Ibid.*, p. 15.

[5]*Ibid*, p. 16.

The Meta-model distinctions fall into three natural groups:

> Gathering Information
> Limits of the Speaker's Model
> Semantic Ill-formedness

Gathering information refers to gaining, through appropriate questions and responses, an accurate and full description of the content being presented. Again, this process assists in reconnecting the speaker's language with his or her experience. There are four distinctions in this category:

> Deletion
> Lack of Referential Index
> Unspecified Verbs
> Nominalizations

Deletion: Recognizing when a deletion has occurred and assisting in recovering the deleted information aids in restoring a fuller representation of the experience. To recover the missing material the Meta-modeler asks: ABOUT WHOM? or ABOUT WHAT? For example:

"I don't understand."
(Response) "You don't understand what?"
(Or) "What don't you understand?"

"I'm afraid."
(Response) "What or whom are you afraid of?"

"I don't like him."
(Response) "What about him don't you like?"

"He's the best."
(Response) "He's the best what?"

"He's the best listener."
(Response) "He's the best listener amongst whom?"
(Or) "Between whom?"

In the case of deletion, asking the question, "How, specifically?" will give information concerning the representation system being used by the client.

"I don't understand."
(Response) "How, specifically, do you know you don't understand?"
"It's just not clear to me" (i.e., visual representation).

Lack of Referential Index: Lack of referential index is a case of generalization that limits a person's model of the world by leaving out the detail and richness necessary to have a variety of options for coping. With this process a person takes an experience and generalizes it in such a way that it's totally out of perspective or out of proportion. To challenge a lack of referential index, ask: WHO, SPECIFICALLY? or WHAT, SPECIFICALLY?

"No one wants me."
(Response) "Who, specifically, doesn't want you?"

"They are obstinate."
(Response) "Who, specifically, is obstinate?"

"This is hard."
(Response) "What, specifically, about this is hard for you?"

Unspecified Verbs: Unspecified verbs leave us in the dark about clearly understanding the experience being described. All verbs are relatively unspecified. However, "kiss" is much more specific than "touch." If someone says he's been hurt, it could have been from a harsh look given by someone important to him, or he might have been hit by a car. Asking for verb specification reconnects the person more fully to his or her experience. To challenge unspecified verbs, ask: HOW, SPECIFICALLY?

"He rejected me."
(Response) "How, specifically, did he reject you?"

"They ignored me."
(Response) "How, specifically, did they ignore you?"

"The children force me to punish them."
(Response) "How, specifically, do the children force you to punish them?"

Nominalizations: Nominalizations are those words that have been transformed from process words (verbs) into nouns. As such, an ongoing process becomes a thing or an event. When this happens we lose choices and there is a need to be reconnected with the ongoing dynamic processes of life. Quoting Bandler and Grinder: "Specifically reversing nominalizations assists the person in coming to see that what he had considered an event finished and beyond his control is a continuing process which can be changed." Nominalizations can be distinguished from regular nouns in several ways. For those who enjoy visualizing, make a picture of a wheelbarrow in your mind's eye. Now put a chair, then a cat, then your mother in the wheelbarrow. Now try putting failure, virtue, projection, statement, and confusion into that wheelbarrow. As you can see, nominalizations are not persons, places, or things that can be put into a wheelbarrow. Another way to test for nominalizations is to check whether the event word fits into the blank syntactic frame, "an ongoing _____."

An ongoing problem   nominalization
An ongoing elephant
An ongoing chair
An ongoing relationship   nominalization

To transform a nominalization back into a process word, use it as a verb in the response:

"I don't get any recognition."
(Response) "How would you like to be recognized?"

"Pay attention."
(Response) "What do you want me to attend to?"

"I regret my decision."
(Response) "Does anything stop you from re-deciding?"

"I want help."
(Response) "How do you want to be helped?"

The next grouping is referred to as *"limits of the speaker's model."* These distinctions identify the limits and by challenging them appropriately you can assist a person in enriching his model of the world by expanding it. The two distinctions in this category are:

Universal Quantifiers
Modal Operators (primarily modal operators of necessity)

Universal Quantifiers: Universal quantifiers refer to the set of words typified by "all," "every," "always," "never," "nobody." Emphasizing the generalization described by the speaker's universal quantifiers by exaggerating it — both by voice quality and by inserting additional universal quantifiers — serves to challenge them. Challenging the speaker's universal quantifiers assists him in finding the exception to his generalization and thus having more choices. Another way to challenge directly is to ask whether the speaker has had an experience that contradicts his own generalization.

"I never do anything right."
(Response) "You absolutely never ever do anything right?"
(Or) "Have you ever done anything right?"

"You're always lying to me."
(Response) "I'm always lying to you?"

"It's impossible to get what I want."
(Response) "Have you ever gotten something you wanted?"

Modal Operators of Necessity: Modal operators of necessity refer to those words which indicate there are no choices: "have to," "must," "can't," "it's necessary." Challenging these modal operators takes a person beyond the limits he has heretofore accepted. There are two excellent responses that serve to challenge these limits: WHAT STOPS YOU? and WHAT WOULD HAPPEN IF YOU DID? The response "What stops you?" serves to take the person into the past to find from what experience this generalization was formed. "What would happen if you did?" demands that the client go into the future and imagine possible consequences. The importance of these responses in assisting someone to achieve a richer and fuller model of the world is greatly emphasized.

"I can't do it."
(Response) "What stops you?"

"You have to finish by Tuesday."
(Response) "What would happen if I didn't?"

"I have to take care of other people."
(Response) "What will happen if you don't?"

"I can't tell him the truth."
(Response) "What will happen if you do?"
(Or) "What stops you from telling him the truth?"

The third distinction of the Meta-model is concerned with *semantic ill-formedness*. "The purpose of recognizing sentences which are semantically ill-formed is to assist the person in identifying the portions of his model which are distorted in some way that impoverishes the experiences which are available to him" (Bandler and Grinder). By changing these portions of his model that are semantically ill-formed, a person achieves greater choices and freedom in operating upon the world. It is these portions which frequently stop the person from acting in ways he would otherwise choose to act. The three classes of semantic ill-formedness are:

Cause and Effect
Mind Reading
Lost Performative

Cause and Effect: Cause and effect involves the belief that some action on the part of one person can cause another person to experience some emotion or inner state. As such the person responding experiences himself as having no choice concerning how to respond. When this is challenged it allows the person to explore and question whether the causal connection is indeed true. He can then begin to wonder what other choices he can generate for responding. The challenge is one of asking: "How does X cause Y?"

"Your writing on the wall bothers me."
(Response) "How does my writing on the wall bother you?"
(Or) ". . . make you feel bothered?"

"You frustrate me."
(Response) "How do I frustrate you?" "How is it possible for me to frustrate you?"
(Or) ". . . make you feel frustrated?"

"His ideas annoy me."
(Response) "How do his ideas annoy you?"
(Or) ". . . make you feel annoyed?"

"I'm sad because you're late."
(Response) "How does my being late make you feel sad?"

Mind Reading: Mind reading refers to the belief on the part of the speaker that one person can know what another is thinking or feeling without a direct communication from the second person. In other words this is a way to recognize when someone is acting on delusions rather than information. Obviously, mind reading can do much to inhibit the usefulness of a person's model of the world. The listener responds to mind reading by asking: "How, specifically, do you know X?" This provides a way for the speaker to become aware of and even to question those assumptions he may have previously taken for granted.

"Everybody thinks I'm taking too much time."
(Response) "How, specifically, do you know what everybody is thinking?"

"I'm sure you can see how I feel."
(Response) "How, specifically, can you be sure I see how you feel?"

"I know what's best for him."
(Response) "How do you know what is best for him?"

"He never considers the consequences."
(Response) "How, specifically, do you know he never considers the consequences?"

Lost Performative: The lost performative refers to those statements that are in the form of a generalization about the world itself rather than a statement recognized as belonging to the speaker's model of the world. Usually these are judgments. The speaker is using the lost performative when he takes rules that are appropriate to him and his model of the world and puts them on others. Phrased in the vernacular this is called "laying your trip on somebody else." The purpose in challenging this is to assist the speaker to own comfortably his own rules and opinions while allowing the rest of the world to have its own. Frequently with lost performative there is no indication that the speaker is even aware of other options or possibilities. To challenge lost performative, ask: FOR WHOM?

It's wrong to be on welfare."
(Response) "It's wrong for whom to be on welfare?"

"This is the right way to do it."
(Response) "This is the right way for whom to do it?"

"That's a sick thing to do."
(Response) "Sick for whom?"

Thus the Meta-model asks the questions What, How, Who in response to the specific form of the speaker's language.

Source: Leslie Cameron-Bandler, *They Lived Happily Ever After* (Cupertino, Calif.: Meta Publications, 1978), pp. 174-80.

One caveat I would offer in using the Meta-model in a client/consultant relationship is that OD consultants need to be aware of an additional set of issues that therapists do not. People come to therapists because they have defined themselves as needing therapeutic help. They consequently place themselves in a dependent position with respect to the therapist and usually try to respond positively to the therapist's guidance of the discussion.

Consultants, on the other hand, work with many people who do not think they need help in the way they express themselves. They may withhold information quite consciously and make statements full of deletions, generalizations, and distortions in order not to reveal certain data on the details of their thinking. Thus requests for specification, gentle challenges to universal quantifiers, and so on may be taken as unwarranted intrusions that put the client on the spot rather than help this person deal more effectively with his or her world.

For Meta-modeling to work in any situation, a strong trusting relationship has to be established first. Following the guidelines of the subsequent sections of this chapter can help one do this. Suffice it to say here that Meta-modeling is an intriguing new technique that helps both client and consultant transform their experiences into highly concrete terms; ones that maximize mutual understanding and enable logical communication be pursued with the confidence that, at least cognitively, each party is operating on the same wave length.

Representational Awareness

When attempts at structuring logical communication prove unfruitful, what is getting in the way may not be the client's inability to articulate conceptually his or her experience or yours. Rather, the problem may lie in differences in the way the two of you are organizing and perceiving your experience in the first place. This is also a matter of transforming experience into language, although on a more subtle level. Once again, Bandler and Grinder have something useful to offer. These authors argue that people vary in the particular senses (sight, sound, touch) they rely on most to take in and organize data about the world. Moreover, individuals' reliance on different senses for representing the world in their thinking can get in the way of effective communication.

Specifically, people differ according to whether they represent their experience internally in visual, auditory, or kinesthetic terms. Those who represent the world internally in visual terms literally think in terms of pictures—like viewing a television set with the sound turned off. Persons who represent the world internally in auditory terms think in terms of voices and conversations. The past is relived in terms of the sounds experienced and the future is conceived in terms of what one might hear. Finally, those who are kinesthetically inclined think in terms of movement and touch. To remember is to relive the bodily sensations one experienced—feeling, touching, grasping, discovering softness, warmth, roughness, and so on.

Behind these representational preferences is the fact that all of us take in data from all our senses as we go through life. Thus, we all record somewhere in our brains the sights, sounds, touches, smells, and so on of every event. However, while we grow up we learn to think consciously primarily in terms of one of our senses, and what happens in terms of the others is stored but tends to remain beyond our awareness.

This condition can create problems when, as adults and presumably even as fairly young children, we attempt to communicate with other individuals who use representational systems that are different from our own. For our representational systems manifest themselves in both what we attend to in interacting with others and in how we talk about our experience.

For example, I, as someone who is quite visually oriented, may be having a conversation with you, who, for the sake of argument, let us say, are auditorially oriented. We are talking about a meeting that I just attended and I am describing in vivid pictorial detail the way people dressed, the looks on their faces when various events happened, and the inferences to be made from the data presented on flipcharts and in handouts. I am quite excited about what happened but cannot seem to convey my excitement to you.

Finally, I show you one of the data sheets that was handed out, and you ask me, "What did so-and-so say about that figure?" I cannot remember the exact words and go on to do my own interpretation based on what I had seen. You remain pleasant but somehow complacent over my interpretation until Harry, another auditorially oriented colleague who also attended the meeting, walks into the room and gives you a word-by-word replay of the conversations that accompanied the data presentation. At last you brighten up, and the three of us make plans for what is to follow.

In retrospect, you wanted me to help you "hear" what happened in that meeting because you process your world in terms of voices. And you were not able to experience my interpretation until Harry helped you do this. I, on the other hand, wanted you to "see" what happened because that is how I process my experience. I could not repeat the words you wanted to hear or the tone of voice that Harry replicated for you, because I did not attend to voices carefully in consciously making sense out of my world.

Obviously, differences in representational systems are not always major deterrents to effective communication. We all develop at least some facility in all three major systems, and modern society demands that we learn visual processing with considerable acuity. The point is that each of us tends to have a preference for one representational system over the others, and the problems that arise from this condition are probably greater than is currently recognized. Bandler, Grinder, and their colleagues have reported its importance in therapeutic relationships with individuals, couples, and whole families. My own experience in the field of consulting is that its importance varies with the intensity of any relationship and, in particular, with the degree to which people work with each other on emotionally important issues and rely on each other for information and mutual support.

Consultant/client relationships in an OD project fit clearly into this category. It is critical for both parties to achieve a comfortable state of rapport with each other where they feel as if they are "talking on the same wave length." I am convinced that problems in structuring logical communications do arise when these two people use different aspects of experience to understand each other while attempting to describe, form opinions around, and plan action on a particular problem.

The task for the consultant in dealing with this problem is to identify the client's dominant representational system, assess it against his or her own, and adjust his or her way of presenting data to the client to match the latter's preferences.

Attending to the Client's Language.   The most direct way to spot a person's representational system is to be attentive to the words he or she uses. Visually oriented individuals pepper their language with pictorial imagery:

> "Do you *see* what I'm saying?"
>
> "*Picture* this."
>
> "That *looks* good to me."
>
> "That's hard to get a *focus* on."
>
> "There's a person with real *foresight*."

Those whose representational preferences are auditory often deal in the language of sounds:

> "Am I *hearing* you right?"
>
> "Her statement was *music* to my *ears*."
>
> "How does this *sound* to you?"
>
> "There's a lot of *noise* in the system."
>
> "We've got to maintain *harmony* in the ranks."

The kinesthetically inclined make frequent references to touch, texture, temperature, and movement:

> "That was a *slap* in the face."
>
> "You're getting *warmer*."
>
> "She plays *rough*."
>
> "Here's something I can *get my arms around*."
>
> "We *went back and forth* on the subject for quite awhile."

Having spotted a client's preferred representational system by the kinds of verbs, adjectives, adverbs, and idioms this person uses more frequently than others, one deals in the same medium in return.[6] This may be difficult in the early stages of a relationship when one might need this knowledge the most, because when the atmosphere is most formal, a client's language may be almost devoid of imagery. Our bureaucratic heritage encourages us to speak as machines to each other and thus to use "unspecified" predicates such as think, know, consider, difficult, important, promising, thoughtful, and so on. The same basic skill that enables us to match predicates allows our clients to converse in these antiseptic terms. We assume, however, that both client and consultant continue to use their preferred representational systems in organizing their experience.

One might argue that if the conversation is proceeding smoothly in this unspecified language, why bother to search further for the client's representational system? The point here is that making the translation into this mode requires the client to use energy that the consultant could release by dealing directly in the client's preferred medium. The transcript that follows shows how a consultant can adjust his or her phraseology to match the client's representational system:

Consultant: So far I understand that you're interested in a training program on interpersonal skills for your desk personnel and secretaries. Can you tell me how you arrived at this goal?

Client: Well, it all started when we received complaints from some very important people in the community who were having surgery at the hospital. One of our trustees asked us to *look* into the problem [visual predicate]. When we did, we didn't like what we *saw* either — patients being left on beds in the hallways without attendees, irritable responses to inquiries over the phone . . . We *looked* around for a consultant and discovered you.

Consultant: This may seem like an impertinent question, but how do you *see* training as the answer?

Client: Well, if they're not *looking out* for the patients' comfort, they need to be taught how to. I know their superiors have made it *clear* that this is a number one priority. It comes through *bold as day* in almost every memo we distribute.

Consultant: Suppose they know already how to attend to patients, but something is preventing them from doing this. For instance, they may not *see* how it makes a difference in the way they are evaluated. Perhaps there is more to the *picture* than just inadequate skills.

Client: Oh, I *see* what you're saying. I heard some gossip in the hallway the other day about one of the administrators yelling at a porter in front of a patient.

Consultant: How do you feel about that incident?

[6]By now, you should have developed some hunches about what your preferred representational system is, having just read this part of the chapter. If not, apply the same techniques being presented to your own behavior or ask some friends to do this for you.

Client: Pretty bad. We had just hired this fellow and thought he was perfect for the job. Well, you're the consultant, if training isn't the answer, perhaps you can *enlighten* us as to what we should do.

Adjusting one's language to the client's representational system is only one of the many strategies a consultant can employ to establish an effective relationship. Moreover, while there is much anecdotal support, there are few rigorous research studies to support the model. Regardless of technical effects, however, the strategy has the added value of keeping one attuned to how the client is thinking as well as to the content of what this person says. And in the long run, as OD consultants it is "how" the client operates that we want to enhance.

Active Listening[7]

So far we have discussed some blocks to logical communication that deal with the mechanics of human dialogue itself. While these are important, their utility is based on the assumption that both client and consultant are willing to communicate in ways conducive to the logic of the task, and that they are not attending to some important requisites for doing this effectively.

The other two blocks we want to discuss in this chapter focus on conditions where both parties may know how to communicate logically, but competing priorities prevent them from doing so. The latter draw time and energy away from the task. They also limit the extent to which each party is willing to follow the logical communication process completely.

One of these competing priorities is the maintenance and enhancement of one's self-concept. As the reference point through which one interprets one's experience, one's self-concept plays an important role in determining both why one is participating in the task, in the first place, and what is acceptable behavior for one's self in this situation. These assumptions, in turn, help to determine what one actually attends to as the task progresses and how one feels about what is going on.

For example, if I see myself as a beginning consultant and I am working in the field with a senior colleague, I am likely to pay as much attention to how my colleague is behaving toward our client as I am to how our client is behaving toward my colleague. My self-concept is that of a learner who needs to understand how the interaction is played out on both sides.

Likewise, when our client pays more attention to my colleague than to me and looks at him or her when asking important questions, I feel comfortable because I am not supposed to be at the center of the action. In fact, if the client were to ask me an important question, I might feel threatened and become so upset that I might not be able

---

[7]The term "active listening" was first formulated by Carl Rogers and Richard E. Farson. While it has been interpreted in a variety of ways in countless management seminars, the earliest publication on the subject that this author was able to locate is Carl R. Rogers and Richard E. Farson, *Active Listening* (Chicago: Industrial Relations Center, The University of Chicago, 1957). The following summary of the technique of active listening is based on this document.

to give a satisfactory answer that I was actually quite capable of creating. My self-concept as learner and junior colleague might be violated if I were to do so, and it is this concept of myself that makes it comfortable for me to be sitting there in the room, witnessing important events, and frequently not having the slightest idea about what to do next.

By the same token, my senior colleague might be giving much more attention to the client than to me because this person sees himself or herself as my representative and assumes that, for the most part, I will keep quiet. He or she may become upset if our client pays more attention to me because part of his or her self-concept involves being the center of the consulting team. My colleague's self-concept as team leader and my teacher is what makes it feel all right to invite me along even if I am not making much of a contribution.

One can see from the foregoing that one's self-concept is a two-edged sword. It makes some experience legitimate, equitable, or logical and simultaneously makes other kinds of experience illegitimate, inequitable, or illogical. It causes one to focus one's attention on some aspects of the situation, and simultaneously draws one's attention away from other aspects. The problem with this is that *how* it causes one to feel and *what* it causes one to attend to may not always contribute maximally to the logical task at hand.

Suppose, for instance, that in the example above the client did ask me an important question and that the answer I was capable of giving (but did not because of my emotional state) was far more appropriate than the one my senior colleague eventually intervened with in my behalf.

Or suppose later on the conversation that, in attending equally to my colleague and the client, I was not observant enough of the latter to detect a subtle shift in his or her mood (tiny tears in the corners of his or her eyes, softer voice tone) and subsequently made a basically harmless, but under the circumstances, flippant remark that was out of tune with the client's emotional state and temporarily hindered rapport between us.

We have been talking about the consultant's experience, but this applies equally to the client. This person may not be responding logically to the task because his or her self-concept is pointing toward other issues as well:

Consultant: Do you think you have a clear enough idea of the plan to get George on board?

Client: Self-Concept — Responsible for consultant's budget.
Assumption — Enough time in light of the budget has been spent on this matter.
Perception — Consultant is taking more time on this matter.
Feeling — Anxious.
Behavior — "Don't worry about George . . ."

Simultaneously, the client may be experiencing still other emotions that are getting in the way of continuing logically with the task:

Consultant: Do you think you have a clear enough idea of the plan to get George on board?

Client: Self-Concept—Competent manager, capable of quickly assimilating others' ideas.
Assumption—I should know the plan, but I am not sure I do. We have been discussing it long enough.
Perception—Consultant is challenging my competence.
Feeling—Mildly confronted.
Behavior—"Don't worry about George" (intended as a mild putdown, a way of avoiding further inquiry).

Active listening is a well-known behavioral strategy that has traditionally been used for helping people discuss sensitive issues, especially ones that threaten their self-concepts and that they feel uncomfortable talking about because the act of doing so appears to them as threatening in and of itself. The technique does this by placing the listener/helper in an appreciative yet responsive role that demonstrates both a willingness to listen unevaluatively (thereby reducing the threat of self-disclosure) and a commitment to help the client articulate more fully what is threatening about a situation so that this person can make more informed choices about what to do next. In the process, the consultant gains new data about the nature of the client's self-concept, and thus greater awareness about how the client is likely to respond to still other issues.

The technique can best be described as a series of behavioral dos and don'ts complemented by a particular emotional posture toward the client. The posture involves placing the client emotionally at center stage and defining one's self as an empathic tool for helping this person articulate, appreciate, and explore his or her unique definition of the world and his or her self in it.

The dos and don'ts identify specific behaviors that highlight this posture and minimize alternative definitions of the listener. Listed below are some of the guidelines I have found most helpful.

Search for the total meaning of what the other is saying and acknowledge all parts of the message. This, in particular, requires that one look for the feelings that someone is expressing as well as the cognitive message. For example, "I think I played a useful role in that meeting" means roughly the same thing cognitively as, "I finally got a chance to show what I can do in that session." But the latter contains the additional affective messages of pride and relief.

"That's fantastic; isn't it satisfying when you can make important people sit and listen" acknowledges both messages in the second statement and would probably help the attendee to discuss what is really on his or her mind. On the other hand, a response such as "Could you tell me what you did that you thought was useful?" would be a logical response to both statements, but only on a cognitive level. Thus, it probably would be appropriate only as a response to the first statement.

Acknowledging the total message, and especially its affective component, is useful because of the stigma in our culture against articulating feelings explicitly when working with business colleagues. Since the feelings are there nonetheless and people want to let others know what they are, they tend to piggyback them onto cognitive messages, as in the example above. A consultant's taking the risk of such articulation for the client both confirms that the total message has been received and identifies the consultant as someone who is not beholden to this traditional but rather stifling norm.

Try to restate the speaker's message in your own words. In many cases, the message another is trying to convey might not be totally discernible even to a very skillful listener. Attempting to restate the other's message in one's own words is a basic but frequently overlooked tactic for coping with this. People avoid it because of another cultural norm, that is, the prescription against revealing one's own incompetence. Adults, after all, are supposed to be able to understand what others say to them. To test out whether one has succeeded in this most basic of activities, especially if the speaker appears to have used correct pronunciation and sufficient volume, may be seen as a revelation of one's own incompetence.

But just as people have feelings that cannot be legislated away, they also communicate almost everything imperfectly. Words, body language, and so on are not meanings in and of themselves, but only containers of meaning, and imperfect ones at that. The active listener who dares to test whether he or she got the other's message not only does both parties the service of maintaining effective communication, but also acknowledges to the other that the process is difficult and that he or she is willing to risk losing face in order to make it work.

Invite clarification of incongruent communication. Frequently, when the topic is sensitive, people say two things at the same time that contradict each other. One message is conveyed by the words they utter, the other by how they utter them—for example, tone of voice and body language. For instance, suppose that, in response to a question about whether a feasible next step in developing a project would be to talk with a client's boss, a respondent says, "Yes, that's a good idea. I'm sure he will give us a fair hearing." But while he is saying these words, his voice turns gruff and his eyes shift away from you toward the floor.

You as the consultant are stuck with contradictory messages. Is the client really enthusiastic as his words suggest, or is he anxious about such a move as his body language implies? Our knowledge of human behavior suggests that both messages are likely to be true in some degree. They are simply coming from different parts of the speaker's thinking. Since the messages contradict each other, it is likely that the speaker is not aware of the more subtle message he is conveying. Putting him in touch with what he has done can help bring this second message into consciousness, where he is in a better position to deal with it and clarify the totality of what he would like to say.

For instance, the consultant might respond, "Well, Harry, your words say we should bring him in now, but the way you said it has me puzzled. You sounded like you were warming up for a fight, and I noticed your face dropped a few inches. Is there something more we should discuss about your boss before we go ahead with this?" The client's response might explain his behavior in a variety of ways—for example, he thinks his boss is really enthusiastic but the two of them have just had an argument; he does not like having to gain his boss's approval even if it will not be difficult; his boss says he is fair, but the client knows he is actually uninterested in this project.

Regardless of what the content of the response is, the consultant's acknowledgment of the second message helps to uncover important additional data for the decision and indicates the latter's regard for the client as a total person, not just his "business" side.

Searching for and acknowledging the total meaning, restating messages in your own words, and spotting incongruent communication all help a client discuss sensitive issues by demonstrating your commitment to try to understand his or her experience. Several other self-explanatory reminders about what *not* to do suggest the requisites for demonstrating one's willingness to treat what the client reveals with a sense of respect and acceptance:

- Refrain from telling the client how he or she should think or feel and from belittling the importance of the issues he or she is discussing. Your construction of the world is unique and so is your client's.

- While it is helpful to acknowledge your ability to identify with aspects of the client's experience, do not discuss your own experience in detail once you have committed to exploring the client's. This shifts the focus of attention to you and away from the client.

- Do not attempt to use humor to ease the tension unless you are adept at this. Most humor is based on some form of double message that might be hard to interpret as intended under tense conditions, and, therefore, its results are difficult to predict.

Awareness of Interpersonal Needs

We want to turn now to a third barrier to logical communication, one that takes the form of a concomitant agenda that often competes with task performance without adding anything to it. This is the satisfaction of interpersonal needs.

Behavioral scientists have long since accepted the notion that almost all human interaction serves multiple ends. The latter can be separated into ends that are instrumental to yet other ends, such as the management of a project or business, and those that are intrinsically rewarding to one or more parties, and thus are ends in themselves. The satisfaction of interpersonal needs of all sorts—for example, companionship, love, recognition, dominance, and esteem—falls into the latter category and is an important if sometimes ulterior motive for engaging in almost any kind of human interaction.

Clinical psychologists spend much of their time helping people to become untangled from the ways in which they attempt to satisfy these needs when their attempt gets in the way of their effective and efficient contribution to more instrumental ends. The objective is not to deny either their existence or the pursuit of their satisfaction but to help people find ways of satisfying them that are at least not harmful, and hopefully helpful, to accomplishing the basic instrumental tasks of everyday life—for example, maintaining life and limb, social respect, self-composure, job, and career.

OD specialists, because they choose to connect with the members of an organization on an interpersonal level, also need to pay some attention to this aspect of human dynamics. An OD consultant need not be trained as a clinical psychologist, but one does need to be trained in some of the basics in this area. For people who are mentally healthy and who in general do not need therapeutic assistance also seek to satisfy interpersonal needs in the context of their work lives. And in the context of a client/consultant dialogue, this can easily get in the way of the process of logical communication.

A wide variety of conceptual schemes are available for understanding and managing interpersonal needs. The one we will offer here is elementary but elegant. The basic elements of this particular model were developed by William Schutz, and they have been used in countless management and Organization Development programs.[8] We will consider a variation of Schutz's model that was first introduced to me by my colleague, Suresh Srivastva.

To begin with, Schutz posits that all interpersonal needs can be classified into three categories: inclusion, control, and friendship. Each of these types of needs, moreover, has a passive and an active state. *Inclusion* in its passive form encompasses needs for popularity, visibility, centrality, recognition, prestige, and acceptance; in essence, being seen as a someone who is valuable, relevant, and worthy of attention. The active form is the need to create these conditions in others—for instance, by including them, organizing them, praising them, recognizing them, keeping them informed, and so on.

The active form of the need for *control* encompasses wanting to influence others, to be in charge, to dominate, to determine the course of events, to lead, and so on. The passive form is simply the converse of this, whether it be as masochistic as the desire to be dominated or as benign as the desire to be led, coached, guided, or simply influenced by others.

The need for *friendship* in its active form is the desire to share one's personal feelings and thinking with others: to open up emotionally, to be friendly, close, warm, vulnerable, and intimate. The passive form is the desire for others to behave in these ways toward oneself.

Schutz posits that people feel most comfortable in relationships where the parties have complementary interpersonal needs. For instance, my need for being included, informed, and so on is matched on your part by the complementary need to include others, keep them informed, and so on. Simultaneously, my need to influence others is matched by a similarly strong need for you to be influenced. In the most comfortable relationship, all three types of needs display complementarity.

Analyzing the current state of a relationship with these ideas in mind can start a useful dialogue around trouble spots in it.[9] For our purposes, however, it is more important to think about *how* two people work toward complementarity as they interact with each other.

In order to do this, Srivastva has suggested that one think about each need satisfying behavior as a commodity or good that one wants to obtain from another individual or that, alternatively, one might provide for the other under the right conditions. Such goods are discussed and bargained over as a normal part of human conversation. Sometimes such bargaining can be extremely explicit.

[8]William Schutz, *FIRO: A Three Dimensional Theory of Interpersonal Behavior* (New York: Holt, Rinehart and Company, 1958).

[9]Schutz has developed a simple, copyrighted, paper-and-pencil questionnaire that provides suggestive quantitative measures for each dimension and is available through University Associates, Inc., 7596 Eads Avenue, La Jolla, California 93037.

A.   I have no intention of letting you run that project on your own unless you keep me better informed. (I will not let you influence me more unless you include me more in return.)

B.   How can I keep you better informed if I don't know what you're doing and what data you need (wants inclusion in return for inclusion)?

A.   Look, I've tried keeping you up to date, but it's like talking to a brick wall. You just don't seem interested in me as a person (wants intimacy in return for inclusion).

B.   I know we've been through that one before, but it's still hard for me to listen to all your tales of woe when you cut me off as soon as it's my turn (intimacy for intimacy). If you want a good listener you better be prepared to take the time to listen to me (intimacy for influence).

More typically, however, the bargaining is much more subtle:

A.   You know, what you people do with your surveys is what I do day-to-day, just by keeping my ears tuned (possibly a bid for recognition/inclusion).

B.   That must keep you really busy (acknowledges other's efforts thereby expressing inclusion). Have you ever tried the survey method to see whether what you're picking up from a few individuals applies to the whole group (bid for inclusion and potential influence)?

A.   No, I've usually considered surveys a waste of time (mild attempt to reduce other's status, rejects inclusion bid). I must say though that what you found in the other group has me a little concerned (bid for intimacy).

B.   Really . . . in what way (acknowledges intimacy, asks for more)?

A.   Well, there is a subgroup in my division, like the one you talked about that seems okay when I'm with them. But I get vibes every once in awhile that everything isn't right and they're not owning up. I'd hate to discover that they've got some real beefs like the group you talked about did (more intimacy, mild recognition/inclusion).

B.   Where do you get the vibes from, anything in particular (more intimacy)?

A.   Well, there is this weekly meeting we have, and . . . (more intimacy). Say, how about some lunch . . . (bid to include the other).

B.   Sure, where do you usually eat (accepts bid, thereby potentially nullifying exclusion statement expressed earlier)?

As one can see from the foregoing, this more subtle form of bargaining tends to be purposively vague, easily open to misinterpretation (alternatives could be offered to my own interpretations), easily defended against, often beyond each party's immediate awareness, and ultimately verifiable only in terms of each party's actual behavior.

Because of all the qualities listed above, it is often easy to read too much into the unspoken side of a conversation. Nonetheless, I have found that this model often keeps me in touch with an aspect of the dialogue that the other techniques discussed thus far miss. Perhaps even more than the other techniques, it requires an unusual degree of self-awareness. For as consultants we are naturally attempting to become included, influential, and intimate with our clients for instrumental as well as intrinsic ends. Thus, our most natural responses to rejection on any of these dimensions are apt to surface at the most inopportune times, and likewise our own manipulative tendencies are likely to become manifest.

For example, it is very easy to feel defensive when your favorite techniques are downgraded, your attempts at influence as an outsider ignored or rejected, and your patient encouragement of initimate dialogue shunted off into trivia. It is also very tempting to become manipulative when you discover that your client is easily hooked on praise or power or intimacy. Coping effectively with these feelings is a major task of the consulting process. For if you cannot handle them, how can you expect your client to?

Two basic strategies are available. First, one can talk about one's own needs, thereby offering them as relevant data to be considered in the logical communication process, and implicitly making a bid for the other party to respond in kind. Second, one can use one's awareness of the underlying dynamics of the situation to discover ways that are likely to meet the needs of both parties and then act accordingly. The objective in the latter case is to reduce unilaterally the tension around satisfying interpersonal needs so that logical conversation around the officially shared task can proceed.

My own preference is to use the second strategy more in the beginning of a relationship and develop a more self-disclosing approach as the relationship progresses. Thus, if a client seems to need praise and recognition, I give it to him or her as authentically and skillfully as I can. If I am feeling needy of the same things, I share my appreciation of myself and give the client a chance to reinforce me in kind. If he or she wants to exert influence over me, or more typically, to imply his or her capacity to do so, I parry these efforts only to the extent that they might eventually get in the way of project objectives and my own integrity. If I feel the need to exert my own influence, I channel my energy into returning the dialogue again and again to the logical format. If my client wants to share his or her personal thoughts and feelings in detail, I welcome this to the extent that I feel capable of listening and responding authentically. And I respond in kind to the extent that I have a need to do this and my client seems to be comfortable with it.

A key question is, How much responsiveness is too much? Certain minimum and maximum amounts of inclusion, influence, and intimacy are critical for the development of an effective relationship. While I suspect that different consultants and consulting styles have their unique requisites, here are some guidelines I try to follow.

1.   Focus on what you like best about your own skills and what you see as your client's potential as a colleague in the OD process, and take pride in expressing these things openly.

Dale Carnegie stereotypes notwithstanding, mutual admiration is the cornerstone of any meaningful relationship. My sense is that clients want to see themselves as hiring confident and successful people, and they want to feel that way about themselves. The more attractice you are to your client, the more this person is likely to want to include you in his or her world, and the more welcome are your own expressions of *inclusion* toward him or her (praise, recognition, avowals of availability and willingness to help, bids to bring the other into a particular activity, briefings on what is happening in the project).

Do not lie about your expertise and experience but play up what you are, what you represent, and what you have done positively, and refrain from discussing past failures and current uncertainties about what you can do. The idea is to stay honest, positive, and optimistic. Simultaneously, try to help your client do the same. Clients' conversation, their body language, their offices and work areas, are filled with signs of past successes. Look for them, ask about them, ask yourself if you can appreciate them, and if you can, then do so.

We and our clients play games, of course, and some of them center around trying to get and give praise manipulatively. For instance, a client may parade his or her successes before you and get your praise only to downplay what you give, either with some uniquely personal outcome in mind or simply the intent of seeing what you will do next. For me, however, the games do not matter if the praise I give is authentic, something I really believe. Then I am just being true to myself.

Being true to myself is a difficult task. I have to check to make sure that I am not "being nice" just to develop the relationship. What makes me a consultant who is often included in the client's world is my willingness to discover and express my appreciation fully and in a way a client can understand. This provides important modeling for the client. If my client is equally or more skillful than I am at it, then it is simply a way for both of us to broaden our awareness of the range of things about each other and our worlds that we can appreciate.

> 2.   Avoid commitments, implied or explicit, that are likely to lock in a generally vertical relationship in either direction. Barring this, "Render unto Caesar what is Caesar's." Base your influence on charisma, expertise, and the spirit of your contracts. Avoid dependency games based on implied connections with other parts of the client system.

Influence issues in OD consultant/client relationships can be especially difficult. The ideal is mutual influence and collaboration, but this needs to be viewed as a long-run gestalt. Moment to moment, each person pushes and pulls in different directions; both client and consultant declaring what he or she will or will not do, suggesting, challenging, kidding, reopening issues, and so on. Sometimes this is done very subtly and sometimes very explicitly. Officially, the client always has the upper hand, but the more the consultant is included by the client system and the more intimate the material that the client shares with the consultant, the more the latter can gain a great deal of influence as well.

The most basic principle I follow with regard to influence is to keep matters clean and above board. I try to justify my attempts to influence the client either in terms of my expertise as it applies to achieving our shared objectives, or in terms of the spirit of the contract we have agreed to. If there are times when the client openly depends on me for guidance, I may offer advice whose rationale he or she may not understand, but only if I am convinced that this person believes in me, and if I can justify the advice to myself. Usually, however, I pursue a shared understanding of the reasons behind whatever I suggest.

At the same time, I make a point of staying out of situations that might imply that I have become part of the formal authority system. It is often tempting to behave toward a client as if his or her boss and I know what is best. In the long run, this only leads to trouble. For then I become identified with the hierarchy and am obliged to live with others' perceptions of it rather than my own record as a collaborator. Line orders, implied or explicit, need to come through the line.

Likewise, I will not act as a subordinate client's advocate per se to senior clients. If I believe in his or her cause, I may present it in the context of project objectives in the presence of more senior clients. This can increase a subordinate's identification with me and thus further the cause of the project, but it is up to the subordinate to declare his or her agreement with my position. It also paves the way for the subordinate to disagree with me later in the service of his or her own perception of the project objectives. We are tied together ultimately through the project, not one-on-one. I stand on my own ground and let the other do the same.

> 3. Test your capacity to pursue intimacy with your clients around their organizational lives. This requires that you learn to care for them as individuals as well as role players. Be clear, however, about your own sense of your skills and energy when encouraging personal disclosure that is not immediately relevant to the task.

Intimacy in a general sense is not a primary goal of OD consultancy relationships. But getting clients to share how they feel and think about the dynamics of their organization and their personal experiences of it, and sharing one's thinking in kind, are the first steps toward experimentation and change. This is extremely hard to do for any extended period of time without caring authentically at least for a client's organizational life. Thus, a kind of bounded intimacy is necessary.

To become an effective OD consultant, I think one has got to like people in general, especially their day-to-day joys and frustrations as organizational participants. This requires a certain degree of personal vulnerability. The more you care, the more your energies become entangled with your clients' lives, and the more you can be hurt. This to me is a major cost of being a practitioner in this field. I am convinced, however, that learning to care, actually suffering with one's clients' defeats and learning how to heal one's self, is more fulfilling in the long run than learning to behave skillfully without caring.

Clients are bound to spot the latter eventually and, while they may still see a consultant who remains aloof as having been helpful, the relationship is likely to lose much of its vitality.

What this implies for the client/consultant dialogue is that, as a consultant, one has to be willing not only to express what one appreciates in the client (in order to maximize inclusion) but to let the client know what aspects of his or her experience strike truly resonant chords in one's own experience. This does not imply that one always should reveal the flipside, that is, the ways in which the client's experiences and thinking are alien to one's own. However, that is apt to come out as well, and often can strengthen the relationship. The client comes to know the consultant better as an individual, and can feel safer in sharing his or her own lack of connection with the consultant's experience and perspectives as well.

Interacting on this level is, in general, a riskier business than responding to influence attempts, and clearly more so than being appreciative of what the other has done and what this person represents. Thus, early attempts at intimate dialogue are likely to be superficial and quite clearly related to kinds of organizational events that fellow professionals in our culture tend to feel similarly about. But as a relationship develops, each party's sense of safety is likely to rise. This, in turn, encourages disclosure of experiences, feelings, and perspectives that one identifies as more uniquely one's own and that are, therefore, more private and more vulnerable to attack or ridicule. Clients who have had little experience in doing this with professional colleagues, as opposed to spouses and close friends, may not know where to draw the line. This, in turn, can create situations in which one finds oneself as an OD consultant listening to clients discuss their family lives, and even their deepest feelings about their own self-concepts.

If the client cannot draw his or her own boundaries, it is up to the consultant to do so. Consultants who are also therapists may choose to make their boundaries fairly expansive, thereby essentially combining the OD task with personal counseling of a more holistic nature. Others with less training can simply signal politely their lack of desire and/or capacity to deal with more personal issues. Ultimately, however, some level of personal disclosure beyond that which the client is used to working at in day-to-day relationships with colleagues is likely to be necessary if client and consultant are to surface and deal collaboratively with the real issues that are critical for the client's and the organization's further development. This, then, is what requires the consultant to care.

CONCLUSION

Some important caveats are in order before ending this chapter. First, none of the behavioral strategies we have just considered are easy to master in a short period of time. Each takes practice to get the hang of and to integrate with one's unique personal style. Rather than try to become skillful immediately at all of them, explore one or two thoroughly and simply remain aware of the possibilities that lie in the others.

Second, each strategy does not work unidimensionally from consultant to client. Rather, each has the delightful quality of inducing changes in you as you learn to change the quality of others' dialogue with you. Each brings attention to what one normally does not attend to in typical conversation, and thereby helps you discover new things about your own thinking and behavior. This makes it doubly important not to rush through your exploration of any one of them. As you try any one of them, remain especially aware of its effect on you as well as on your client.

Finally, the strategies presented by no means comprise an exhaustive list of what might be useful for the OD consultant on an interpersonal level. They do provide some idea of the range of strategies one might follow, however, and the fourfold table used here to organize them represents a simple roadmap for considering the types of problems one might want to address. What is important is to have a variety of options to pursue in attempting to enhance the quality of one's interaction with a client. If you are trying to pursue logical communication and the conversation bogs down, shifting your attention to Meta-modeling, or matching representational systems, or active listening, or spotting and trying to deal with interpersonal needs is first and foremost a way of getting yourself unstuck, of seeing what is happening in a different light, so that your own creative energies are released. The strategies allow one to behave purposively in doing this. Any one of them is a clear advance over floundering around, but none of them is likely to provide the perfect solution to the situation you are facing.

The following chapters continue with the subsequent stages in the OD cycle. While each stage has its unique interpersonal problems and opportunities, all of them require an ongoing dialogue with one or more clients that can be enhanced through the use of the strategies presented in this chapter. Keep them in mind as you read along, and try to spot particular situations where important conversations with the client will make these tactics especially useful.

CHAPTER NINE

GATHERING DATA

Once a contract has been agreed to, it is time to start the formal data gathering process. We want to emphasize the word *formal* here, because the consultant has been gathering relevant information throughout the first three stages. What happens now is that data gathering becomes the public task of the relationship.

The data gathering stage serves a number of functions, the most obvious of which is providing the raw material for achieving a collaborative analysis. On the consultant's side, the necessary data for understanding the organization from a theoretical perspective are gathered from interviews, observations, questionnaires, and organization records. Likewise, data from the same sources allow the consultant to, learn the informal language of the organization, to build inductively models of how the organization's members think their system operates, to identify both the issues around which there is energy for change within the organization and the political forces for and against such change, and to begin to develop a model of a productive change program that takes all of the foregoing into account.

From the client's perspective, the formal data gathering activities enable a significant proportion of the membership to develop their own models of how the consultants operate, to begin to learn their language, to size up how useful they might be to their own and the organization's interests, to review and clarify their own models of their organization, and to begin to develop their own models of a productive change program.

Finally, these activities enable both parties to begin the dialogue whose result is hopefully a merging of their respective worlds and a shared analysis upon which successful change activities can be based.

But if this is all that was involved, the project probably would not get very far. A shared understanding of the system is not enough. Not just shared ideas but important relationships have to be developed between the consultants and as many potent people within the client group as possible. When it is time to take action, people's organizational lives may be at stake. No plan can foresee all the contingencies that might arise, and thus guarantee personal security and fulfillment beforehand for each participant. It is the pattern of relationships between the clients and their consultants, feelings of mutual trust and confidence, that ultimately allow both parties to begin the change process.

Thus, it is equally important to conceive of the data gathering stage as an important relationship building process. Formal data gathering is the public side of what is going on. Relationship building is the private, informal side. Both have to work hand in hand if the project is ultimately to be successful. It is primarily the responsibility of the consultant, moreover, to make this happen.

CHOOSING A DATA GATHERING STRATEGY

When one takes into account both the formal and informal functions of the data gathering stage, particular reasons become clear for choosing what data to gather and what methods to use in gathering them. If all one were interested in were the data themselves, one might use as an underlying principle the notion of gathering only those data that are relevant to the conceptual models you and your client have in mind, and only those data gathering methods that are most cost efficient in terms of the importance of the data gathered. But when relationship building is identified as an equally important objective, then other rationales become important as well. One needs to gather data whose generation and transference from client to consultant facilitates the development of a positive relationship between the two parties, and to do so in ways and under conditions that also facilitate this outcome. In other words, relationship building requires attention to process and context as well as to content.

Four basic data gathering strategies are generally used in OD projects: interviews, questionnaires, observation, and analysis of organization records. Of these, interviews and questionnaires tend to be the primary tools. Interviews are by far the most costly in terms of data gathered per person, but they have the advantage of providing an arena for relationship building and collaborative problem solving as the data are gathered. They are the primary vehicle for the style of OD discussed in this book, and we will devote the bulk of this chapter to them. The other three methods are less costly and can be used to good effect in particular situations. We will review their main features after exploring the interview.

The Interview

The advantages of the one-on-one *interview* as a data gathering device include:

- being able to state and continuously restate the goals and methods of the project and thereby to clear up any confusion on these issues before data gathering begins;

- being able to provide an additional opportunity for a particular client to air his or her concerns about the project and to respond to these concerns as best one can before proceeding further;

- having the opportunity to make sure that each research question is understood and explored fully;

- having the opportunity to discover and explore important issues one had not anticipated during the planning stages;

- having the opportunity from the very beginning to participate in problem solving and stimulate action in ways consistent with project objectives and philosophy;

- having the opportunity to begin to build a relationship with another member of the client system that will facilitate further problem solving and experimentation in later stages of the project.

Setting the Stage

Every interview can be conceived as a miniature OD project in and of itself. The major difference is only that this smaller project takes place in the context of a much larger one, and the latter sets important boundaries about what can and cannot be done. For instance, one has already established that a series of interviews will be done with a particular sample of the client group, that particular kinds of questions will be asked, that the data will be fed back under particular guidelines, that certain rules of confidentiality will be followed, and so on. But to this point in time, one only knows for sure that one's primary client or clients know and have agreed to this. The person you are about to interview may have been informed of the project and his or her role in it in a variety of ways (memos, group or individual meetings, passing comment in the hallway), may have absorbed this information with varying levels of accuracy and completeness, may have additional concerns not covered in earlier meetings with the organization's leadership, and may feel everything from widely enthusiastic to highly coerced by your presence.

Consequently, it is useful to think of oneself as conducting some important scouting, entry, and contracting activities before getting down to the interview itself. The first task is to establish who you are, who the interviewee is, and why the two of you are meeting at this time. I usually make a point of telling a brief history of myself and the project to date at the very beginning of each interivew. This can become extremely tiring in a large project, but even people I have already met several times seem to welcome this. It provides the interviewee with a chance to get focused, to size me up, to remember any questions he or she might have already and to discover new ones for me to answer, and to have answered questions this person might feel uncomfortable about asking, without having to reveal this. By the same token, it gives me a chance to present the project in my own words and to highlight both my aspirations for the project and my understanding of how it will be conducted.

Once I have done this, my task now is to respond as well as I can to any other concerns the interviewee might have. Quite often, people want to know a little more about the field of OD, to let me know of any past experiences they have had of this nature, to clarify questions of confidentiality, and to state their own views of the project and its possible outcomes. My emphasis in responding is both on being as clear as I can and on trying to put the interviewee at ease, and I try to use the same interpersonal techniques we reviewed earlier to do this.

The foregoing can take as long as half an hour when a client seems particularly nervous or resistant. While this can reap havoc on an interview schedule, it is well worth it to ensure the integrity of the interview itself, and the time problem can be reduced by scheduling at least 15-minute breaks between interviews. Almost always, however, such introductory activities take less than 10 minutes. The end result, ideally, is an informal contract to engage in the interview in the spirit and form agreed to by the larger organization.

The Interview Schedule

The ultimate form of an interview schedule (the list of questions and issues to explore with each interviewee) depends to a considerable degree on the concerns of the leading client or clients. The critical issues to cover are typically identified in the entry meetings and, if the client so desires, can be elaborated on in follow-up meetings after a contract has been agreed to. But unlike data gathering through questionnaires (where such follow-up meetings are especially important because one only gains responses to what specifically is asked), the one-on-one interview provides an opportunity for a broad-based inquiry that not only addresses the concerns of the leadership but also helps to reveal the unique concerns of every interviewee. Tapping into the latter can be especially useful, because it helps to reveal where the energy for change is within the system as a whole, and thus where the leadership's concerns may support or run counter to those and the rest of the organization.

There is a series of general questions that lend shape to such a broad-based inquiry that cover the individual level elements in the analysis model discussed in Chapter Six. These are the same questions that we used in the South City Chemical project. Each of them can be followed up with probes that highlight either particular leadership concerns and/or those of the consultant. Taken together, they also provide a very comfortable format for getting to know the interviewee as an individual, how he or she experiences the organization and his/her role in it, and where this person would like his or her own career and the larger organization to go. Thus, they also set the stage for building a relationship in which the interviewee feels that the consultant understands his or her perspective and has important knowledge for acting in his or her behalf. In the following paragraphs, we will take each question in turn and discuss how one can use it to help the interviewee unfold his or her experiences.

1.   *"Perhaps you might begin by telling me about your job."*

When asked this question, some people dive right in with a fairly detailed job description. Others may say, "What do you want to know about it?" In any case, what I am really after here is a pretty vivid description of what this person does all day. I do not just want to know what is written in this person's official job description. The real task is to develop a comfortable sense of how this person places himself or herself in the work flow of the organization and the concrete kinds of day-to-day activities that he or she undertakes. If someone says, "I'm in charge of the word processing operation here,"

I might follow with, "What does that involve?" If I get a list of duties—for example, processing work requests, assigning jobs to each member of the team, maintaining morale—I might ask for a little elaboration on each. I try to stay away from extreme detail. The idea is to tap into the total configuration.

Starting off as above, further questions might be, "Which of these activities take the most time?"; "Which are the most important for doing your job effectively?"; "Which do you like most/least?"; "Why is that?"; and "What does a typical workday look like?"

Some people can be amazingly vague about describing what they do, in which case I try to get a sample of activities from them. Others are short and to the point and I push gently for more detail. Others are extremely descriptive, and I respond by trying politely to shift our attention to still other elements of the job.

Two things guide my behavior. First, I want to make sure that I am getting data on all the particular issues related to the topic of the job itself that I, my colleagues, and the primary client have agreed are important. Second, I want to come away with the feeling that I am at least beginning to know how this person conceives his or her job and how he or she is currently experiencing it. My efforts regarding the latter vary from person to person and are guided by my own interests, energy, the time of day, past interviews, and so on. It is not a rigorous inquiry nor do I mean it to be. I do it for the sake of getting to know this person, and through this interview and every other, for the sake of filling myself with the gestalt of the organization.

> 2. *"Before we talk further about your work today, could you fill me in on how you got into this position? What has your career been like so far?"*

Having established the interviewee's current job as a reference point, the next task is to gain some historical perspective. This is helpful for several reasons. First, the latter parts of the interview will require the interviewee to comment on the wider organization and its environment. Some people respond with a variety of qualifiers— for example, "I really don't know what happens on a policy level"; "The only area I feel confident to speak about is _____"; or "I have only had contact with this group once or twice." Others speak so authoritatively one might think that they knew positively everything about the organization's operations. Still others seem unusually naive about even their immediate job environments. A little personal history early in the interview helps to place these things in perspective.

Second, most people find talking about themselves intrinsically rewarding. Asking them explicitly to do this often stimulates their involvement in the rest of the interview and lets them know that you indeed are interested in them as individuals. Third, the request for personal history is indirectly an invitation to elaborate on one's self-concept, which is just as important for the interviewer to understand when interpreting the data as past experience per se. Fourth, discussing personal history provides a comfortable opportunity for getting or confirming basic data on age, education, seniority, country of origin, and so on. Finally, the question provides a natural entry point for discussing career satisfaction and long-term job commitment, both of which are important variables in most organizational diagnoses.

3.   *"Whom do you work with most closely on a day-to-day basis? What do they expect from you, and what do you expect from them? How well are these expectations being met?"*

These three questions, in essence, invite the respondent to map out his or her important social networks, to comment on the social contracts both explicit and implicit that hold them together, and to identify the points of tension and cohesiveness within them. They mark the first important transition point in the interview. Up to now, the focus of the conversation has been on the individual respondent. Now we begin the process of surveying larger and larger spheres of activity that surround the interviewee and shape his or her work environment. The first step outward from the self addresses one's interpersonal relationships. The results are often startling because a surprisingly large number of people have never given much systematic thought to at least some of the issues involved.

People find it easy to rattle off whom they work with very closely. Some of the latter will probably already have been mentioned in the answers to the preceding questions, and an easy point of departure is to clarify what they do and how frequently they interact with the respondent. Then one can move on to other people the respondent interacts with frequently, but not as intensely. It is also important to establish which of these people are in a long-term relationship with the respondent, and which are more temporary or intermittent colleagues in various projects. How detailed you should get depends upon how important the topic is to your own theorizing and to your primary client's concerns. For example, if you and your client are especially interested in the dynamics of a particular 12-person team, you might want to get a reading on how closely the respondent interacts with each of these people. Left to their own devices, most respondents will mention between three and eight relatively close associates, and then start questioning you regarding how exhaustive you want them to get.

The fun part comes when you start to ask a respondent to specify what he or she expects from each of these people, and vice versa. Quite often, the individual has not thought about it. If this is the case, it is especially important to give the respondent time to think and to use your interpersonal skills to help this person come up with clear answers. This is another part of the interview that can take an unanticipated amount of time. The topic is an important one, however, because it is a norm in most organizational cultures that people should know what they expect of each other. Respondents may feel embarrassed when they realize these data are not at their fingertips. Consequently, they are likely to appreciate your help in clarifying these expectations. Your successful assistance here can make the interview more than an act of service to the larger project, and thus may help you establish a potentially meaningful relationship with the respondent.

Interviewees' perceptions of how well the expectations involved in their immediate relationships are being met often surface as they describe what the expectations are. Thus, the third question in this series often gets at least partially answered in the context of the other two. Nonetheless, it is important to push for some clear evaluations in concluding this section. Here again, the exercise in and of itself can create new insights and problems to work on for the respondent. It is up to you, the interviewer, to decide whether to try to be helpful at this time. Sometimes, useful suggestions are obvious to an outsider. At other times, the conversation reveals issues that you can legitimately promise to work on at a later time as part of the larger project. If you make such promises, however, be sure to remember them. Subsequent events may make the treatment of particular people's issues less feasible, and it is important to get back to them personally if this happens.

> 4. *"How do the structure and policies of the larger organization (division, institution) help or hinder you from doing your work effectively?"*

Having covered the interviewee's concept of self, role, and interpersonal relationships, the stage is set for inquiring into how this person thinks about the larger organization. The focus is on the organization as a vehicle for accomplishing work-related objectives, that is, as a means to particular ends. This is likely to make sense implicitly to the interviewee, because organizations are conceived in our culture as social instruments, as vehicles for achieving objectives collectively that cannot be achieved individually. Talking about them explicitly in this way reinforces this notion and sets the stage for problem solving around ways of making the organization even more effective as a social instrument.

Note, moreover, that the concept of work can refer to many things. In its broadest sense, work is any activity in which one exerts strength of faculties to do or perform something. Thus, it can refer to activities designed to maintain and enhance one's self-concept, or to enact a particular role, or to maintain and enhance particular relationships, or to accomplish any other objectives, including the maintenance and enhancement of the organization itself. Consequently, the conversation can move in many directions, depending upon how a particular respondent interprets the concept of work and on how the interviewer chooses follow-up questions.

Many interviewees tend to respond initially by using their formal roles as reference points, by pointing to negative features of the organization rather than positive ones, and by identifying what the organization does well or poorly rather than how it works—"Project leaders like me are not given the authority necessary for fulfilling their responsibilities"; "The outpatient scheduling system is creating havoc for me"; or "Even though I am a senior professional in this organization, I end up having to do an endless amount of paperwork."

The challenge for the interviewer is to help the client think about *how* the organization has evolved so as to create these conditions, to help this person appreciate the positive aspects of the organization as well as the negative, and to broaden the issues covered to include both highly personal (ego-related) objectives and more collectively shared objectives.

For instance, a logical follow-up to the complaint listed above on lack of authority for project leaders might be, "What stands in the way of your being given more authority?" If the respondent points to the idiosyncrasies of a particular leader you might ask further, "How do you think he or she justifies this position to the rest of the leadership?" The tenet being used here, of course, is to focus whenever possible on *what* is the problem rather than on *who* is the problem. This encourages the client to think in systemic terms, which in turn facilitates inquiry into how the organization has created particular conditions.

Systemic analysis almost invariably leads to the identification of important tradeoffs in organization design, and thus recognition of the positive as well as the negative features of the respondent's organization in its current state. For instance, an appointment secretary in an outpatient clinic may feel frustrated by the way physicians are allowed to juggle their schedules, but the positive side may be maximum use of the physician's time, and patients who feel their needs are being responded to, and thus a productive work environment for the appointment secretary. This is not to say that something cannot or should not be done about the problem. Indeed, finding a solution to it would probably fit well into a project's objectives. The point to be made is that any action program needs to take these tradeoffs into account.

Finally, this kind of analysis helps the interviewee to come to grips with differences between his or her own personal needs, the rational demands of his or her role, and the necessary costs of pursuing larger values. For example, a senior professional in a community service organization may feel frustrated over the amount of paperwork he or she has to do, but through such dialogue it might become clear that this person's colleagues share the same frustration, and that to create a cadre of assistants for the convenience of people at this level might rob the organization of its image as a tightly run operation where everyone puts in extra effort in the service of community goals.

Probing into how an interviewee explains the dynamics of the organization and its impact on his or her own work can be especially exciting for several reasons. First, this is where one begins to collect a list of issues that can become the public focus of subsequent phases in the project. Others can be derived from the preceding questions, but the latter tend to be more personal and require the additional step of first being recognized as issues shared by many individuals before collective action is taken on them. By contrast, the issues gathered under this question are about the organization per se and thus are open to public dialogue immediately. In fact, one is likely to locate most of the issues that the members of the system have been discussing openly with each other for the past several years.

Second, one begins to get an idea of the general level, quality, and value orientation of the conceptualizing that the members of the system are used to engaging in with respect to their organization. Responses vary from thoughtful and thorough to cursory and superficial, from sophisticated to naive, and from militaristic to humanistic in their underlying assumptions. As one interviews across the top of a particular client group and down its ranks, it is often fascinating to discover variations along each of these dimensions. Such data, moreover, are critical for designing effective feedback formats and problem-solving sessions in subsequent phases of the project. Third, this question provides both the consultant and the client with important opportunities to influence each other's thinking, and thereby to begin to change both the organization and important aspects of the project. As the interviewee tells me his or her theory of what is going on, I chime in with my own ideas and the two of us often develop new perspectives. Moreover, both of our thinking can continue to evolve after the interview is over.

I do not share my own interpretations until after I have learned what any interviewee has to say on a particular subject, so my data are not tainted directly. But I am not beyond sharing a theory about a particular organizational issue, which I have developed with one interviewee, with another in a subsequent interview (although I make a point of not sharing the first contributor's identity). And it has frequently happened that I will be told new variations on a theme from the colleague of someone I had interviewed a few days before.

Pure researchers might blanch at this particular tactic, since over the course of an interviewing activity, the thinking of the client population might have changed considerably from what it was before the consultants entered. But I consider this quite legitimate in Organization Development activities, because the ultimate objective is a shared, collaborative analysis of the client system and not an unbiased picture of a particular group's viewpoint, which might be more useful for research purposes. Ideally, the interviewing activity in and of itself stimulates people into thinking about their organization in new ways and even entices them into new problem-solving activities quite apart from what the consultants are doing. And ideally, for the consultants, this same activity helps them discover new ways of thinking about the organization and a language for doing so that will maximize the chances of devising meaningful change activities that are both consistent with their values and exciting for the client system.

5.   *"What trends do you see in the way the organization has been evolving over the past few years?"*

This question asks the interviewee to consider his or her experience on the broadest level to be addressed in the interview. For to talk about the way one's organization is evolving requires at least some attempt at identifying with the organization as a whole, even if it is only for the purpose of contrasting it with one's own experience or with that of some other group either inside or outside the organization. The question also has the effect of encouraging the interviewee to think about the organization's external environment and the interaction between the two.

Respondents typically start out by describing conditions that, in their opinion, have either gotten better or worse: "This place used to be like a family. Everybody knew everybody else on a first-name basis and we all knew what was going on. Now we are so big that the left hand doesn't know what the right one is doing." "Until last year, we had been operating under really tight budget constraints. Now things have loosened up a little and life around here is more exciting."

As with the question immediately preceding this, one can get a sense of the interviewee's organizational models by asking for an explanation of why these conditions have developed. This, in turn, creates an opportunity for joint theorizing and the development of an even richer model of the organization's dynamics. Once again, one can see the distribution of people's preoccupation with and sophistication regarding these matters as one interviews various segments of the system, and this too is helpful for planning later parts of the project.

With few exceptions, the higher the rank of the person interviewed, the more that he or she has to say on this subject. The question is excellent for identifying who is and who is not actually included in discussions of broader policy issues. For while the members of particular subgroups tend to have unique party lines that are easy to spot regarding how the organization treats them, only those actively involved in policy making tend to share the same language and focus on the same issues when discussing the direction of the organization as a whole. By the same token, it is often possible to spot some interesting and often valuable alternative perspectives from people who are on the periphery of the main policy-making group. Melding their perspectives into subsequent feedback sessions often creates some very stimulating dialogue, and occasionally provides a way for some of these people to gain or regain recognition as potentially valuable contributors to the system.

> 6. *"Suppose you had three magic wishes about how to change the organization in any way you wanted. What would they be?"*

Now that you have inquired into a wide range of the interviewee's experience (job, career, relationships, the organization as hindrance or help, the organization as a dynamic entity by itself), the time is ripe for addressing action issues explicitly. The preceding dialogue is likely to have generated a whole list of possible change activities. This new question allows the respondent to identify still others, and then to begin to reveal his or her priorities.

This is an important turning point in the interview. My focus as the consultant is on identifying where the interviewee's energy for change is. It is as if we have just collaborated in laying out a grand banquet, and now I am waiting to see where my client will dive in. Coming where it does in the interview, the question would logically elicit suggestions about organization-wide policy. For people near the top of the system, this might easily be intertwined with all of the other issues covered thus far. Those further down in the system have a clearer option of focusing on the whole organization or on particular parts that are more relevant to their immediate experience, including their roles, relationships, and careers. In either case, it is useful to explore with the interviewee how each of this person's "wishes" might affect all of the levels discussed thus far.

My personal objective here is to help the interviewee identify ideal changes that might advance the interests of both the individual and the organization, and, simultaneously, to clarify the ways in which particular desired changes might benefit one of these entities at the expense of the other. Clarifying the latter is important in my view, since such one-sided outcomes would be out of place in the context of the project's integrative ethos. Further dialogue can often lead to ways of framing the issues involved so that both the individual and the organization benefit.

Pursuing such integration is often hard work but well worth the effort. For it forces the interviewee to confront the fact that he or she has chosen to act as part of a larger system. To act congruently as an organization member, one has to take the larger system's interests into account. By the same token, to commit oneself to the welfare of the organization when this stands clearly in the way of one's personal needs, raises the question of whether one should remain a member of this larger system. Ultimately, a particular individual's choice to leave the organization or some segment of it, and to seek membership in another that is more congruent with one's needs, may be just as valuable an outcome to the project as the discovery of new ways in which the needs of both the individual and the organization can be met.

Beyond this particular issue, an important payoff to this question is the identification, through comparison across interviews, of the major themes around which there is energy for change. Typically, there is a great deal of convergence among the concerns of particular groups, and even of the organization as a whole. For example, I have found that desires to do something about conditions such as poor superior/subordinate relationships, poor lateral relationships, poor career counseling or advancement opportunities, ineffective decision making, and feelings of inertia or stuckness, surface near the top of the hierarchy and cascade down through the membership. It is as if any system has only so much energy at a given point in time to invest in change efforts and, regardless of the diversity of individual perspectives, collective experience creates a focus of its own. It is up to the consultant to bring this into system-wide awareness, for while shared concerns may exist, this may not be at all apparent to the members themselves.

> 7. *"What do you personally want to do more of or start doing, continue to do at about the same rate, or do less of or stop doing completely?"*

This three-part question represents the other side of the coin to the preceding one. While the former emphasizes collective change, this one puts the emphasis explicitly on personal change. Once again, the ultimate objective is the same, that is, to integrate individual and organizational concerns. But here, if one has not done so already, one can explore where the respondent wants to move now with his or her personal life.

Every organizational role can be enacted in a myriad of ways, each of which might benefit the organization as well as the individual. As the interview comes to a close, it is useful to ponder the unique interests of the respondent in this regard. The data one receives might not be immediately relevant to prospective change activities, but it is useful to record and keep in the back of one's mind. Action alternatives often arise later on that fit a particular individual's emerging interests or that might facilitate the latter if formulated in a particular way. This is where the consultant's knowledge of each participant's personal objectives can come in handy.

Sharing such data, moreover, helps to strengthen the client/consultant relationship. At subsequent meetings, the client knows that the consultant knows what his or her personal objectives are. Even the meagerest attempt by the consultant at facilitating their pursuit in the context of more broadly shared goals, can solidify a relationship and create a strong ally for the project as a whole.

> 8. *"What kinds of things would have to occur in order for you personally to consider this project a success?"*

This question helps to put the total interview into perspective. A good interview contains a great deal of expansive thinking, and it would be foolish to think that every ideal might be achieved. Asking the interviewee for his or her minimum criteria for success helps both parties put the previous conversation into perspective. It also helps one in creating a list of the most important issues to address when analyzing the data and creating a feedback process.

Tailoring the Interview to Suit Your Needs.   As mentioned earlier, these questions tend to cover the full range of an individual's organizational experience. However, all of them need not be covered in complete detail in a particular study. This depends on the study's primary focus as agreed to by you and your primary client. For instance, a project that focuses heavily on firm-wide issues of structure and policy might not require delving deeply into role expectations. Likewise, one that centers on a particular team might not need heavy emphasis on firm-wide issues.

I would suggest, however, that at least some attention be given to each of the topics in the schedule for two reasons. First, it helps to build the relationship. And, second, it provides for an additional scanning of relevant issues that one's primary client might not be aware of.

Perhaps the most important quality of the list itself is the sequence in which the questions are asked. In any study, some questions can be truncated and others can be expanded to meet particular inquiry objectives. But this does not prevent one from moving from the individual's immediate role and career, outward to larger organizational issues, and then back to more personal issues around ideas for action. I have found that most respondents are quite comfortable with this progression, and that there is a minimum of backtracking necessary in order for the interviewer to understand the context of each response.

Questionnaires

Data gathering through *questionnaires* is less costly than interviews. A single questionnaire can be administered to hundreds or even thousands of individuals at a small fraction of the cost of interviewing a similar number. Questionnaires that use structured response categories—for example, rate the level of your satisfaction from 1–low to 5–high—are also amenable to summary statistical analysis. The larger the group being studied, the more useful such analysis is. Most large-scale OD projects consequently use questionnaires for major data gathering efforts.

Many organizations also use questionnaires to gather data on other issues—for example, general climate surveys and preference testing with respect to current or proposed policies. Consequently, using questionnaires has both the advantages and disadvantages of doing something that fits easily into an organization's culture. On the positive side, employees are more likely to be familiar with their administration and, if this has been handled well in the past, less anxious about this aspect of their involvement in an OD project.

On the negative side, employees, especially in large organizations, are likely to have had the experience of filling out questionnaires and being disappointed for one or more of the following reasons:

1.   lack of feedback — not being told what the results are, or not having a chance to discuss the results with important people;

2.   lack of follow-up — regardless of the quality of feedback, nothing happens of significance with respect to the issues covered;

3.   poor questionnaire design — the specific questions asked or the response categories provided for answering particular questions do not allow the respondent to convey what he or she thinks is important on the subject being covered; and

4.   insensitive administration — being herded into a room to fill out a questionnaire without being given a thorough explanation of its intent or how the results will be used.

All of these pitfalls can be avoided through sensitive administration and design. For example, when used in the context of an OD project, questionnaire design is usually done by an action group made up not only of the consultant and primary clients but also individuals from the groups whose opinions are to be tapped. This helps to ensure that the questions will be experienced as relevant by the respondents, as does pretesting a new questionnaire on a small sample of the subject population. Likewise, insensitive administration can be avoided through careful introduction of the questionnaire in the context of the larger project. Guards against failure to feed back the results and lack of follow-up can be built into initial contracting sessions and publicized widely.

Questionnaires can also be used to good effect in conjunction with an interviewing program. For example, if a primary client wants summary data on particular issues that are easily codified — say, job satisfaction or level of agreement with particular policies — a short questionnaire can be handed out and explained at the end of an interview.

Yet another strategy is to build a questionnaire from interview data. For example, a client might be interested in tapping the concerns of several hundred people but is not sure about what these concerns are and therefore what specific and easily codifiable questions to ask. Some strong hunches can be developed by interviewing a representative sample of the group and using these data to construct the questionnaire.[1]

Observation

Few OD projects rely primarily on *observing* the members of an organization at work as a primary data gathering method. Nonetheless, this technique is invaluable as a source of additional data. Observing one's clients' nonverbal behavior while conversing with them enhances understanding both of what they are saying and what they are hearing. A great deal can also be learned about a client from the way this person dresses, the location and furnishings of his or her work space, and the conversations with other organization members that he or she might have while in the consultant's

---

[1] For a more complete treatment of questionnaires in OD projects, see David A. Nadler, *Feedback and Organization Development: Using Data-Based Methods* (Reading, Mass.: Addison-Wesley Publishing Company, 1977).

presence. General observation of the physical setting and activity of the client system as a whole, likewise, is an important part of scouting and entry.

Observation can also be used systematically to enhance one's understanding of interview and questionnaire data. For instance, the interviews I did while working with departments in a large health care center, revealed that the receptionists' desk was a critical source of tension. Moreover, I got different versions of what was going on from nurses, physicians, patients, attendants, and the receptionists themselves. Spending several days in a waiting room chair next to a receptionist's desk and taking notes on what I saw and heard, proved to be essential in making sense out of these reports.

Observation can also be combined occasionally with limited forms of participation. In the same health care study, my colleagues and I wanted to know how a patient experienced his or her interaction with a particular department. The easiest way to find out was for one of us to make an appointment to see one of this department's physicians. After gaining all of the physicians' agreement, we picked an especially busy day and let a new member of our team, whom the staff had yet to meet, be introduced to the department in this way.

Finally, observation can be combined directly with interventions. This happens in process consultation, where the consultant comments on a group's activities as they unfold and helps its members discover more effective ways of working together. We will have more to say on this strategy in Chapter Eleven.

Analysis of Organizational Records

Written organizational data are useful both for understanding a client system's current state and the impact, if any, of one's interventions. For example, if a client is particularly concerned with turnover or absenteeism, recorded data on these parameters can be used to assess the severity of the situation at the beginning of a project and any progress made toward resolving it.

The minutes of meetings, policy directives, performance reports, written job evaluations, statements of job objectives in an MBO system, and biographical data on project participants are just some of the many documents that can prove equally important in understanding the current state of a system and how it is evolving.

When working, for instance, with a task force to resolve issues surfaced in a collaborative *analysis*, I find it especially useful to obtain copies of the minutes of each meeting. Progress or the lack of it is clearly evident when decisions are recorded on paper. The group's written record, moreover, is an excellent vehicle for sharing its progress with both the group itself and the rest of the organization.

Collecting organizational documents during interviews can also be useful. Suppose a client complains about the way he or she has to write job descriptions, job objectives, or progress reports. Asking for a written example that both of you can look at as the client elaborates on this issue can improve your understanding of this person's concerns and provide you with an additional piece of data to reflect on when writing up your conversation.

Too great a preoccupation with documentation, of course, can have undesirable effects, as anyone familiar with accounting procedures in a large organization can tell. My own experience, however, is that most OD consultants underutilize the typically vast amount of written material their clients produce day-to-day, rather than the reverse.

CONCLUSION

The formal data gathering stage of an OD project involves both the collection of data from the system as a whole for conceptual analysis and the broadening of the consultant's relationships with members of the organization beyond the initial entry and contracting groups. Four methodologies are typically employed: interviews, questionnaires, observation, and analysis of organizational documents.

The one-on-one interview is the preferred method because of the opportunities it provides for relationship building as well as clear communication. Interviews are less costly but provide for less client/consultant contact. Nonetheless, they are almost a necessity when dealing with very large systems. Observation and analysis of organizational records are secondary methods that can be used to enhance interviews and questionnaires.

While we have focused most heavily on the interview in this chapter, it is important to stress that all four strategies are useful. An ideal data gathering strategy is one that uses each to its best advantage. Other than questionnaires, moreover, each methodology can be used throughout an OD project. Scouting, entry, and contracting involve interviewing and observation at a minimum, and are greatly enhanced with organizational records. As we will see in the following chapters, all three are equally important in feeding back data and developing action programs.

CHAPTER TEN

FEEDING BACK DATA
AND DEVELOPING
A PROJECT AGENDA

In Chapter Six we discussed a four-phase approach to analyzing an organization. The chapters that followed dealt with the mechanics of relationship building and data gathering necessary for doing such an analysis. In this chapter I want to take up where we left off analytically at the end of Chapter Six and present concepts and procedures for sharing one's analysis with clients. The last part of the chapter will deal with managing the transition from the analysis process to planning action.

Let us assume that you have already gathered your data and analyzed it according to the four-phase process outlined in Chapter Six. You now have some appreciation for: (1) why the organization (or the segment of it you are studying) is as successful as it is; (2) the problems it is now facing; (3) the direction it seems to be heading in; and (4) the way its various members relate to each other in the context of their day-to-day activities. Having achieved all this, it is important to remember that this analysis is yours alone. It is not a collaborative analysis. Your clients provided the data, but you did the analyzing.

This is not to say that such work is unfruitful. On the contrary, it provides you with a kind of membership in the client system, in the sense that you now carry with you a data-based perspective on the organization. Thus you can talk its language, identify the cast of characters and their relationships, and present your own views on issues you know are of concern to many members.

Your task now is to facilitate a series of activities in which you and your clients can develop a *shared* analysis of the organization and its culture. This analysis hopefully will be distinguished by the facts that: (1) it is based to a strong degree on data gathered in a novel way (compared to daily operations); (2) it involves inputs from more members of the organization than is typical of other internal analyses conducted by the organization; and (3) you with your relatively unique skills, values, concepts, and professional identity are a party to it.

Developing a shared analysis involves first and foremost a commitment to retread the path one has already taken alone. One has to begin again by sharing at least some of one's descriptive data so that clients can question their validity, correct them, add to them, and subtract from them. Also, shared analyses and action planning require a consensually validated data base. The chances of developing such a data base are enhanced when various members of the organization see the data in a particular sequence, with particular formats and degrees of detail, and with particular immediate objectives in mind. The following sections cover each of these points.

SEQUENCING THE SHARING OF THE DATA

Two criteria are important in determining the order in which data are fed back. The first is rank. Put simply, unless the contract stipulates otherwise, more powerful people get to see the data before less powerful people do, or at least they have the right to demand this. This is often quite useful from both the organization's and the consultant's viewpoint. It allows those at the top of the hierarchy to anticipate and prepare for their subordinates' responses to the data. It also allows superiors to act as a final check point for the consultant regarding the suitability of the format being used to present the data and regarding the use of words, phrases, ideas, and so on that have a particular meaning to organization members that the consultant may not have anticipated. Finally, feeding back data from the top down allows the consultant to enlist the aid of leaders at each level in conducting meetings with people below them in the hierarchy.

The second criterion is the general relevance of the data gathered to particular subsets of the membership. Often, this cannot be determined beforehand because discovering what is relevant to whom comes from the analysis itself. Thus, within the constraints of hierarchy, considerable freedom to arrange feedback meetings with different groups of people is essential. For instance, upon analyzing the data the consultant may find that there are some issues that are of general concern to the membership, regardless of rank or function, and at the same time, that particular functions or work units have other concerns that are clearly different from each other. It might make sense, therefore, to hold two sets of feedback meetings: one for general issues, where it does not matter who attends a particular meeting, and one for the concerns of particular groups, to be attended only by the members of those groups.

To the extent that one differentiates the feedback process by sharing data at different times with different people, it is also important to work out beforehand how the outputs of these meetings will be integrated with each other. For example, at South City we fed data down the hierarchy initially and then held an integrative meeting in which the leaders of various subgroups reported the responses of their subordinates back up to the rest of the leadership. In other projects I have found it useful to hold separate feedback meetings with different work units, where at least part of the data concerned their relationships with the other groups. Knowing this beforehand, I would preschedule a meeting of all the groups whose relationships were at issue as a follow-up to these initial meetings.

This kind of planning is not only necessary for the logical conduct of the overall project, but also useful in showing the participants of any one meeting how their responses will be dealt with by others in the organization. People who know that their inputs will be made use of in other meetings are more likely to be active participators than those who are prevented from seeing the plan of the total project.

CHOOSING A FORMAT FOR PRESENTING DATA	Three kinds of presentation formats represent a continuum from emphasis on descriptive data alone to the inclusion of the consultant's own diagnostic concepts and interpretations.

The Oral Presentation.   By far the simplest format to work with is an *oral presentation* that reviews at least the first two phases of the consultant's analysis, that is, the system's strengths and recurrent problems. Flipcharts or overhead transparencies are presented to the audience in terms of a series of themes and supporting quotations (see Figure 10-1).

FIGURE 10-1
Sample Flipcharts from an
Oral Feedback Presentation

AGENDA*

> I.   Introductions
> II.   The Project
> III. Things You Like
> IV.   Problems
> V.   Wishes
> VI.   Discussion

THINGS YOU LIKE*

Theme: A Stable Work Force

- "We have built up a strong camaraderie over the years."
- "We have very low turnover for this industry."
- "Many of the hourly work force have been here from the beginning."

Theme: Pride in Past Accomplishments *

- "We were the first division in the company. It was our success that let it expand."
- "This has been the flagship. We have always led the way in new methods and products."
- "This division has always been known as a class place to work."

*New page in the actual presentation.

FIGURE 10-1 *Continued*
---

*Theme: Ability to Work Under Pressure**

- "The greater the pressure, the harder we work together."
- "When something needs to be done, we stop bickering and get the work out."
- "This organization is at its best in crisis situations."

PROBLEMS*

Theme: Communication

- "I need to have more information on what's going on in other departments."
- "Not only are we not given information, we are blamed for not knowing."
- "Things go in one ear and out the other [no follow-through]."
- "You can't talk to your boss and you can't go around him [or her]."
- "This is a 'grapevine' company."

*Theme: Consistency in Management/Policy**

- "I have three bosses, and they each tell me to do different things."
- "Standard policies have too many exceptions."
- "Lots of changes were started but not followed through on."
- "One day you can do it for the customer and the next day you can't."
- "Departures from policies are identified but not corrected."

Theme: Lack of Mutual Caring and Respect

- "They treat us like children, as if we want to break the rules."
- "People don't care about my opinion."
- "When you've done something right, no one praises you."
- "When someone gives you something to do and then things go wrong, they say, 'It's your problem, not mine.'"
- "I was promised _____ when I came here, and nothing has happened yet."

*Theme: Lack of Professionalism in Management**

- "Managers don't need to be cruel."
- "Do as I say, not as I do."
- "There's no need to use rude, abusive, coarse language with employees."
- "Reprimanding employees in front of others is out of place."

*New page in the actual presentation.

FIGURE 10-1 *Continued*

Theme: Elitism / Favoritism / Politics*

- "Executive committee is more equal."
- "Promotions are based on relationships rather than performance."
- "All energy was directed toward the executive committee, and not down through the ranks."
- "We used to be a family and now we have cliques and many battles."

Theme: Training at All Levels*

- "The organization recognizes training but it's still in the 'lip service' stage."
- "They said they'd get me in a training program and nothing happened."
- "No one knows what they're doing; we keep working around in a circle."
- "People are promoted without being trained for the job."

Theme: Excessive Management Change

- "They come and they go and we're still here."
- "Where do we stand now, who are we going to get now—nothing is ever stable."
- "Changes can be demoralizing and frustrating if policies and philosophies change."
- "There's so much change, I don't know if *I'm* next."
- "Turnover in management has always got people talking."

WISHES*

Theme: Communication

- Increased information for departments, more cooperation, monthly speak-out meetings.

Theme: Training

- Orientation program with introduction into all areas, more training for front-line employees, need for consistent, ongoing training.

Theme: Benefits / Compensation*

- Bonus programs—management level.
- Incentive programs—hourly level.

*New page in the actual presentation.

FIGURE 10-1 *Continued*

- Higher/more fair salaries.
- Pay for sick days without a doctor's certificate.
- Educational benefits (company pays).

Theme: Employee Relations *

- Find out what employees are thinking on a regular basis.
- Improvement of human relations skills at management level to enhance employee relations.
- Recognition and appreciation for a job well done.
- Equal treatment for everyone—no special privileges.
- Keep the people we have—they're good.
- More trust in one another.

Theme: Management Practices *

- Want an understanding boss.
- Consistency in style of management.
- Stability in the management group.
- Management should know what they are doing.

Theme: Policy *

- Abolish demeaning rules.
- Let department heads run their departments.
- Seniority should count for something.
- Consistency in the enforcement of rules/policies.

*New page in the actual presentation.

Starting with the system's strengths builds bonds with the audience that are likely to be appreciated later when the system's problems are introduced. This also tends to get the meeting started on a positive note, provided the observations are experienced as accurate.

Once the subject of problems in general has been broached, it is also useful to start with minor ones and to separate major issues with minor issues in order to give people time to absorb them.

Regarding the quotations themselves, I try to make those written down, simple, to the point, and as accurate as my notes and the demands of disguise allow. These are the words people are staring at as I elaborate orally, and if they are not an accurate reflection of the sentiments of a good many of those present, the credibility of my work as a collator of the data can be questioned. In talking around the quotations, I try to refer to concrete examples that I think many members of the audience can empathize with.

Beyond addressing strengths and problems, this kind of presentation can also include short sections on members' action suggestions. This may or may not be appropriate, depending upon how much additional dialogue around the problems themselves is anticipated. Ending the presentation by talking about remedial actions tends to dampen intense problem elaborations and discussions within the audience. On the other hand, it does have an upbeat quality to it that can generate action planning when problems are clearly understood and collaboration around their resolution is the more pressing issue.

One of the most difficult factors to contend with in a largely oral presentation such as this is data overload. I have had the privilege of facilitating dozens of training teams through a role-play of this format, based on their analysis of a very small amount of data, and the vast majority have overwhelmed their clients with data. As a rule-of-thumb, few groups can successfully absorb more than about 40 minutes of dialogue; around 25 seems to be ideal.

This limits the utility of this format to two kinds of situations: large meetings where only the highlights of an analysis are presented, and small group meetings (usually involving several sessions) where a large body of data can be broken down into several presentations with time for discussion in between.

In any case, plenty of meeting time needs to be planned for discussion following the presentation, since dialogue is the medium through which the data are digested and, in the process, modified by both clients and consultants.

The Quotation Package.   The second format to be discussed is the one we used in our work at South City Chemical. Instead of presenting the data orally, the themes and quotations are written down and distributed to clients several days before the feedback session. This allows for greater depth of coverage and much greater scrutiny by clients.

The actual mechanics of making a *quotation package* are straightforward but time consuming. One assembles all of one's data that involve the client's own words—whether they cover interviews, observations of group meetings, or written documents. One then reads through them again, and again, and again, looking for recurrent themes regarding any aspect of the organization that can be related to the core issues being addressed and that fit somewhere into the four-phase analysis process.

Having identified the themes, the next step is to select a series of especially cogent quotations that reveal the variety of opinions held about each theme, and to arrange them on paper in a way that allows the reader to see their similarities and differences easily. Care needs to be taken here to avoid quotations that can easily be attributed to a particular individual or that target a particular individual for either praise or blame (see Figure 10–2).

When using this format, clients almost invariably spend some of their time

FIGURE 10-2
Sample Section from a
Quotation Package

Status Differences Among Major Job Groupings

Several individuals observed that discrepancies in status, monetary rewards, and ability to advance in the organization existed among the science ladder, the technical marketing ladder, and the managerial ladder.

On the whole, the managerial ladder was viewed as having the most prestige of the three; and that the marketing ladder allowed an individual to reach higher positions faster than the science ladder. The science ladder was viewed as being the least defined and least visible of the three, in addition to having the lowest status with the lowest monetary rewards.

Individuals expressed frustration at having to abandon the research or bench work they loved, to advance in the system or to gain a high salary level and more status. The reaction was expressed in terms of the company placing a lower value on the work of those who chose science careers.

*   *   *

"People who are viewed as technical specialists don't have the same status as managerial people."

"There is not as much value placed on technical work as managerial work—this is a common complaint. Although people say this is not really the case, certain behaviors reinforce this assumption. For example, if advisors are added to the management group they are managers, not technical people."

"The way it seems to me is that the company believes that the people who are outward facing are the bread and butter of the company and should be rewarded as such."

"The technical ladder is not as visible for advancement as the management ladder. People don't generally know the difference between Chemist I and II. The ladders are not really equal in money or status. But then I'm not sure that management needs such a high degree of technical help."

*   *   *

"I would like to see that I can go into higher positions in the company, yet stay on in the technical line. [Right now, to move into higher positions, you have to leave the technical ladder.]"

"People who just want to be research scientists have no way to improve their salaries."

"The managers need to remember that they can't do anything without the bench workers. Management is just another area of expertise and they shouldn't be paid more and have more status."

"We should be able to do the type of work we want to do and still be able to advance without becoming a manager."

"I wish we had more top-notch science people around; we are not fostering opportunity to develop them the way we are recruiting. People who are expert oriented stick

FIGURE 10-2 *Continued*

around on the bench for a short while, then get frustrated and change to the management ladder, or go into tech service or sales."

*   *   *

"There is a problem of there not being a technical career ladder. It's not so much a matter of money as it is of prestige. I would like to see a ladder system in which there are as many levels for technical people to pass through as there are for people in marketing and management."

"There is a discrepancy in the technical marketing ladder and the science ladder in terms of dollars. That is, senior researchers make less than market development specialists."

*   *   *

"There are two functional tracks, one in marketing, one in science. Depending on where you enter the division on what track, it determines how fast and the way and how far you will be able to rise in the division. This is job level as well as salary differential."

"The first step on the ladder in marketing is higher than the first step on the science ladder."

"There may be comparable positions on each side, science and marketing, but it may be easier to reach one position via one track as opposed to the other. On the science technical side, you may not be able to reach what you could reach via the marketing side at all."

both prior to and during the feedback session in trying to figure out who said what. Most of the time they are wrong, and I think there is an important reason for this. People pick the person whom they feel would be most likely to say such a thing, and indeed that person may have been the original author of the idea expressed. But the question was picked for inclusion in the document because it expressed an idea currently held by at least a few and often many people in the organization. In essence, it has become part of the organization's culture and we as the consultants are just as likely to have heard it from people who heard it second- or third-hand and found it to fit their own thinking, as we are from its originator. In fact, its source in this respect really does not matter.

When I am dealing with a fairly large group of people—for example, more than 30—I often find it useful to create several quotation documents with slightly different purposes—for example, a general one that addresses issues of concern to the entire system, plus additional documents that focus on the issues that are relatively unique to particular subgroups. The group-specific documents, which are usually considerably shorter than the general document, are especially helpful when the latter is more than about 20 pages in length. This is about the limit in terms of document size that I have found most people can prepare for adequately and use as the focal point of one- to two-hour meetings. Longer documents can be used as reference sources, but do not expect them to be thoroughly digested by more than a few especially interested clients.

With the data presented beforehand under this format, something else needs to be substituted for the consultants' presentation as the initial means of getting discussion going. I find it easiest, after introductions have been made and the meeting's purpose clarified, to ask each person to identify the two or three issues of greatest concern to him or her in the document. I summarize these comments on flipcharts as each person speaks. Then I invite the group to help me identify shared themes in these concerns, make a summary list, and invite suggestions as to which theme to begin with. By this time, the current social structure in terms of who talks most is sufficiently evident for me to first draw out the talkers and then elicit comments from the quieter participants.

A slight variation on this format is to enhance the basic quotation package with concepts for interpreting the data. One can do this either with short lecturettes at any time during the feedback meetings or with short written documents accompanying the quotation package. In any case, once presented, the consultant needs to show the group how to use the concepts and work with the group to discover their utility in analyzing the data. The consultant may have already done this individually, but if the concepts are to become part of the collaborative process, the clients have to learn to do this as well.

The Written Report.   The third format to consider is a *written report* in which the consultant not only summarizes the data gathered but also offers an analysis of them. This comes rather close to the traditional consulting report, which includes a set of action suggestions in addition to description and analysis. But it can be made a vehicle for collaborative analysis and action planning if the consultant includes enough descriptive data to allow clients to offer alternative analyses, and if the analysis itself is couched in tentative terms rather than dogmatically.

Such reports are most useful when the analysis is well focused initially. For instance, suppose a client is convinced that people's roles are not sufficiently defined for them to coordinate their efforts efficiently. The data collected support this position, and the consultant's primary task is to help the organization develop guidelines for defining roles in more useful terms. In a case such as this a well-documented description of several roles, accompanied by a clearly explicated analysis of the problems, can set the stage for clients and consultants to work together in developing new role definition procedures. The meeting itself can use any issue in the document as a starting point, although once again it is useful to start out with a discussion of the validity of the data, then the analysis, and finally, action planning.

Criteria for Choosing a Format.   Deciding which format to use in a given situation requires consideration of what one has learned from one's own analysis. Clients whose worlds are largely oral, where only the trivial and the unusually important are written down, tend to prefer oral presentations and, at best, short, well-focused documents. Those whose worlds are dominated by the written word—for example, researchers and staff personnel—often like a written document to ponder. Action-oriented people may not appreciate a great deal of description and analysis that is not tied to specific action suggestions, but, given the lack of action suggestions, they seem to prefer as much analysis accompanying descriptions of the data as possible. As in writing contracts, the closer one's format shows an appreciation for the way the organization would like to see itself operate, the easier it is to focus attention on the collaborative process itself.

On the other hand, one should not overlook the fact that a feedback format can represent an important intervention in and of itself. While choosing a format that fits an organization's culture can make initial dialogue easy, one might also consider using an alternative that does not, in order to encourage a different kind of thinking in the client group.

For instance, a group of highly action-oriented managers might prefer a concise report containing a minimum of descriptive data and focusing heavily on action suggestions. One's data might indicate, however, that one of the problems this group is suffering from is lack of systematic problem solving, where the description–analysis–action planning sequence is being short-circuited. Presenting data in terms of a quotation package, as opposed to a report, might irritate this group. Their natural tendency, if one's assessment were right, would be to avoid discussion of the validity of the data in the document and jump immediately to action planning. Having the document there, however, would provide important opportunities for challenging the group to check out its assumptions and for questioning particular assumptions based on one's own reading of the material. In this way, one can model a more rigorous problem-solving process and provide important reasons for pursuing it.

Meeting Objectives

Beyond developing a plan for sequencing feedback meetings and choosing a presentation format, one needs to establish a set of specific objectives for each meeting taken by itself. The purposes of a specific feedback meeting depend on the answers to several questions:

1. How much attention should be given to validating the data and venting feelings about them, versus analyzing their implications?
2. Should action suggestions be pursued, or is it better to end the meeting with the analysis in progress?
3. How much attention should be given to appreciating the organization for its successes versus exploring its problems?
4. To what extent should the meeting be used to convey the commitment and philosophy of the formal leader and/or the consultants and/or other participants?
5. To what extent should the meeting serve as a vehicle for opening up issues and creating energy for change versus bounding issues and channeling current energy in particular directions?

6.   To what extent should the consultant focus on *how* people are working with each other and try to gain new understandings about these dynamics versus focusing on the content of the material discussed?

There are no pat answers to any of these questions, and again they require consideration of what one has learned from one's own analysis of the data. At a minimum, it is important to agree with the organization leader of the meeting beforehand as to what at least some of these objectives will be, and to plan with this person on how to accomplish them. My own preference is to have this person actually run the meeting in a way we have planned together, so that I can attend to the process and suggest adjustments along the way as I learn more about what would be useful from the progress of the meeting itself.

UNDERSTANDING AND ANTICIPATING CLIENT RESPONSES

Feedback meetings are a kind of midway point in the OD process. They require a lot of preparation and a well-established relationship with the client system. They are also starting points for a whole new phase of activity. Consequently, they can be used both as tests of one's knowledge of the organization and as new data for predicting the course of future activities. Both of these functions are important and a careful exploration of them can provide additional insights into the mechanics we have just discussed.

Client Reactions and Group Orientations

We have already seen in Chapter One how clients' reactions to feedback activities can be related to particular values and their attendant group orientations. Specifically, in an interview/feedback project with a large health care organization (we called it the Northern Medical Center), my colleagues and I found that different subsets of the client group had different reactions to both the feedback process and the data presented. (See Figure 10-3). Some clients viewed the process with a lively interest and inquired readily into the validity and meaning of the data. Others mouthed platitudes toward the process and then spent a good part of the time grumbling about people whom they thought had said negative things about them. A third subset expressed outrage toward the process and then went on to deny the importance of the data in the first place. And a fourth subset expressed apathy about the process and were skeptical that the data revealed through it would be taken seriously by those who were in a position to act. Further analysis of the backgrounds of the people who made each kind of response, our subsequent experience with them, and with other individuals who responded in similar ways, led us to conclude that each of these response patterns can be related generically to a particular group orientation in our OD paradigm (see Figure 10-4).

People who share a clear affinity to the consensus orientation, which we as OD consultants try to model, will see the feedback process as consistent with how they prefer to work in general, and will find the results interesting and useful. The consultant is

FIGURE 10-3
Types of Reaction
to Feedback Data

OUTRAGE TOWARD THE PROCESS
DENIAL OF THE DATA

"I think this is dangerous."

"You should never have printed things like this."

"Why wasn't I told to my face?"

"We don't really have any problems."

"There are just a few complainers here."

INTEREST IN THE PROCESS
INQUIRY INTO THE DATA

"It's useful to have the quotes without authors, any of us could have said this."

"The comment about _____ was something I never thought of."

"I don't agree with the statement that _____."

"Can someone help me understand why someone would say _____?"

APATHY ABOUT THE PROCESS
SKEPTICISM ABOUT THE DATA

"I could have said more but I didn't think it was worth it."

"Everyone knows this already."

"Just watch, nothing will happen."

"Are they really going to act on this?"

PLATITUDES TOWARD THE PROCESS
ATTACKS ON IMAGINED QUOTERS

"Glad to have things out on the table."

"We needed this."

"What they need is a good stiff kick in _____."

"Most of this is _____'s own fault."

Source: Adapted from Eric H. Neilsen, "Reading Clients' Values from Their Reactions to an Interview/Feedback Process," in *The Academy of Mangement Proceedings 1978* (Academy of Management, 1978), p. 309.

seen as a potential collaborator with a fresh viewpoint that might enhance these people's own goals and those of the organization.

The interview/feedback process itself is consistent with the values of candidness and self-responsibility because the data collection and dispersal procedures facilitate the sharing of personally meaningful data, the kind of data one would share naturally if one were always candid. It does so, moreover, in a way that disassociates particular people from the issues, thus enhancing the sense of safety needed to discuss such data openly and making it possible for people to respond to the data as autonomous actors, responsible for their own behavior, and not tied to particular leaders or groups whose ideas demand support or attack.

However, the interview/feedback process is also at least partially amenable to the concerns of individuals holding other combinations of OD values and their opposites. They simply view and use the process in different ways.

Thus, individuals who prefer a dependence orientation may view the process as desirable if their leaders want to engage in it. The consultants become surrogate leaders in the interview process, if it is sanctioned by the formal leaders. Thus, the propensity toward being candid is maximized. However, individuals who follow this

FIGURE 10-4
Group Orientations
and Responses
to the Feedback Processes

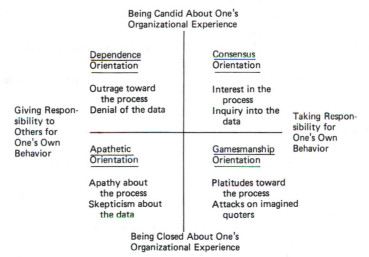

Source: Adapted from Eric H. Neilsen, "Reading Clients' Values . . .," p. 310.

orientation will also rely heavily on their leaders to interpret the results. Feedback data that reveal problems that they think their leaders should have been responding to, or that reveal leaders' dissatisfaction with their followers' performance, will produce anxiety. Such responses threaten the other assumption upon which this orientation is based, that is, that it is safe for one to give responsibility for one's behavior to others. This can lead either to pleas for help from the consultant (as an alternative leader) and/or an outright rejection of the activity and the consultant, as happened with one group temporarily in the Northern Medical Project.

Clients who prefer the gamesmanship orientation, by contrast, may welcome the process if they can conceive of ways in which it can serve their personal interests. Data, however, are offered strategically and feedback sessions revolve around hidden agendas. The consultant is viewed as just another gameplayer, intent on serving his or her own interests. The data generated by the process are used to further individual goals. The consultant can easily be trapped into responding to particular needs if he or she is not aware of what is happening.

Finally, followers of the apathetic orientation respond perfunctorily to the process if an authority figure has sanctioned it. The consultant is just someone else they have to comply with in order to survive. The consultant's initial attempts to create excitement and commitment to the process are viewed with a profound skepticism.

In line with this formulation, one can argue that clients' reactions to the interview/feedback process represent a useful way to identify important trends in underlying values. Clients who react either with outrage and denial or who invite the consultant to do all the work of interpreting the data for them can be hypothesized tentatively as unwilling to take responsibility for their own behavior. Subsequent interventions can be aimed at showing the merits of a more self-responsible posture. Clients whose reactions appear to be strategic and self-oriented can be hypothesized as devaluing candidness, and subsequent activities with them can be oriented toward enhancing more open communication. Clients who react apathetically can be viewed initially as devaluing both candidness and self-responsibility, and the consultant can choose follow-up activities that highlight both of these values. Finally, those who react most quickly with interest and a spirit of inquiry can be viewed as potential collaborators in designing and implementing follow-up activities in general. All of these hypotheses of course need to be corroborated with the rest of the data that one gathers. The point is that client reactions are themselves valuable data in the ongoing analysis process.

Problem Types as Determinants of Client Reactions

Recently, I have discovered a second way to explain the same patterns of client reactions. This explanation complements the initial one quite nicely. It is equally anecdotal in its data base, but once again I would encourage the reader to try it out as a heuristic guide.

While individuals who respond in a particular way frequently embrace the predicted value orientations in the rest of their work, this is by no means always the case. Clients who are basically collaborative and consensus oriented will occasionally become just as manipulative, skeptical, or outraged as individuals holding contrasting values, and vice versa. Part of the reason, I believe, lies in the nature of the specific problems apparent in the feedback data.

Two qualities of the data fed back are central to this second explanation. The first is whether or not the data point to problems that those being fed back to are already aware of. The second is whether or not they point to problems that the client has an immediate interest in trying to resolve. Figure 10–5 indicates four possible types of problems that can be derived from different combinations of these aspects of the feedback data and gives an example of each type.

The connection between this array of problems and people's reactions to the feedback process can be easily grasped by thinking about how one might respond to hearing about each type of problem in the presence of one's peers. If it is a problem you and your colleagues have been unaware of and would like to resolve, what could be more natural than showing a strong interest in the details of data and appreciating the process that surfaced the problem?

By contrast, suppose you and others had long been aware of a problem presented in the data and had been trying to resolve it for some time without success. Here it would be natural to expect a good deal of self-protection and scapegoating. Failure to resolve the problem would be a source of embarrassment, like having one's dirty linen aired in a public forum. At the same time, it would be hard to fault the interview/feedback process openly since it did indeed surface an important problem.

Next, suppose that the problem revealed was one you and your colleagues already knew about and had chosen not to attempt to resolve. Skepticism would be the

FIGURE 10-5
Types of Problems Surfaced

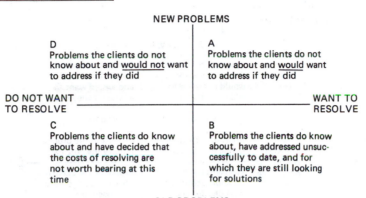

NEW PROBLEMS

D
Problems the clients do not
know about and <u>would not</u> want
to address if they did

A
Problems the clients do not
know about and <u>would</u> want
to address if they did

DO NOT WANT
TO RESOLVE

WANT TO
RESOLVE

C
Problems the clients do know
about and have decided that
the costs of resolving are
not worth bearing at this
time

B
Problems the clients do know
about, have addressed unsuc-
cessfully to date, and for
which they are still looking
for solutions

OLD PROBLEMS

Examples:

A.   Several valued people are thinking about leaving the organization in the near future. They are saying that their career paths are blocked, when, in fact, they are not.

B.   The production scheduler is performing poorly, the person in her position has been replaced four times in the past two years, but no one seems to do well in this job.

C.   There is high turnover among field sales personnel. While the problem is annoying, studies have shown that reducing turnover would require more training and home office visits. This solution looks more costly than the current cost of replacement.

D.   Turnover among newer people is extremely high. Current interviews indicate that this is because people were attracted to the firm due to management's portraying an image of rapid growth, implying opportunities for rapid advancement. The company continues to posture itself this way, although recent growth has been slow, and advancement nil. Management does not want to recognize this because such an acknowledgment would require major rethinking of the firm's prospects and potential loss of morale and stakeholder support.

natural response, almost by definition, since the utility of addressing the issue has already been identified as low. Apathy about the process would also seem natural if all it had to offer were problems of this variety.

Finally, suppose you and your colleagues were made aware of a problem none of you wanted to address, such as the fact that you were still advertising yourselves as a growing enterprise, something that kept all of your spirits up, when the data clearly confirmed that this was no longer true. Denying the data and rejecting the process would be a natural, if not a particularly ideal, way to deal with this revelation. Figure 10-6 summarizes the hypothesized relationships.

Explaining the reaction patterns of clients to the interview/feedback process in terms of their underlying values orients the consultant toward the potential long-term

FIGURE 10-6

Types of Problems Surfaced
and Responses
to the Feedback Process

NEW PROBLEMS

	Problems the clients do not know about and would not want to address if they did	Problems the clients do not know about and would want to address if they did	
	lead to	lead to	
DO NOT WANT TO RESOLVE	Anger at the process Denial of the data	Interest in the process Inquiry into the data	WANT TO RESOLVE
	Problems the clients do know about and have decided that the costs of resolving are not worth bearing at this time	Problems the clients do know about, have addressed unsuccessfully to date, and for which they are still looking for solutions	
	lead to	lead to	
	Apathy about the process Skepticism about the data	Platitudes toward the process Scapegoating and self-protection	

OLD PROBLEMS

problems and opportunities in the relationship with the client group. But often, however, this is not of much use as an immediate guide to action in the feedback meeting. Explaining the same reaction patterns in terms of the specific qualities of the data fed back may cause one to ignore their long-term implications for the relationship, but this approach has the advantage of directing the consultant to some potentially useful action steps in the short term.

First, to the extent that the clients' reactions are products of the kinds of problems the data reveal, one can use them as guidelines for framing the meeting itself or the relevant part of it as an opportunity for helping the client in specific ways (see Figure 10-7).

A.   Discovery of new problems that people want to act on is likely to set the normal problem-solving process of the client group into operation. This gives the consultant an opportunity to observe what this process is and to suggest improvements in the process that are consistent with OD values.

B.   Having to discuss problems that have already been addressed and not resolved can be frustrating, but it also presents a chance to try new approaches. Focusing on "*what* is the problem," not "*who* is the problem," offering systemic models through which to do this, and providing expertise on how other groups have resolved similar problems are ways in which the consultant can be helpful.

C.   When certain problems have existed for quite awhile and people have given up attempting to resolve them, either because they do not think they have the resources to

FIGURE 10-7
Types of Problems Surfaced
and the Opportunities
They Represent

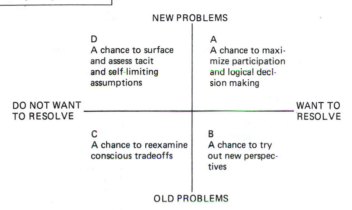

do so or because they choose to use these resources elsewhere, surfacing them again can be demoralizing. The consultant can be helpful by presenting the activity as a chance to reexamine and affirm one's priorities and resources. Perhaps conditions have changed or people's energy has changed. Often the suggestion of a "breakthrough" project is useful, that is, an all-out effort to resolve a particular problem and build new confidence and knowhow in the process.

D.   Finally, broaching problems that people do not really want to acknowledge, much less deal with, can be very touchy. But doing so presents a chance to face the devil head on. The consultant can show that taboo topics can be treated gracefully, can highlight the costs of avoiding such issues, and can give the group courage and emotional support for dealing with them.

Second, discussing each type of problem may be facilitated by my focusing on a different one of the interpersonal skills presented in Chapter Eight (see Figure 10-8).

A.   Structuring one's communication so that it moves from description to analysis to action planning, models the logical problem-solving process for clients and helps to combat poor decision-making procedures. Participation can be enhanced as well through conscious attention to silent members and the maintenance of more equal air time.

B.   Making process observations on what is happening interpersonally in the session and encouraging others to do so helps to get people to come to grips with their self-protectiveness. Trying out new approaches is not just a cognitive issue. Typically, it means behaving differently toward each other as well.

C.   Meta-modeling challenges people to clarify their assumptions behind long-held positions: "What, specifically, leads you to conclude that reducing turnover through more training would not be cost effective?" Changes in important underlying conditions that support such assumptions might have gone unnoticed.

FIGURE 10-8
Types of Problems Surfaced
and Interpersonal Skills
That Facilitate Their Discussion

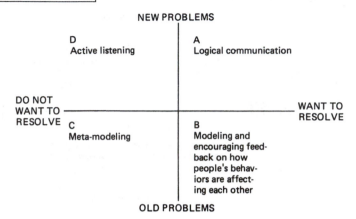

D.   Active listening helps people get in touch with how their need to protect their self-concepts is preventing them from dealing with important problems. For example, acknowledging that one's organization is no longer growing, especially if one played an important role in its past growth, can be bruising to one's ego but necessary for long-term survival. Being listened to empathically and being helped to articulate the feelings involved is a first step to addressing such problems realistically.

Third and finally, different types of problems invite different kinds of prework with the senior clients who will chair the feedback meeting (see Figure 10–9). This requires that one predict how one's clients will respond before the meeting takes place. Careful analysis of the data using the diagnostic scheme in Chapter Six sets the stage for doing this.

A.   Under a participative format, one can start by giving each person a chance to offer comments on the feedback data, summarize on flipcharts, prioritize, and allocate set blocks of time to discuss specific items. The leader conducts the discussion. The consultant records and guides interaction.

B.   When self-protectiveness is likely, it is important for the leader to stifle destructive interactors, after they have had their say, and are just working their issues. The leader should focus on what is the problem, not who is the problem, and say so at the beginning of the meeting. It is also helpful if the leader owns up to his or her own defensiveness and commits to a new approach. The leader can also sanction group critiques and invite and accept personal feedback.

C.   When apathy is predicted, it is useful for the leader to start with news of what is being done or planned with respect to certain problems, to state his or her commitment to explore particular areas and desire for others' help, and to clarify areas where action will still not be taken.

FIGURE 10-9
Types of Problems Surfaced
and Appropriate Prework
Activities with the Group Leader

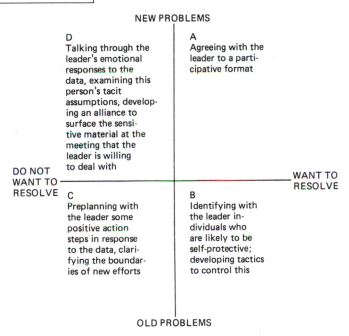

NEW PROBLEMS

D
Talking through the leader's emotional responses to the data, examining this person's tacit assumptions, developing an alliance to surface the sensitive material at the meeting that the leader is willing to deal with

A
Agreeing with the leader to a participative format

DO NOT WANT TO RESOLVE

WANT TO RESOLVE

C
Preplanning with the leader some positive action steps in response to the data, clarifying the boundaries of new efforts

B
Identifying with the leader individuals who are likely to be self-protective; developing tactics to control this

OLD PROBLEMS

D. Finally, it is especially helpful for the leader to take an active role in exploring heretofore taboo issues, to express confidence in the group's capacity to cope with them, and to share his or her own experience in dealing with these issues.

Following any of these strategies may not lead immediately to the desired results, if what is causing the clients to react in a particular way are their basic values around candidness and self-responsibility rather than their immediate responses to the problems surfaced. But, as we have suggested elsewhere, many people hold different positions on these values, depending upon their interpretation of the situation at hand. All of these strategies represent ways of both legitimizing and showing the utility of candidness and self-responsibility in the feedback process. Thus, they maximize the chances of such clients interpreting the situation in the desired way.

MAKING THE TRANSITION FROM FEEDBACK AND ANALYSIS TO ACTION PLANNING

Once data have been formally fed back to the client system and the themes in them collaboratively examined, validated, modified, elaborated, and analyzed, the stage is set for developing action plans. When the client system is small (8 to 10 people), and the data not too complex, the beginnings of action planning can follow naturally from analyzing the data presented for the first time. One simply identifies the key issues of most concern to those present and uses them as an agenda for subsequent problem-solving sessions.

More often, however, the data are fed back in several sessions, and further meetings are necessary to synthesize the outputs of these sessions into a workable agenda. In situations such as these, it is useful to get a consensus of each group's conclusions and preferences regarding future problem solving, so that its leader has something to take back to the integrating sessions with other leaders.

Separate integrating sessions are also useful when a lot of data have been fed back and clients have needed time just to talk and think about them both during and after the feedback meetings. For example, in situations where the data have already been discussed at least once, I find it useful to use the following procedure to help people draw their findings together and build an agenda for action planning.

The procedure is a modified version of Delbeque, Van de Ven, and Gustafson's nominal group technique.[1] Start by asking those present (ideally, no more than 8 to 12 people) to think about the feedback data and their discussions regarding them to date, and to draw up two lists of three to five items each. The first list should indicate what they have now come to see as the most salient aspects of the current state of their organization, or those parts or aspects of it being analyzed. For instance, in working with a community fund raising agency, I asked a group of its executives to list the three to five most important features of: (1) its lay leadership, (2) the executive staff as a group, and (3) the administration supporting the executive staff. The second list should then indicate what each person sees as the three to five qualities that the systems just referred to should have *ideally*.

Once the participants have written these lists by themselves, ask them to contribute to a shared picture in the following manner. Starting with any person and moving in sequence around the room, each person offers one item per turn on his or her list that the consultant writes verbatim on a flipchart. Contributions and the discussion surrounding them should follow these ground rules:

1. One may not repeat an idea already offered. Usually after about two rounds of contributions, people start to run out of items not already on the charts. They may think up additional items if they like or simply say "pass."

2. People may ask for clarification about an item being offered, but they may not evaluate its merits or disagree with it. They may, if they so desire, offer an item representing an opposing position when it comes to their turn. An important feature of this process is that it prevents invidious comparison and argumentation before all the data are shared.

3. The procedure continues until the participants have no new items to add.

Do this first with the items dealing with the current state and then proceed directly to the ideal state lists. Once all the items are up on flipcharts, the next step is to ask people to focus their attention on the ideal items and look for overlaps in them so

[1]Andre L. Delbecq, Andrew H. Van de Ven, and David H. Gustafson, *Group Techniques for Program Planning: A Guide to Nominal Group and Delphi Processes* (Glenview, Ill.: Scott, Foresman and Co., 1975).

that a mutually exclusive list of items can be created. Then ask people to compare the ideal state items with those describing the current state and check off those ideals the group thinks have already been achieved.

The remainder of the ideal list now needs to be prioritized in terms of how important people think the achievement of each ideal state is over the next few years. A simple method for doing this is to allow each person to distribute five votes among the items in any way he or she wants. (I usually hand out several magic markers and let people mark the votes on the sheets themselves.) The votes are then counted and the items relisted in the order of their popularity.

The final step is to make an initial categorization of the items in terms of their amenability to being resolved in the near future by the group's efforts. This tends to require some clear inputs by the formal leaders present. I encourage them, with as much discussion as they want from the group, to place each item in one of three categories.

> 1.   Ideal states that the larger organization will not help the group pursue or that simply cannot be achieved under present circumstances.
> 2.   Ideal states that might be achieved were cooperation obtained from other (usually powerful) members of the organization or its constituencies who are not present.
> 3.   Ideal states that members have a feasible chance of achieving through collaboration with each other.

Items in the first category are then acknowledged and set aside. The most appropriate people for following up on items in the second category are identified and assigned the task of approaching those individuals whose help is needed. The items in the third category become the group's problem-solving agenda for future meetings.

The whole procedure can take anywhere from two to eight hours. With very few exceptions, I have found it an excellent activity for gaining the commitment of any group to follow up its feedback experiences. It has a "building" quality to it. The participants are often surprised to see how much they have accomplished and, in particular, how many things they can agree on.

EVALUATION AND NEXT STEPS

The total process, from the initial scouting sessions to this point, has led to the creation of a list of items that both client and consultant think are the most important aspects of the organization to experiment with. They are also items around which the client system as a whole has the most energy to act and that are within the client's power to change. If the process has been managed adequately, the consultant is in general agreement with the client's thinking and through their interactions the parties have established comfortable, collaborative working relationships that will allow a considerable amount of mutual influence to occur in subsequent activities.

Completing the collaborative analysis and developing an action agenda is a major watershed in any OD project. A discrete piece of work has been accomplished that in itself represents the essence of the OD process. It is useful at this point to ask oneself and discuss with the client whether the continuation of the relationship would be worthwhile. If the answer is yes, this is also a good time to lay the groundwork for evaluating future interventions. The analysis just completed often provides excellent base line data regarding the current state of the organization around any issue. Before major interventions are made, more data can be gathered to confirm the current state so that the success of each subsequent intervention can be evaluated more concretely.

For example, if the analysis has indicated that the specific procedures of a management-by-objectives system need to be improved, it might be useful to start the improvement activities with a list of the system's current faults and quantitative indicators to back them up—for example, frequency of incorrectly completed forms, missing progress reports, and Likert scale measures of current satisfaction with the system. Then several months later, when the system has been changed, there is a clear reference point with which to assess the results of the change effort.

The same can be done with various qualities of the client/consultant relationship. Suppose client and consultant agree to continue to work together but one feels the other does not keep him or her sufficiently informed, while the other wants the first person to be more available. Both parties can agree to try to meet each other's needs in the future, and simultaneously to check each other's progress in doing this several months hence.

CONCLUSION

Completion of this phase of the project also tends to be a turning point in the nature of the consultant's contacts. By this time, the consultant has become acquainted with a great many people but has worked with few of them very closely. Conceptually, he or she has learned something about the total system but not a great deal about any particular feature of it. Technically, a relatively homogeneous set of procedures has been applied to everyone he or she has worked with. The creation of a specific action agenda invites developing stronger relationships with specific groups of people, gaining a detailed understanding of specific organizational features, and working in different ways (or on different agenda items) with different groups.

In particular, work on discrete problems rather than on the organization as a whole tends to involve three kinds of activities:

1. counseling particular individuals—for example, in order to accomplish a shift in leadership style or develop a new skill;

2. acting as a process consultant to ongoing groups as they deal with the items on their action agendas—for example, working with the physicians at Northern Medical as they tried to develop vertical groups, a new residency recruitment program, a new physical layout for their offices; and

3. facilitating the development of task forces to deal with specific action items—for example, the task forces at South City.

In the last two chapters we will offer some basic concepts and techniques for executing each of these activities. We conclude this chapter with a review of the critical steps in the feedback process:

1.   Analyze the system you are studying using the procedures outlined in Chapter Six.

2.   Based on your analysis, decide which people need to hear and see what kinds of data, in what sequence, and with what end results in mind.

3.   Decide on a format for each session and get the help from particular organization members (leaders, etc.) to make the meeting a success.

4.   In light of your analysis, think about how the participants in a particular meeting are likely to respond and prepare strategies for dealing with the responses you anticipate.

5.   As you participate in each feedback session, consider what new insights can be gained from the interaction itself. Did people react the way you thought they would? Are your strategies for managing their reactions working? Are there basic value differences evident that you will need to be sensitive to in the future?

6.   As the feedback meetings progress, consider what the best way will be to integrate the results. Is your initial plan still valid? How could it be modified to respond to any new learnings?

7.   Hold the necessary meetings for moving people's attention from understanding and analyzing the feedback data to developing an agenda for future change and experimentation.

8.   Assess your relationship with your clients, make contracts for follow-up activities, and build in procedures for evaluating their effects.

CHAPTER ELEVEN

BUILDING
CONSENSUS ORIENTED GROUPS

Collaborating with one's clients in an organizational analysis and feedback process may seem like an extremely lengthy prologue to making important changes. Such an effort is worthwhile, however, because so much more gets done than the analysis itself. Before discussing some of the basic interventions that logically follow this activity, we would do well to review certain things that are likely to have happened by this time. While they may not always make one's follow-up activities easy, they stack the odds in favor of success. Simply realizing this and understanding the conditions one has created sets the stage for thoughtful, parsimonious, and efficient action.

To begin with, by the time you have completed the analysis and feedback phases, you and your primary clients know each other quite well. You have either learned to work together comfortably by this time or the relationship, quite appropriately, will have ended with a minimum of harm done to the client system. Second, not only do you and your clients share a common analysis of the problems and opportunities facing the organization, but you are also aware of where the energy for change lies. Therefore, projects can be chosen that many people want to succeed.

Third, you as the consultant have developed a distinct identity within the client system. Not just your primary clients but many organization members have begun to learn the approach you are advocating; what other people, especially powerful people, think about it; what your interpersonal style is like; the general extent of your interpersonal skills, something about your conceptual skills, and your technical skills in handling project work. In short, you are now a known technical entity in the life of the client system. As such, your actions are likely to be quite understandable to others, and this in itself is a giant step toward collaboration around critical change projects. Likewise, you have come to know many of the organization's members in similar ways, and thus are in a position to know not only what you would like to do but how your clients are likely to respond.

Fourth, you are not only a known technical entity (a tool with particular strengths and weaknesses), but also a political entity in the life of the client system. If you have done your work carefully, you have developed a support system for your efforts as well as some idea of your potential as a source of influence. There are people in the system who know that you know what they want, and some of these people may be willing to support you in return for your support of them. Sad to say, you are also likely to have developed a few enemies or detractors as well, but such is the price of entry into any complex social system.

Fifth, the analysis itself has probably set numerous streams of activity in motion. People do not always wait for formal phases of an OD project to be completed before taking action on issues already within their province. And if only a modest number of these initiatives have begun to create favorable results, you have made some important friends. The converse is also likely to be true, and to the extent that you have experienced help and growth through others, you are likely to see yourself as having true friends within the client system as well.

Thus, through the analysis process, you have become a bona fide member, however temporary, of the organization, and as such are in an excellent position to act on your intuitions as well as on your formal plans. Your own and others' actions now make sense technically, politically, and socially. What you are able to accomplish now will still be determined in large part by your special skills, new learnings that you continue to accumulate, and the endless patterns of change that the client system is experiencing from many other directions. But you have also developed some momentum. The challenge now is to learn how to use it in a productive manner.

Look carefully at the momentum you have created. What are its primary features? To the extent that you have followed the guidelines in preceding chapters, its most salient quality is that it represents a living experiment in collaborative management. Your actions have embodied equality and holism in relating to others at an interpersonal level, candidness and self-responsibility in collective decision making, and a commitment to the welfare of the total organization plus an acknowledgment of all members as important resources in achieving this end. Hopefully, what you do next will be viewed at least initially in these terms, and you are likely to achieve your greatest success by continuing to advocate activities that are understandable in terms of this approach.

This chapter treats two kinds of basic interventions that can be used to continue your modeling of OD values in the context of the organization's tasks. Each intervention involves group activities that are natural steps in responding to the action agenda produced by a collaborative analysis. These are (1) developing task forces, and (2) facilitating group process. Like all other group activities, each can be pursued in ways that are consistent with different values. What I will attempt to do here is to provide guidelines for accomplishing them that are consistent with the consensus mode.

This does not mean that everything needs to be decided through consensus decision making, but that the dominant orientation of the participants is toward candidness and self-responsibility. Any way of making decisions or of performing any other group function is fair game so long as the participants take personal responsibility for their own behavior while engaging in it and are candid with each other about their experience. Building consensus oriented work groups means developing their activities in ways that keep these values in the forefront.

DEVELOPING TASK FORCES

A *task force* is a temporary system in the life of an organization. It is usually created to perform a specific task that cannot be done either as efficiently or as effectively through current structures and policies. It is temporary because it is usually disbanded once the task is completed. It is conceived as a task *force* rather than, say, a task *group*, because it tends to have a single focal purpose, a finite objective that justifies its total existence, rather than an ongoing function that a group might perform.

Task forces are used in organizations to address wide varieties of infrequently occurring objectives—for example, to resolve a particular crisis, to plan or implement a major change in structure and/or policy, to follow up on an organizational analysis or any other kind of consulting activity. Three things are especially important to consider when using task forces to follow up the kind of analysis covered in this book. First, despite the frequency of their use, it is dangerous to assume that most managers know how to establish and run a task force with much skill. However temporary, task force building requires skills in structural design and change, and most managers do not get a great deal of practice or training in this area. Second, task forces, like interview feedback processes, can be developed to enhance the pursuit of wide varieties of organizational values, and not just those related to OD. Consequently, by the way people are chosen, goals are set, procedures are established and sanctioned, and so on, a given task force can promote dependency, gamesmanship, and apathy as well as the consensus orientation that fits our interests. In the following paragraphs, we want to provide some guidelines that are particularly amenable to developing a consensus oriented task group, or at least one that encourages this orientation more than others.

Finally, it is important to note that a task force is not only a temporary system in the life of an organization, but also a potentially major interruption in the normal pattern of its everyday events. It takes its members out of their everyday roles. Its operation temporarily changes prevailing patterns of communication and influence. And often its outputs are designed to alter prevailing ways of doing things. Consequently, its composition, goals, and operating procedures can be of major concern to many organization members.

Care needs to be taken not only in the selection of participants and the development of effective ways of working together, but also in maintaining supportive relationships with other members of the organization who are in a position to hinder either a task force's operations or its effectiveness. In fact, one might argue that, in many OD projects, a task force's external relationships are the primary determinants of its success or failure.

Steps in Developing a Task Force

Let us assume that a prior analysis has defined some clear goals for a task force to pursue and that there is broad-based support, at least in principle, for their accomplishment. Under these conditions, it is not unlikely that your primary client will ask you for suggestions about how to develop and make the task force a success. Here are some steps I have found useful in helping a client do this.

> 1.   *Begin by considering where in the organization's hierarchy and division of labor the expertise, information, influence, and energy exists for achieving the desired goals. Draw up a list of potential members using these criteria.*

The critical issue is to locate the people who are ideal for the job both technically and interpersonally (not everyone works well in groups), and who simultaneously have the necessary energy and time available. Quite often, the impetus for a change is either at a rank above or below the group ideally suited for making it. For instance, the top management of a nursing staff (director and associate director) may have concluded that greater delegation and decentralization are necessary, but they may face a group of head nurses (a level below) who, while agreeing in principle with this need, are generally satisfied with the benefits of relying on their superiors for all sensitive decisions. And yet, the development of a more participative system might logically reside at the head nurse level. Or the situation might be reversed, with the head nurses excited about the change, but the top group reticent about letting go of key prerogatives.

Situations such as this usually require a task force membership that combines some members who have the energy with others who have the resources. The task force, thus, becomes a microcosm for working through the details of a problem area being faced by the larger system.

> 2.   *Draw up a list of other people in the organization who are likely to have a major stake in the task force's operations or its outcomes.*

While this list may overlap with the list you created in step 1, it may also include people who are more in a position to react to the task force's activities rather than actually to provide impetus for them. They represent the task force's immediate social environment, and much of the group's work needs continuously to take these people's needs into account. You may want to include some of these people on your list of prospective task force members even if they cannot be proactively helpful, because getting their responses to ideas as they emerge is so important.

Besides developing a list of these constituents, it might also be useful at this time to begin to think about what the particular needs and concerns of these people are. Jot down your hunches for each individual, and then consider two questions. First, how sure are you of whether your assumptions are correct. And second, just how important do you think each of these concerns are — for example, how strongly might the individuals involved react if their concerns were not responded to?[1]

> 3.   *With the lists above in mind, identify your choices for the leader of the task force.*

---

[1]See Mason, Richard O. and Ian I. Mitroff, *Challenging Strategic Planning Assumptions: Theory, Cases and Techniques* (New York: John Wiley and Sons, Inc., 1981).

The primary client with whom you have been working on developing the task force may be the ideal person to lead the group but, just as often, he or she is too high in the hierarchy to fit the criteria of access to relevant data, relevant expertise, and available energy. Thus, the two of you may need to pick someone whom your client is willing to support politically and who is otherwise ideal for the job. While your client will usually have his or her preferences, you can draw on your experiences in the analysis activities to suggest people who are especially interested in the task and who your client may not think of without your input. Ultimately, your client's willingness to support someone is probably the most important criterion, since few task forces succeed without continuous support and buffering from above. The second most important criterion would probably be the leader's potential for getting along with other important stakeholders in the organization.

Once a prospective leader has been identified, approached, and committed to the task, other members of the group can be selected with this person's help. Having the actual leader's inputs considered is preferable to selecting the entire group unilaterally, because it enhances this person's commitment and can minimize the selection of members who may be ideal technically but who are not likely to accept the designated leadership easily. Task forces are tender enough phenomena to begin with, and it is worthwhile to avoid sensitive internal relationships that are not required by the politics of the task itself.

All of this sets the stage for actually inviting the other members to join the task force. Preferably, this should be done by the task force leader, with appropriate ground work (phone calls and chats with prospective members' bosses) done by this person's superior.

4.   *Clarify the mandate for the task force with its leader and the person he or she will report to, and then work on establishing guidelines within which the task force must work.*

Even before the membership of the task force has been finalized, it is useful to work with the leader and his or her immediate superior to clarify the mission of the group and to set up key operating parameters. Here the current quality of relations between these two people warrants attention. If it is excellent to begin with, little needs to be done. Effective superior/subordinate relations are marked by clear communication, sensitivity to the boundaries of delegation, and easy mutual access during crises. However, when the relationship is relatively new and/or has had a difficult history, it is useful for a consultant to be present at the initial planning session to help each party hear the other.

A subordinate who is psychologically in the business of proving his or her competence or autonomy may miss important information in the mandate. Likewise, a leader who is not totally sure of the subordinate may truncate what needs to be said in order to make the process seem smooth, or alternatively create more boundaries than necessary in order to satisfy his or her own control needs.

While some relationships are so good that little needs to be said, it rarely hurts to make sure that the following issues have been covered:

- nature of the desired end product (usually a series of recommendations plus supporting analysis);

- desired deadline for completing the project;

- frequency and form of progress reports and whom to keep informed;

- people whose advice and/or approval needs to be sought in order for the group to succeed both politically and technically;

- the boundaries of the group's decision-making powers and the kinds of outputs that will be taken seriously (eg., we *will not* resolve the problem by adding additional staff but recommendations regarding changes in roles are fair game);

- guidelines regarding confidentiality in the gathering and exchange of data;

- expectations regarding the level of involvement of members' regular superiors;

- resources available in terms of funds, organizational data, each member's time, and support services; and

- particular problems/issues to look out for.

5.   *Work with the leader of the task force to plan the first meeting.*

The first meeting of any group can have a major impact on its subsequent history. I have sat in on task forces where words spoken inadvertently in the first 10 minutes set the stage for conflicts and tensions that dominated the proceedings of the group for several months. Thus, careful preparation by the leader is critical if only for the sake of avoiding social blunders.

Considerable work of a purely informational nature needs to be done. First, the basic mandate of the group needs to be stated. While each member has probably been told this in the process of being invited or assigned to the task force, restating the group's purpose is important for making sure that everyone has heard the same thing when in each other's presence. In the context of OD, it is often useful to review briefly the entire project so that the mandate can be affirmed as having arisen out of a broadly based, participative analysis project, and thus represents the interests of a large constituency within the organization.

There is symbolic power in doing this as well as efficiency in technical communication. As we noted earlier, a task force is usually comprised of people from different parts of the organization. Thus different members are likely to have different personal agendas, and the groups they represent may have competing interests and rivalries in a number of areas. The existence of the task force is a symbolic recognition that certain common interests exist that are sufficiently strong to override these differences, or at least to dampen them in this context. Starting off the first meeting with a statement of the shared goal, mandated by powers greater than any particular member's, is one way of highlighting this condition.

Second, it is helpful for the leader to clarify his or her role as being bounded by the logic of the task, and not specifically by his or her formal authority or prerogatives. For example, it is one thing to say that *I* will be calling on each of you to put in approximately 30 hours over the next two months or as many as required (with the "for what" unstated), and quite another to say that it looks as if *we* will need to put in about 30 hours apiece to have a report ready for the planning committee (or Mr. X) by such-and-such a time.

In short, if the task force is to work as a team, overt status differences need to be dampened from the beginning. At the same time, task force members rarely object to the official leader doing much of the administrative work and even delegating tasks with considerable directiveness, once objectives and task logic have been agreed to. Their own superiors rarely provide them with the time that the work of the group actually requires. Thus, tasks clearly mandated by the leaders help to justify time spent away from their regular jobs.

Following the leader's statement of the mission and some of the basic parameters of the group's operation, the next logical step is to allow every other member to state his or her interest in the task and, in particular, any personal goals he or she might have. This gives people a chance to assess each other's level of commitment and interest. Some members may be there because they have been ordered to while others actively sought membership in the group. While these things may not be stated overtly, a lot comes across through tone of voice and body language. This also gives the leader the chance to interact a little with each member and to affirm publicly the qualities in each person that he or she is seeking in behalf of the group's goal. One advantage of doing this is that someone who does not want to be there may brighten up a little when praised for the particular expertise he or she can offer the group.

Such introductions also provide a short break in the formal aspects of the leader's role, so that this person does not do all the talking from the beginning. Once completed, members are likely to be ready for more of the technical details. The leader can proceed to lay out the rest of the parameters that his or her superiors have placed around the task (see item 4 above) and invite group discussion of these. Having had a chance to talk already, members are more likely to state their views on each item and explore issues that might have been overlooked had a participative norm not been created.

From this point, the group can get down to the business of creating its own internal structure and doing the work. Typically, some planning is appropriate for dividing the task into reasonable components, assigning roles for particular kinds of work, establishing a timeline to prepare for externally imposed deadlines, and settling meeting schedules and locations. This, in turn, often sets the stage for taking a look at whose cooperation outside the group will be necessary for getting different kinds of sub-objectives accomplished, and contact roles for pursuing these people's cooperation can be created.[2]

While all of these issues warrant consideration when planning the first meeting, all of them rarely get covered when the task force actually meets for the first

---

[2]For readers wanting a clear program to follow in dealing with these issues as well, Rubin, Plovnik, and Fry have created an excellent manual for task team development. Their procedure takes a group systematically through establishing goals, roles, decision-making methods, and work procedures. It is especially good for new groups whose members have not worked together before. See Irwin M. Rubin, Mark S. Plovnik, and Ronald E. Fry, *Improving the Coordination of Health Care: A Program for Team Development* (Cambridge, Mass.: Ballinger Publishing Co., 1975).

time. A number of things might happen that can and, if they do, should slow down the process. Members may want to discuss past aspects of the project to reaffirm their understanding of what has happened. (Some members are almost invariably more informed than others.) Different members may have different interpretations of the group's mandate and these differences need to be hashed out, even if this requires further interaction with individuals who are not present.

Upon meeting them, it may become obvious that some of the people in the room are not really appropriate for the task. I have found, for instance, that popular or revered members of an organization are often asked to join important task forces because of the sense of solidarity they create, and in spite of the fact that their technical skills do not fit the task. At the same time, once the conversation starts, it may also be obvious that other people not present are really needed. The latter need to be brought on board if possible before anything else happens.

Finally, while getting a structure in place is important, establishing a favorable climate is equally so. The follow-up activities to a diagnostic project are usually not crisis situations. Consequently, momentum for getting things done has to come to a sizable degree from within the group and from the enthusiasm created by the larger project. The leader has to balance the need for an appropriately crisp procedure with the need to make members feel welcome, appreciated, and convinced that their task is truly important for the organization's future. This usually requires that more air time be provided for each member to state his or her views and for people to connect with each other around larger issues, than would be the case were a crisis at hand. As a consultant, I often find myself attending to these issues, while the leader keeps an eye on the clock and on the official task. Once on board with each other, most groups can complete the rest of their startup work at the beginning of the second meeting and still make significant progress on the task itself.

6. *Once a task force has begun its work, its leader needs to perform four functions: (a) maintain and enhance group commitment and individual contribution in the face of changing demands on member's time and energy, (b) maintain focus and internal coordination, (c) maintain communication and rapport with those who sanctioned the task and others who are concerned with its outcomes, and (d) keep the peace internally. The consultant's job is to help the leader remain attentive to each of these duties and provide support where desired.*

Several months can pass between when a task force is set up and when the final report is due. As a temporary system with few stable organizational supports to bolster its operations, any task force is vulnerable to disruption from a wide variety of sources. Crises or simply increased work loads for some members in their regular jobs can drain their energies away from the group's tasks. Subgroups within the task force that are working on different subtasks can lose rapport with each other due to unforeseen problems in coordination and lack of ongoing communication with other members. Important constituents whose continuing support is critical can lose interest as other issues change their priorities. Important stakeholders can grow impatient for results, even though they have agreed to a particular series of deadlines. New strains in relations between units represented in the task force can affect members' capacity to collaborate.

Divisive cliques may develop within the group as the work progresses and conflicting approaches to the task emerge. Without the traditional supports of stable structure and policy, the burden of dealing with these issues falls on the shoulders of the leader.

While most people selected as task force leaders tend to be pretty well rounded, I have found that few are equally good at all of these functions. My task as a consultant is to discover where the leader's weak points are and suggest ways to compensate for them. Role therapy (to be discussed in the next chapter) is often useful for dealing with both internal and external relationships, and this can be bolstered by concrete suggestions about administration and planning, as well as process consultation (to be covered in the next section) in group meetings.

Working with different leaders consequently requires attention to different issues, and there is no sure formula for being successful as a helper. However, the following guidelines for task force leaders may prove useful on a general basis:

- Agree on a regular meeting time, when possible, so that members can build this into their routines. A given meeting can always be canceled if there is nothing to do. More often than not, however, even brief meetings are useful for keeping each member informed, affirming the vitality of the group, and alerting people to problems before things get out of hand.

- Divide into subgroups when this makes sense in terms of the task, but make sure to agree on a way to share the ongoing progress of each subgroup with other members before the work is divided up. Problems in coordination can be avoided when everyone knows what is happening on a general level, even if they are not involved in all the details. Agreeing to a progress report procedure early on sets norms for open communication and avoids embarrassing situations where subgroups that run into trouble are afraid to use the rest of the group as a resource.

- Keep an eye out for interpersonal tensions within the group, and model candid confrontation by dealing openly with one's own interpersonal issues at group meetings.

- Keep your own leader informed of what is happening, especially when major problems are being encountered. Task force leadership is not an ideal arena for displaying rugged individualism. Ultimately, what is important is successful task performance from which everyone will benefit, not individual stardom.

- Maintain personal contact of some sort with each member outside the meetings. This provides an additional avenue for surfacing problems and opportunities and enhances the contribution of individuals who prefer to be silent in groups.

- The watchwords for the internal work of task force leadership are, "How can I help you get your part of the job done?" The leader in this setting is primarily a communicator, coordinator, and supporter, not a judge or controller. In this context, it is also important to praise the group for every success it creates. With so little going for it structurally, mutual appreciation of the progress the group is making toward its one and only goal is a critical source of cohesion and stability.

7. *As the task force begins to reach conclusions, and especially as the time for reporting out approaches, run important positions by key constituencies and attempt to work through politically sensitive issues.*

If the intent of this kind of task force is to implement the will of the broader membership, there is little utility in secrecy. The watchwords for external work are, "Consult widely." The more that all the relevant members of the larger organization have been involved in the task force's activities, the more its visibility and sense of importance are maintained, and the more likely it is that its outputs will have broad-based support.

> 8.   *Design presentations to other groups in such a way that there are few surprises for those on the receiving end.*

This goes hand in hand with the preceding suggestion. Formal presentations of a task force's work serve three purposes that can be hindered by unanticipated disclosures. First, they are opportunities for publicly confirming the group's accomplishments, accomplishments that the audience is likely to feel good about if they already know about them and have had a part in making them possible. Second, formal presentations are opportunities for displaying excellence in teamwork and preparation. A polished presentation reinforces the hoped-for assumption that the task force was appropriately staffed and managed. Surprise positions may indicate that some people have not been kept properly informed and thus question this assumption.

Third, formal presentations are also formal transition points in the larger process of solving organizational problems. Few task forces have more than the power to formulate and recommend solutions. Their formal reporting activities signal the organization as a whole that at least an initial pass at this phase of the problem-solving process has been completed. The next step is for those reported to, to weigh these suggestions against other organizational priorities and sanction specific actions. Surprises in formal presentations can prevent such transitions from taking place smoothly.

All this is not to say that task force reports should not be innovative or controversial. Task forces themselves are out-of-the-ordinary mechanisms, and out-of-the-ordinary outputs are expected. The point is that formal presentations are not the place to air the extraordinary for the first time. Innovation is a political process that needs to be managed throughout the life of the task force. By the time a formal report is made, potentially controversial issues should already have been shared with relevant stakeholders. If a controversy does develop and cannot be resolved by the time of the formal report, this is a signal that the task force has gone as far as it can in creating such a resolution, and it is now up to more powerful bodies to deal with it.

> 9.   *Avoid the temptation to seek new goals and maintain the life of the group after its mission has been completed.*

Success breeds solidarity and a natural desire to continue working together. Thus, there is impetus for making something permanent that was intended to be temporary. This may be justified in particular circumstances—for example, people discover that there is an ongoing stream of problems similar to the one that the task force was originally assigned. More often than not, however, the team's solidarity is the more powerful factor in its members' desire to continue working together. There is a strong temptation to create problems that fit the team's talents rather than to accept the fact that, from the organization's viewpoint, the team's usefulness has ended. Facing up to this fact can be difficult. Formal wrapup meetings, attended by the organization's leadership, social gatherings, and lauditory letters can help create the necessary symbolic closure.

PROCESS CONSULTATION

Besides helping to set up task forces to address items on the project agenda, an OD consultant can play an important role in helping client groups in general to improve their moment-to-moment interaction. This is known as *process consultation*, and it is equally as useful in ongoing work groups as it is in temporary task forces.[3]

Process consultation is an important subspecialty for many OD consultants. It involves intervening skillfully in *how* a group is operating as opposed to contributing to the content of what its members are discussing. Its purpose is to bring people's attention to conditions that are getting in the way of their effective interaction, and to model behaviors and provide insights that help them deal with these conditions in candid and self-responsible ways. Attention may be brought with good effect to a number of issues—for example, patterns of communication, member roles and functions, problem-solving and decison-making styles, group norms, leadership and authority relations, and intergroup competition and cooperation.

Process consultation is best learned by attending laboratory training programs where one first starts out as a participant in a T-group, and then proceeds in stages to the roles of cotrainer and senior trainer. Such an extended learning program is important, because one rarely finds opportunities to experiment freely in developing one's process skill outside of groups designed specifically to do this. Unlike learning one-on-one consultation, where many people are open to someone else's efforts at being attentive and helpful, helping roles in a group tend to be reserved for leadership positions. Group air time is a scarce resource because it has to be shared among several people, not just you and the other person, and the impact of one's statements, both positive and negative, is greater because several people are listening. Thus groups, especially work groups, can easily become critical of process comments that are not on the mark. New consultants working in real task groups often become paralyzed by trying to say something "perfect." More often than not, after a few unsatisfying attempts, they end up saying nothing at all and feeling very frustrated.

Nonetheless, there are some basic process skills that one can begin to master without the help of an especially cooperative group. Many of them are direct extensions of some of the one-on-one skills discussed in Chapter Eight. They involve saying things any member can say and be appreciated for, because they are not far from the realm of normal task contributions. What matters is their timing, rather than their insightfulness or provocativeness, or the personal modeling that might need to follow to make them effective. In the rest of this chapter, I want to review a number of these potential inputs in the context of a conceptual model of group process.

[3]For a more rigorous treatment of the technique of process consultation, see Edgar H. Schein, *Process Consultation: Its Role in Organization Development* (Reading, Mass.: Addison-Wesley Publishing Co., 1969).

A Model of Group Process

When acting as a process consultant, I find it useful to think of the members of a group as performing one or more of three functions at any point in time (see Figure 11–1).

FIGURE 11-1
Three Functions
of Group Life

SATISFYING INDIVIDUAL NEEDS	RESPONDING TO TASK DEMANDS	MAINTAINING THE GROUP AS A SOCIAL SYSTEM
Communicating Effectively	Defining Problems	Participation
Maintaining and Enhancing One's Self-Concept	Analyzing Problems	Membership
	Seeking Solutions	Informal Roles
Gaining Inclusion, Influence, and/or Friendship	Action Planning	Influence Patterns
	Taking Action	Norms

Very simply, groups are arenas in which individuals can pursue objectives intended to benefit only themselves (individual needs), as well as objectives designed to benefit the group as a whole (shared task demands). The pursuit of each kind of objective, if left totally unchecked, can get in the way of the other, and therefore lead to confusion and frustration. Consequently, groups develop mechanisms for coordinating these two streams of activity, and occasionally they take the time to monitor and modify them if they are not working properly. This involves maintaining the group as a social system. At any point in time, some members of a group may be preoccupied with satisfying one or more individual needs. While other members may be focusing on responding to needs shared by the group as a whole, and still others may be concerned with the group's condition as a social system. All three activities are going on at the same time, although typically a large proportion of the group is focusing on one of them. Moreover, who is doing what is constantly changing, as is whatever it is that the bulk of the group is attending to.

The fact that some shared focus of attention tends to be maintained is a group's saving grace, for it means that one or more of these activities can be acknowledged specifically and enhanced if someone such as a consultant can enter this sphere of attention. In the following sections, we will elaborate on each activity and discuss what some useful process comments/interventions might be.

Satisfying Individual Needs

By individual needs, I am referring to kinds of objectives that are experienced at the moment as unique to a given individual, and not necessarily shared at that moment by other group members. These can include: the desire to make a specific task contribution, to communicate one's point effectively, to influence particular people or a particular activity, to achieve a certain status in others' eyes, to gain emotional support or intimacy from particular individuals, and so on.

Satisfying any one member's individual needs, at least to some degree, is important for the group as a whole in order to gain that person's attention and energy for satisfying other members' needs, as well as those of the group as a whole. An individual whose personal needs are not being met is likely to have less energy to give to others, unless he or she can be given viable reasons for why this is not occurring.

Moreover, continued frustration frequently leads people to sabotage the rest of the group's activities either intentionally or inadvertently. And this, in turn, can lead to frustration for the membership as a whole.

A process consultant, therefore, can make important contributions to the group's operation by paying attention to each member's behavior, looking for signs of individual dissatisfaction or frustration, and finding ways to respond to them. The latter can be done either directly, as one member of the group to another, or by bringing the group's attention to the individual's concerns, so that others can also acknowledge and respond to them.

Individual dissatisfaction and frustration can be spotted from behaviors such as changes in voice tone, body posture, and facial expression, lack of attention to what other members are doing, frequently leaving the room, holding side conversations, disruptive joking, and use of sarcasm. One can also infer such discomfort from situations where a person's comments are ignored, belittled, or interrupted, or where he or she seems to be having trouble in being understood or in understanding someone else.

The techniques discussed in Chapter Eight for talking with clients, when used judiciously, can be employed to respond to these phenomena. Logical communication is an effective response to situations in which a person does not seem to be able to get his or her point across. Meta-modeling and active listening can be used as backup strategies and also as ways of bringing a person back into the conversation and explicating his or her concerns. Direct expressions of valuing others, acknowledging their influence on one's thinking and identifying with their plight can be used to respond to needs for inclusion, influence, and friendship.

Care should be taken, however, not to embarrass a person by encouraging or making personal disclosures that might damage the very image he or she is trying to create. An important principle to follow in exploring personal frustrations is to begin with as mild an intervention as possible, such as simply inviting a person back into the conversation.

For example, suppose that, during a meeting, you notice that a person's facial expression becomes distorted and that he or she withdraws from the conversation when someone speaks disparagingly of a particular individual or topic. One might begin by asking for his or her views on the topic or individual in question. This gives the person you are trying to help the opportunity to disclose his or her views, with follow-up help through Meta-modeling and active listening on your part, or alternatively to politely deflect your invitation.

Occasionally, the person may offer a third alternative, which is to ask you why you wanted an opinion. This presents you with a multitude of choices. For instance, you might politely deflect the response yourself—"Oh, I was just curious." Or you might give the person some personal support — "I have found your views really thought provoking on other topics and would really value them here." Or, becoming a little more intrusive, you might share your behavioral observations — "Well, I noticed that your face scrunched up a little when X offered views and that you have been silent ever since, and I was wondering whether you have got some important opinions yourself on this matter."

How you make this choice represents the art of process consultation. A multitude of factors might be taken into account: your relationship with this individual to date, your knowledge of the issues involved, the person's character and interpersonal style, your status and image in the group, what else is happening in the group at the moment, how you are feeling at the moment, and so on. In my experience, different process consultants might handle this situation in different ways, depending on all of these factors. While some guidelines are almost universal, such as avoiding undue embarrassment and showing respect for the other person's integrity, there is no one correct answer. Through practice, coaching, and feedback in laboratory training settings, and trial and error on the job, one develops a repertoire of responses that are effective in the context of one's personal style.

If one has not had laboratory training, perhaps the most important advice would be (1) to be supportive rather than challenging, finding ways for people to enter and exit from the conversation with your emotional support; (2) to remain as descriptive as possible, pointing to the obvious that others may not want to acknowledge (such as interruptions and incomplete communications); and (3) to refrain from interpreting another's behavior without an explicit invitation to do so. A great deal can be learned initially, moreover, by discussing incidents with group members after a session is over, while saying relatively little in response to personal needs during sessions. In this way, one can check one's hypotheses after the fact and begin to build one's analytic skills and supportive relationships with a minimum of risk. Done conscientiously, the time is likely to come when choices to be more intrusive during sessions feel right because the emotional support is there from those who need your help.

Responding to Task Demands

A considerably less risky area to work on is to bring a group's attention to the way in which it is pursuing its publicly acknowledged goals, and to offer suggestions for enhancing its problem-solving strategies. Groups have been found to solve problems most effectively when they proceed from:

1. describing both the problem and the conditions that have created it; to
2. analyzing the problem and considering a variety of ways to resolve it; to
3. developing criteria for a satisfactory solution and applying them systematically to the potential solutions considered; to
4. choosing the best alternative and planning action to implement it.

Being attentive to this dimension of a group's activities involves asking oneself questions such as:

1.   Have enough suggestions been made as to the best way to define or tackle the problem, before we start looking for solutions or following a particular analysis procedure? Are there present any potential experts on this subject whose ideas have yet to be tapped?

2.   Is everyone aware of what has happened thus far in terms of the group's problem-solving behavior? Would a summary be appropriate at this time? Should I, the consultant, attempt one or ask someone else to, and if so, who?

3.   As the group turns to proposing potential solutions, is there enough giving or asking for information around each idea? Are people judging particular proposals before giving themselves a chance to see how they stack up against other available alternatives? Are everyone's ideas being sought out or are some people holding back?

4.   Once the search for alternatives has been completed, has the group developed a useful set of criteria for evaluating each of them systematically? Are people giving due credence to their intuition and gut feelings as well as to their technical thinking?

5.   Is the group staying on target, or is it skipping logical steps in the problem-solving process, or avoiding anxiety provoking issues through running away from them, fighting, or depending on a single individual or a subgroup to make decisions that are logically the responsibility of all those present?

There are no perfect answers to these questions, or to any of the many others one might ask about a group's rational processes, but the simple act of asking them self-reflectively keeps one attentive to this aspect of the group's operations and is likely to provide one with a steady stream of pragmatic comments. Quite often, after 20 minutes to an hour of conversation, the simple act of providing a group with a straightforward description of its problem-solving behavior to this point is enough to get several people examining this dimension on their own.

Maintaining the Group as a Social System

During a short period of time, such as a single meeting, much of a group's activity is likely to seem haphazard if not downright chaotic. This is especially true if the group is new or if the one who is observing is new to the group. Research has shown, however, that groups quickly develop certain uniformities that serve to regulate quite stringently the allocation of resources for group and individual objectives.

Subgroup Formation.   To begin with, the distribution of various personal characteristics across a group's membership can frequently encourage the development of cliques or subgroups, whose members in turn feel more comfortable interacting with each other than with the rest of the group. For example, a management group of more than, say, a dozen individuals might display subgrouping between its older and younger members, especially if this difference is reinforced by major differences in seniority, expertise, and formal education. Greater comfort in interacting can in turn lead to greater mutual tolerance for and support of particular personal needs — in the example above, greater support for demands for deference by the senior subgroup, greater support for questioning the status quo by the junior subgroup. Other personal characteristics along which subgrouping might be based would include ethnicity, gender, and one's personal track record.

The impact of personal characteristics on subgroup formation can be reinforced or attenuated in turn by formal organizational characteristics, such as rank, salary, and functional specialty. Suppose, for instance, that the younger members of the group above all held staff jobs while the older ones all held line positions. This would accentuate the subgrouping, while a mix of staff and line jobs within each cluster might alternatively attenuate it.

Norms.   While personal and organizational characteristics foster particular patterns of subgrouping, the values, skills, and life experiences of group members interact with formal task demands to create important norms. Norms are informal rules of personal conduct that the members of a group or subgroup expect each other to abide by. Norms typically represent a group's response to the level of fit between externally imposed demands and the shared personal interests of individual members. For instance, in an organizational setting, when members' values are consistent with senior management's assigned objectives, strong norms are likely to develop around mutual assistance and task accomplishment . Alternatively, when individual values and assigned objectives conflict, norms may develop around restriction of output, lack of investment in the task, and maintenance of antiorganizational perspectives.

Informal Roles.   Subgroup identities and norms work together to create particular types of informal roles. Individuals who are members of the largest and/or the most powerful clique in a group, and who also prove themselves capable of behaving in compliance with norms shared by the group as a whole, are more likely than others to be accepted by all members. They quickly become the group's "regulars" and are given more opportunities to satisfy their personal needs and to influence group-wide activities.[4]

On the other hand, members whose personal resources or characteristics are valued by the group but who do not conform as individuals to its norms achieve the status of "deviants." These are the people in any group who seem to maintain a running battle with their colleagues by conforming just enough to make others' tolerance of them worthwhile but not enough to be seen as reliable, dependable, and trustworthy. In a sense, they make a business out of satisfying their personal needs at the expense of the group, but without doing this to the extent that their net value to the group is negative.

Members who consistently fail to conform to the group's norms and/or who, because of their personal characteristics, do not fit easily into an important subgroup, typically become the group's "isolates." Consider a young (low-status), college educated (high-status) manager of computer services working with a group of generally older, high school educated, line foremen. Because of this person's background, he or she

---

[4]The role designations of "regulars," "deviants," "isolates," and "leaders" used here were first developed by Zaleznik et al. See A. Zaleznik, C. R. Christensen, and F. J. Roethlisberger, *The Motivation, Productivity, and Satisfaction of Workers: A Prediction Study* (Boston, Mass.: Division of Research, Harvard Business School, 1958), pp. 152-58.

might insist on violating group norms, experimenting with standard operating procedures, refusing to confine work to traditional hours, and wearing formal rather than informal attire while on the shop floor.

From this person's viewpoint, experimentation might be an important value, working beyond the usual quitting time of little personal consequence, and wearing a coat and tie at all times a sign of good breeding. But since there is no one else in the group who shares the same background, the rest of the group might see all of these behaviors as acts of defiance, sabotage, and snobbery. After some initial efforts at enforcing conformity through teasing, parental admonishments, open confrontation, and withdrawal of social support, the rest of the group is likely to ignore this person as much as possible and go on about its business as if he or she did not exist.

Finally, individuals who are accepted behaviorally by others as informal "leaders" are typically those who are members of the clique with the greatest resources, who possess the personal characteristics most valued by that group, and who are most adept at conforming to the group's norms and ideals. When several cliques exist, each is likely to have its own leader, and major decisions for the group as a whole are made by these individuals. Such leaders may or may not also possess high organizational status, depending upon the posture of their group toward the rest of the organization. But they are clearly given the greatest freedom to use the group's resources to satisfy their own needs, so long as they also continue to do what is necessary to maintain their leadership roles.

Understanding the Informal System.   Patterns of subgrouping, norms, and informal roles are central characteristics of a group's informal social system. They are important for a process consultant to analyze and understand for two reasons. First, they represent a group's natural way of determining each member's access to group resources for satisfying personal needs in the context of the larger task. A basic formula is involved. The more an individual embodies personal characteristics that others would like to have and behaves in ways that are experienced as responsive to the larger group's interests, the more this person is permitted to satisfy his or her own needs.

Second, while these mechanisms may be the natural ways in which groups in our society have learned to resolve the dilemma of individual versus group interests, they are typically far from ideal when viewed in terms of either humanistic values or technical effectiveness. Isolate and deviant roles may be pragmatic responses to a group's need to create order in the midst of chaos, but they are also a potential waste of human resources. A person who has become an isolate or a deviant may have earned his or her status justly through poor performance in the past, but this does not guarantee that he or she cannot contribute in effective ways to the task at hand. Moreover, if this person's status is due to personal characteristics beyond his or her control (unfortunate combinations of age, gender, ethnicity, race, and education), major resources may be held back from the group due to fundamental prejudices that are inconsistent with humanistic values.

Likewise, group norms that inhibit candidness, self-responsibility, and the treatment of others in a spirit of holism and equality may represent pragmatic responses to important value conflicts, but the OD process represents an alternative way of dealing with these conflicts. Finally, the development of subgroupings based on similarities in personal and organizational characteristics may foster a sense of personal safety, but they also limit the discovery of the totality of a group's resources and encourage an elitist posture toward the governance of any system.

Given these conditions, a process consultant can be helpful to a group by bringing attention to aspects of its social system that are getting in the way of its effectiveness and suggesting alternative ways of dealing with the underlying issues they address. Some descriptive questions for directing one's analysis of a group are provided below.

Participation[5]

Participation (who participates? how often? to what effect?) is the easiest aspect of group process to observe and the key to identifying major subgroups. Typically, people who are higher in status, members of more powerful subgroups, more knowledgeable, or simply more talkative by nature, tend to participate more actively; those who are newer, lower in status, less included, uninformed, or who are not inclined to express their feelings and ideas, generally speak less frequently. Even in groups comprised of people of equal status and competence, and in which subgrouping has not developed, some people will speak more than others; this variation is expected, and is not necessarily a sign of an ineffective group. However, when large disparities exist between the contributions of individual members, it is usually a clue that the process is not effective. Particular individuals or coalitions may be dominating the discussion and blocking out valuable views.

Some questions to consider in observing participation include:

1. Who are the high participators? Why? To what effect?

2. Who are the low participators? Why? To what effect?

3. Are there any shifts in participators—for example, does an active participator suddenly become silent? Do you see any reason for this in the group's interaction, such as criticism from a higher status person or a shift in topic?

4. How are silent people treated? Is their silence taken by others to mean consent? Disagreement? Disinterest? Why do you think they are silent?

5. Who talks to whom? Who responds to whom? Do participation patterns reflect subgroups that are impeding or controlling the discussion? Are the interaction patterns consistently excluding certain people who need to be supported or brought into the discussion?

6. Who keeps the discussion going? How is this accomplished? Why does that person want the discussion to continue in that vein?

---

[5]Portions of the following sections are excerpted from a Harvard Business School teaching note (9-477-029) by Anne Harlan and John J. Gabarro. The note itself was based in part on an earlier teaching note by the author.

Influence

Influence and participation are not the same thing. Some people may speak very little, yet capture the attention of the whole group. Others may talk frequently but their words go unheard. *Influence* is typically a function of status—in particular, a person's informal role. It is normal for some people to have more influence on a group's activities than others, and this fact is not necessarily a sign that a group is ineffective. However, when one individual or subgroup has so much influence on a discussion that others are rejected out of hand, it is usually a clue that the group's effectiveness will suffer and that discussion will fail to probe alternatives in depth. This imbalance is particularly dangerous when minority views are systematically squelched without adequate exploration. Asymmetry in influence can also lead to internal conflict and alienation among those who feel squelched, and this in turn can reduce both individual satisfaction and task performance.

The following questions can be used to assess influence patterns within a group:

1. Which members are listened to when they speak? What ideas are they expressing?

2. Which members are ignored when they speak? Why? What are their ideas? Is the group losing valuable inputs simply because these people are not being heard?

3. Are there any shifts in influence? Who shifts? Why?

4. Is there any rivalry within the group? Are there struggles between individuals or subgroups for leadership?

5. Who interrupts whom? Does this reflect relative power within the group?

6. Are minority views consistently ignored, regardless of possible merit?

Norms

Norms, as we have already noted, are informal and unwritten rules of behavior that group members have come to expect of one another. Deviations from group norms are responded to through challenges, warnings from other group members, and punishments that may vary from kidding to physical harm. The severity of these sanctions usually varies with the importance of the norm being violated and the violator's informal status. Continued failure to comply typically leads to loss of status, social ostracism, isolation, and whatever support and resources a group has to offer. Norms can cover every aspect of a group member's thinking, feeling, and behaving, although obviously only behavior can be monitored easily.

Of particular interest to a process consultant are norms that are related to the basic value paradigms in this book. These are norms that interfere with candidness, self-responsibility, balanced participation, mutual influence, the expression of feelings as relevant parts of one's experience, the treatment of each member as a potentially valuable resource, and the pursuit of shared commitment to group goals. In general, norms that support collegiality, consensus decision making, and collaborative organization are viewed as desirable in the context of OD project activities, while those that support the logic of the other quadrants in our paradigms are targets for change.

Questions that can help in exploring group norms include the following:

1.   What rules or norms does the group act as if it is operating by? Try to be as specific as possible. You might consider apparent rules regarding participation and influence, since observed patterns that indicate subgrouping and status hierarchies are typically reinforced by norms supporting their maintenance. You might also consider norms regarding the group's view of the world outside it, the group's goals and their priorities, the distribution of labor with respect to each goal, decision-making procedures, procedures for dealing with unusual events, the use of humor, and the limits of personal freedom.

2.   What happens when individuals depart from the observed behaviors you have hypothesized as being supported by group norms? Are the departers challenged, shunned, ridiculed, or punished in any other ways? A retaliatory response by the group is evidence that a norm is clearly in force.

3.   What value orientations seem to characterize the norms you have identified? Identification of a particularly strong consistency between the logic of your descriptions and one of the quadrants in the value paradigms can be helpful in anticipating still other norms.

4.   What norms, specifically, seem to be getting in the way of the group doing its work in a spirit of collaboration and coinquiry?

5.   What would be a more preferable norm to replace each undesired one with? How might you model it in a way that demonstrates its value to the group? How might you bring it to the group's attention in a way members might find acceptable?

Some of the actual interventions one can make in order to modify the group's social system are little different from those suggested for increasing the satisfaction of individual or task demands. One simply does them for a different reason. One can invite people back into the conversation in order to broaden participation and thereby dampen the impact of a particular subgroup, in the same way one does this in order to respond to a person's blocked desire to air an important viewpoint. One can suggest that proposals not be evaluated until all are on the table in order to counter the influence of particular people who are trying to railroad their ideas through the group, in the same way that one does this to make sure that an effective problem-solving procedure is followed. Interventions of this sort make use of one's own status and influence as another member of the group.

One type of intervention that is different is to make comments on the group's social system itself and invite members to inquire with you into the viability of particular features. Here are some examples:

Participation and Subgroups.   "I am curious as to why the three people here from the marketing group never say anything during these meetings, and I wonder if something is standing in the way of your joining in."

Influence and Roles.   "I am troubled by what I see happening to Jerry here. In the past hour, he has made three attempts to make a statement and he has been interrupted every time; once by you, Bill, once by Tom, and once by Harry. I recognize that Jerry is the newest person in your department, but I wonder whether you are giving yourselves a fair chance to hear what he has to offer."

Norms.   "I have noticed that, for the past three meetings, the topic of next year's salary increases has been put on the agenda. And yet we have not actually discussed it in any detail. Something else always seems to come up. Have you considered what will happen if this group does not offer its own suggestions in the near future?"

Developing Your Own Style

Attending to individual needs, task demands, and the group as a social system represent three major foci for process consultation. While they can be separated analytically, process comments usually affect all three simultaneously, as one can see from the examples above. What is important is for a consultant to be aware of this complexity without becoming paralyzed by it. I find it easiest to do this by shifting my attention from one arena to another in accordance with my intuitive sense of what is most important to the group at the moment.

For instance, I might spend the first part of a meeting thinking about the group in terms of task demands, until particular aspects of the group as a social system seem to be getting in the way of effective problem solving. After some work at the social system level, particular people's personal needs may seem especially pressing and I will start to focus on them more directly. The feedback I get is that my actual behavior does not shift radically in accordance with the lens I am using. Nonetheless, these differences in orientation are very real to me, and I am sure I use different words to go with the different orientations. My hunch is that the impact I have on a group is largely a product of my own internal consistency or lack thereof, however, rather than the particular formula I use for selecting a conceptual lens.

This suggests, in turn, that what matters in the long run is one's personal style. Schemes such as the one just presented are ways of coping as an individual with a complex situation, just as the one presented in Chapter Eight on talking with clients represents primarily a coping device for keeping one's inquiry process alive in a two-person conversation. What is critical is to have at least some scheme as a guide and to use it conscientiously until it becomes tailored to one's personality. The potential for broadening one's repertoire through examining new schemes and developing new ones on one's own is endless. Thus, what is presented above is only a beginning.

CONCLUSION | Developing task forces and engaging in process consultation are two basic techniques for working with groups of clients when following up an organizational analysis. They set the stage for identifying and implementing a wide variety of more specific interventions for tackling the organization's developmental agenda. But groups are not the only arenas in which more specific interventions can be formulated. One-on-one work with individual clients is often equally if not more important. In the next and last chapter, we will explore role therapy as a basic technique for deepening one's relationships with particular clients and for creating a dialogue for planning future interventions.

CHAPTER TWELVE

BUILDING
COLLEGIAL RELATIONSHIPS

This chapter is about building collegial relationships by means of a technique called role therapy.[1] *Collegial relationships* are ones that exhibit a spirit of equality and holism; equality in the sense that neither party is seen as basically more worthy than the other, holism in the sense that each party treats the other as a multifaceted human being as opposed to the enacter of a particular role.

Equality and holism are important qualities in a relationship, because they discourage self-oriented behavior at the expense of the other and encourage looking outward together at whatever is of concern to either party. This, in turn, lets shared concerns surface and sets the stage for mutual help in problem solving.

Role therapy is a consulting technique that fosters these qualities by making it safe for the client to act as if they already existed, and thus reap their benefits. If it is successful, the consultant gains a colleague for exploring and experimenting with the rest of the organization. The client benefits individually with respect to his or her own concerns and may even develop the incentive to use the technique with other organization members, thereby diffusing collegiality throughout the organization.

In the following sections, we will first look at the theory behind the technique; second, at the actual behaviors involved; and finally, at some general guidelines for applying it successfully.

---

[1]Parts of this chapter first appeared in Eric H. Neilsen and Suresh Srivastva, "Role Therapy as a Modal Intervention in Health Care Organizations," in *Organizational Development in Health Care Organizations*, eds. Newton Margulies and John D. Adams (Reading, Mass.: Addison-Wesley Publishing Co., 1982), pp. 331-56. Quoted with special permission of Addison-Wesley Publishing Co.

| **THE LOGIC OF ROLE THERAPY** | A *role*, for the purposes of the ensuing discussion, is a cluster of obligations and prerogatives related to a collective task.[2] *Role behavior* is what a person does in the |

process of performing these prerogatives and exercising these obligations. Role behavior has three components: (1) role envisioning, (2) role interaction, and (3) role reaction.

1.   Role Envisioning.   This refers to the thinking about one's role that a person engages in prior to attempting to perform that role in a particular situation. For instance, it is what goes through a manager's mind prior to entering a meeting where he or she will have to act in others' presence as a manager. The manager does not know for sure exactly what others will expect or how to behave in order to fulfill their expectations. No one can know this since all human experience changes subsequent thought and, therefore, no amount of planning can predict future expectations perfectly. The essential point is that one begins with some notion, however vague, of what is likely to happen and how one might, can, should, and will behave in order to achieve one's own and others' objectives.

Envisioned roles are complex phenomena since many factors are involved in anticipating how one will act in a given situation. For the purposes of role therapy it is important to note that they include at least implicitly considerations regarding one's ideal self, one's assumptions about what others will expect and how one feels about these expectations, one's impulsive or hedonistic wants, one's assumptions about how much discretion one can exercise in responding to others' demands, and one's own knowledge of how one has behaved in similar situations in the past. These factors remain with varying levels of awareness in the actor's mind as interaction in the situation thus prepared for begins.

2.   Role Interaction.   The second component of role behavior, *role interaction,* refers to the consistencies and discrepancies that arise between an actor's envisioned role and what actually happens while the actor is attempting to act in role. For instance, a manager may enter into conversation with colleagues assuming that he or she will be recognized by them as the senior expert on a particular topic, only to find that others are treating another member of the group in this way. Or the manager may expect that others will treat him or her as the authority on a particular problem and find that others are confirming this expectation by their behavior.

3.   Role Reaction.   Our human inability to predict the future, by definition, causes interaction in role to create an ongoing stream of surprises and disappointments, confirmations and disconfirmations, anxieties and catharses. Consequently, role behavior also involves a third component, that is, how the role player reacts to the discrepancies between his or her envisioned role and what actually happens. We call this *role reaction.*

[2]Harry M. Johnson, *Sociology: A Systematic Introduction* (New York: Harcourt, Brace and World, Inc., 1960), p. 16.

The behavioral components of role reaction are crucial ingredients of role therapy in the sense that a consultant works with the client in terms of this approach to respond to the generative aspects of role envisioning and interaction and the consequences embedded in the behavior identified as role reaction. People's reactions to such discrepancies can be observed and classified in four basic categories: (1) denial, (2) avoidance, (3) adaptation, and (4) coinquiry. Each category has its particular strengths and weaknesses, but only one of them, coinquiry, is a foundation for a collegial relationship and thus Organization Development activities.

Denial.   The strategy of *denial* involves refusing to recognize to oneself that one's envisioned role is considerably different from what one is actually experiencing. For instance, a person may enter a meeting assuming that the preparation he or she has done is what others want. During the course of the meeting this person may get a variety of signals, perhaps even a direct statement, indicating that they are expecting something else. Reacting to this mismatch through denial would mean that the actor in question would refuse to recognize it and continue to behave as if he or she had, indeed, done what was expected and that others were responding as expected.

This example deals with a particular meeting, but the strategy of denial may be used in connection with more enduring dynamics. For example, people may assume that others see them as competent in a given area and that their advice on matters related to it will be both wanted and taken seriously. If they receive signals to the contrary across a variety of interactions and continuously refuse to recognize them, they are using the strategy of denial.

All of us, of course, practice denial continuously in our interactions with others. It is a major means of protecting one's self-concept and, when others go along with it, of avoiding social embarrassment.[3] It seems to be most useful under two conditions. The first is when the mismatches involved are so minor that recognizing them would draw one's attention away from tasks that could easily be completed in spite of them. The second is when the mismatches are so great that recognizing them would rob oneself of the capacity to contribute in any way to a particular activity. For instance, suppose that a project leader has invited several people to collaborate on a given task and discovers immediately that some of those invited are objectively wrong for the job. Provided the leader can get at least some objectives accomplished, recognizing how unsuitable certain people are might create so much anxiety that the leader might not deal effectively with those who are suitable.

Denial is an ineffective strategy, however, when it prevents one from attending to mismatches that one *can* cope with emotionally and that have long-term consequences for task effectiveness. New surgeons in an operating room, for instance, can get off to a very bad start when they refuse to recognize that some of their co-workers, such as experienced nurses, know more about certain aspects of the surgeon's job than they themselves do. Likewise, older physicians who can no longer match their juniors in certain aspects of medical technology, but who can perform credibly in other ways,

[3]Erving Goffman, *Interaction Ritual* (Garden City, N.Y.: Anchor Books, 1967).

may make life difficult both for themselves and their colleagues if they refuse to recognize these emerging differences.

Finally, denial as a strategy for coping with disappointments in role expectations is, in my experience, especially typical of what we have called developmental relationships. Two people who treat each other holistically and yet recognize a clear level of inequality between each other, are bound into a situation in which one person by definition knows better and thus is expected to foresee the future, while the other is less capable and thus is expected not to do this as well. In cases where it becomes apparent that this it not so, denial is the easiest way to cope so as to keep the basic premises of the relationship intact.

Avoidance.   The strategy of *avoidance* involves attempts to prevent others either from recognizing role mismatches or from making them even greater. Suppose, for instance, that a person enters a meeting with the expectation that he or she will have the right to make the final decision on one of the topics to be discussed. Once the meeting starts it becomes apparent that the group wants to make decisions by voting and that, were the actor in question to resist this openly, it might create conflict that he or she does not want to face. The actor might engage in avoidance behavior in any number of ways to prevent others from recognizing the mismatch or to prevent the group from taking this choice away. For example, this person might: (1) refrain from sharing his or her expectations, thus avoiding overt discussion of the mismatch; (2) support someone else's resistance to the voting process, while disclaiming any personal interest in the matter; (3) request postponement of the decision for lack of sufficient data and use expertise to create the confusion necessary to make this convincing; or (4) vote on other issues so as to solidify a coalition that would increase his or her chances of influencing the decision as expected. It all sounds a little dubious but it happens all the time.

Avoidance works when one can get away with it. Its practice provides organization members with an accurate picture of their position in the power hierarchy. The more power a person has, the more adeptly he or she can use it. Thus, by using avoidance behavior, people quickly learn where they stand along this dimension. As a strategy for role playing in the service of collectively held goals, however, avoidance has at least three drawbacks. First, it equates power with morality. Avoidance behavior, when carried to an extreme, creates situations in which the people with the most power get their way in the short run, even where this flies in the face of broadly held social values. Eventually, important constituencies that support these values coalesce and rebellion results. Such outcomes, of course, can be avoided if those with power are also moral. The point is that there is nothing in the avoidance behavior itself to encourage shared commitment and conformity to commonly held values. The emphasis, ultimately, is on the achievement of individual objectives. Collectively held goals and behavioral norms become redefined in terms of the negotiated interests of a ruling elite.

Second, the pursuit of avoidance behavior may be inconsistent with task demands. The role a person expects to play may not be the role needed to get the job done. For instance, one might expect to be given discretion over a task that others can do more effectively. Under these conditions, the more a person jockeys to get his or her envisioned role accepted by others, the more he or she hinders effective task accomplishment.

Finally, avoidance behavior puts a drain on personal energy that might more effectively be used to get tasks done. The more people are preoccupied with avoiding mismatches with the roles they want to play, the less time and energy they have to contribute to the tasks that they and others have come together to accomplish.

Avoidance is the stuff of organization politics. People can use their formal authority, their control over material resources and important information, others' sense of obligation to them, their professional credentials and the deference that goes with them, their charisma and others' sense of being dependent on them to shape activity beforehand and control it as it progresses so that their envisioned roles become a reality.[4] This, by definition, involves the continuous avoidance of openly recognized differences between what an individual expects to happen and what actually does.

Likewise, avoidance as a coping strategy is most conducive to what we have called political relationships in our value paradigm. People who view each other primarily as potential instruments for achieving their personal aims have little incentive to share their unmet expectations, for this might give the other an unwanted advantage. And since, in this kind of relationship, the other is viewed as basically an equal, explicit demands to conform are difficult to implement, while avoidance tactics, even if revealed for what they are, are fairly safe to attempt.

Adaptation. A third behavior for dealing with mismatches between one's envisioned role and subsequent experience is to recognize them privately and revise one's envisioned role to fit the experience. For example, consultants might enter a meeting assuming that their role is to attend to the group's process, only to find that people are expecting them to contribute to the content as well. To take an *adaptive strategy* might be for the consultants to say to themselves, *I guess we are not just process consultants after all; our role is to contribute to content, too.* Note that this is the counterpart strategy to avoidance, where the consultants might say to themselves, *I did not intend or prepare to contribute to the content, but I do not want to reveal this, so I will see if I can structure our interaction so that I do not have to.*

To adopt an adaptive strategy is to go with the flow. It involves continuously updating one's envisioned role in light of other people's behavior, rather than trying to change their behavior to fit the role one envisioned. It is especially useful for people in low power positions who are willing to accept the status quo. It is organizationally useful to the extent that those who practice it are novices who are incapable of envisioning their roles appropriately for task accomplishment. Under these conditions adaptation represents an important socialization process. Each interaction provides data on what one's role should be, until one eventually experiences fewer and fewer mismatches because one's envisioned role is more in line with others' expectations.

The adaptive strategy also has major weaknesses for both the organization and the individual. On the organizational level, individuals who pursue this strategy in-

---

[4]John P. Kotter, *Power in Management* (New York: AMACOM, 1980).

tensely, when they are beyond their initial training, fail to provide their colleagues with the independent judgments they have to offer. Such judgments are important when they concern how best to use one's skills, what one's lasting work and career interests are, and when one feels wronged or mistreated. They are also important when the individual is viewed ambivalently by others. The latter may both want this person's advice and want to argue about and test it as well. Under these conditions, if the individual in question acts adaptively, his or her lack of resistance to others' testing may rob the organization of important learnings.

The strategy is costly on an individual level when it leads people to waste time and energy on activities they are not suited for. This, in turn, can lead to repeated failure experiences that damage one's self-confidence, initiative, capacity to learn, and ability to maintain an integrated identity.

The adaptive strategy is especially conducive to what we have called service relationships, where the two parties recognize a basic inequality between them and also choose to treat each other in strictly instrumental — role defined — terms. The mutually recognized inequality leads one person's expectations to be met more often and thus, *noblesse oblige*, to adapt to the occasional situation when they are not. The less worthy party's expectations are conversely easy to identify as inappropriate when they are not met, thus making the adaptive strategy palatable to this person as well. The choice to relate on strictly instrumental terms, moreover, discourages either party from exploring these conditions openly.

Coinquiry.   *Coinquiry* entails two types of behavior. The first is the open recognition both to oneself and to others of mismatches between one's envisioned role and one's subsequent experience. The second is the invitation to others to share this problem and to collaborate with the actor in developing a new role that is more in line with his or her envisioned role *and* his or her subsequent experience. Suppose, for instance, a personnel manager with an industrial background accepts a job in a large medical center under the assumption that he or she will be allowed to institute a series of uniform, organization-wide policies typical of industrial settings. Suppose, further, that after a few months the manager realizes that the physicians he or she deals with resist uniform standards and insist on departmental autonomy regarding personnel matters. Following a coinquiry strategy here would involve sharing this mismatch with physicians from several departments and inviting them to help the manager establish a new philosophy of personnel policy development. Such a strategy, ideally, would enable the manager to discover new complexities in personnel matters that were not present in industry. Simultaneously, it might lead the physicians to discover some of the benefits to be derived from certain aspects of the industrial model.

The strength of coinquiry lies both in the fact that mismatch problems are shared and that their resolutions are mutually determined. Sharing the problem provides important outcomes both for the actor and for his or her colleagues. The actor has an added incentive for doing something about the mismatch and colleagues can factor their knowledge of this condition into their understanding of the actor. The individual's request for help from others in resolving a mismatch is an act that publicly recognizes his or her mutual dependence with them. Thus, it is an invitation to pool resources and to focus on what is the problem, not who is the problem. Finally, the data provided through the combination of sharing and joint problem solving around this issue are likely to be richer than what any individual could gather alone.

Coinquiry is not without its drawbacks, however. First, the person who practices it is open to misdirection and manipulation by others who are using different strategies. Those who practice denial and thus refuse to recognize their own mismatches may have trouble empathizing with someone who practices coinquiry and label this person as irrelevant. Those who practice avoidance may capitalize on the coinquirer's overture as an opportunity to use him or her covertly, to service their own ends. Those who are adaptive may help a coinquirer resolve a mismatch at the expense of sacrificing the best use of their own skills. Thus, coinquiry works best only when everyone involved uses it.

A second drawback to this strategy is that it can be emotionally taxing. The data one receives from others when one shares one's envisioned role can publicly reveal one's own incompetence. The process may also surface differences in basic values and goals, for others simply may not see one's objectives as acceptable. Thus, it may require important personal choices about whether this is the right setting for one to work in.

Unlike the other strategies, however, both of these drawbacks can be overcome through continued commitment to coinquiry. The maintenance of candidness and commitment to mutual problem solving can model behavior for others to deal with their own denial. This may not be enough to change their behavior, but at least it is a start. Pursued long enough, coinquiry can reveal others' avoidance behavior, since the inconsistencies in behavior that are the inevitable byproducts of the avoidance strategy will eventually be revealed through reporting one's own experience of being manipulated. Once again, this may not be enough to dissuade others from using avoidance in the future, but it does block its effects on oneself and reveals past behavior for what it is. The choice is then up to the actor to decide whether he or she is willing to continue to associate with the other.

The same is true for interactions with those engaged in adaptive behavior. For their continued responsiveness to whatever pressures from others that arise will also be revealed in the reporting of one's personal experience of the other; thus setting the stage for either problem solving or yet another choice about continued association.

Finally, by confronting one's own mismatches publicly and inviting help, the stage is set for a more realistic assessment of oneself and one's choices in the future. Ultimately, coinquiry may result in the disbanding of an organization or one's own departure, but for the very best of reasons, that is, the maintenance of personal integrity.

Alternatively, coinquiry can result in a self-renewing learning process. For no matter what happens, the strategy maximizes the sharing of resources, continued experimentation with the organization in response to new conditions, and confrontation of behavior that is inconsistent with the premises of organized activity.

Finally, of all four coping strategies, coinquiry is most consistent with collegial relationships, where both parties recognize each other as basically equals and relate to each other holistically. On a general level, we have argued that these conditions encourage the sharing of aspirations, problem solving, and confrontation around each party's personal development. Coinquiry around the problems of day-to-day work is a natural extension of this. The assumption of equality makes each party's viewpoint relevant and the holistic posture makes open discussion of one's role legitimate and safe.

THE SPECIFICS OF THE TECHNIQUE

So far we have established that the aim of role therapy is to get a client to practice coinquiry when encountering discrepancies between his or her envisioned and enacted roles. We see this as a key to building collegial relationships because those who have the courage and self-discipline to treat their roles in this way stand the greatest chance of developing a similar philosophy toward other people. In this section, we want to describe the basic techniques for accomplishing this aim.

Three different kinds of activities are involved:

1. *Analysis.* Analyzing the various components of a client's role behavior (role envisioning, role interaction, role reaction) so that one can see the kinds of reaction strategies this person currently uses in response to particular mismatches; and analyzing the client's role set (the cluster of roles within which his or her own role is embedded) and various characteristics of all the role incumbents involved. Both analyses provide important insights into the context within which the client operates.

2. *Modeling.* Using coinquiry in one's relationship with the client so that the latter can experience its effects and picture the kind of behavior it involves.

3. *Coaching.* Problem solving with the client around ways for him or her to initiate coinquiry with colleagues, with respect to particular role-related problems he or she is now facing.

Analysis

The first step in *analyzing* clients' current role behaviors is to gather data on how they have envisioned their roles, experienced them, and reacted to these experiences in the past. In the context of a larger OD program, these data are usually gathered through a series of interviews with as many as possible of the people one will be working directly with. Specific data on role behavior are gathered here through asking:

1. Whom do you work with most closely?
2. What do you expect of each of them?
3. What do you think they expect of you?
4. How well have these expectations been met?
5. What have you and your colleagues done when these expectations have not been met?

By comparing these data across sets of individuals who interact frequently with each other, one can develop a series of working hypotheses about how each person has envisioned his or her role in the past, how well this has fit subsequent experience, and the strategies that he or she has used to deal with the discrepancies.

For example, in the course of interviewing the members of a top management team, one might discover that Mr. Jones is known for ignoring others' negative perceptions of him and that, indeed, in his own interview with you he reports few mismatches in his day-to-day work. Both data points support the hypothesis that he uses a denial coping strategy. At the same time, Ms. Smith may be known for being a hard worker, easy to get along with, and *always* responsive to the group's needs. And simultaneously, in your personal interviews with her, you learn that while she feels accepted by others, she is unsure of her direction, overworked, and frustrated by never having enough time to discover or pursue her own interests. The data here suggest that she prefers adaptation as a coping strategy. While people use different coping strategies in varying degrees, my experience has been that they do tend to have a dominant strategy or two and that co-workers pick this up quite easily.

The next step is to check out one's hunches by observing how one's clients interact with each other when one is with them. One can look at how they behave in feedback meetings, at group meetings where you are working as process consultant or are simply there to observe. One can watch how they interact over the phone, in the hallways, and even at lunch. One can become familiar with current life in their group and discover how various problems are being played out.

Besides observing how clients interact with each other, one can focus on how they interact with you and how you experience this interaction. In particular, it is useful to explore whether a client uses the same behavioral strategies with you that the rest of the data indicate he or she uses with others. For example, if others report that a client is manipulative with them (an avoidance behavior), do you experience him or her in the same way? If not, are there good reasons why he or she might not behave this way with you in particular?

Social Context.   Gaining an initial understanding of a client's favorite coping strategy is only one part of the analysis task, however. Equally important is the need to gather data about the *social context* in which the client operates, in order to develop some ideas about whether this style makes sense for this person's current well-being. It would be ideal for all clients to engage in coinquiry, both with their consultants and with each other. As stated earlier, however, there are many good reasons why another style might make sense, at least in particular relationships.

When dealing with especially troublesome relationships, where one has already discovered that the parties do not engage in coinquiry, one needs to ask the following questions in deciding what role to take as a consultant: (1) Is it realistically safe for each party to step out of his or her role by talking candidly about his or her experiences in it? (2) What forces or conditions exist that might make such activity unsafe for either party in this relationship? (3) What prospects does coinquiry hold in this situation for changing these conditions so that they will support coinquiry in the future?

Ultimately, the answers to all three questions require subjective judgment by the consultant and may need to be modified as one interacts more and more with each party. However, the strength of one's judgments can be enhanced initially by looking

FIGURE 12-1

A Roadmap for Assessing
the Key Forces Shaping
a Relationship

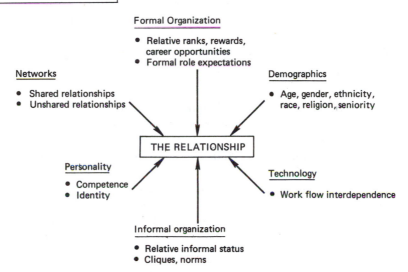

for potentially important factors in a variety of directions. Figure 12–1 represents a roadmap for doing this.

Formal organization, demographics, technology, informal organization, personality, and networks represent six subsystems, each of which can affect the relationship both alone and in interaction with each other. While each subsystem might be explored exhaustively for its implications, the really important dynamics relative to each are usually quite obvious. The utility of the roadmap is in getting one to look systematically in many directions. In the following paragraphs, let us briefly consider each subsystem for the more straightforward insights it can offer.

Organization.   When thinking about whether it is safe for either party to step out of role and talk candidly with the other about his or her experience in it, it is especially important to look at the relative ranks of the two individuals, and in particular at the potential for one party to be able to control the fate of the other. Differences between two people in terms of their hierarchical positions can encourage negative attributions by each party toward the other. These can lead to the more powerful party taking undue advantage of the other and the less powerful becoming self-protective.

While formal rank is probably the most important *organizational factor*, it is also useful to consider other indications of organizationally based differences in power, such as salaries, perquisites, and apparent career paths. Sometimes these can cancel each other out. Consider a superior whose subordinate has been identified as an "up-and-comer" with strong chances of moving into higher positions in the near future. Common sense suggests that the superior is likely to attribute more power to the subordinate than he or she currently has, as a result of this longer term consideration.

Formal, documented role expectations are also important to assess. For instance, as part of an MBO system, one manager may have promised another a certain product or service to be rendered at a specific time. If failure to meet this agreement is likely to be reflected in the formal evaluation system, and if changing the nature of the contract is beyond the immediate control of both parties because of its interdependence with still other contracts, both may feel stressed. Either party may want to blame the other for his or her own poor performance and avoid coinquiry as a matter of self-protection.

Demographics.   By *demographics*, I mean the social indicators that students of population dynamics use to characterize individuals, such as age, sex, race, religion, and ethnicity. When studying the members of an organization, one might also include indicators such as company seniority, department seniority, job seniority, and professional seniority.

Indicators such as these are important to peruse because individuals use them as measures of status and power, on the one hand, and of social similarity and like-mindedness, on the other. In any given region of the country, for example, one is likely to find a status hierarchy in terms of ethnicity, race, and religion. Greater age relative to another person tends to be a general indicator of higher status and, parallel with this, so are all forms of seniority. Likewise, men have traditionally been awarded higher status than women in Western culture, although, of course, this is now changing. Unlike organizational rank, any one of these indicators taken alone is not likely to determine a clear power difference, but when several reinforce one another their impact may be significant. Imagine, for instance, what your initial hunches would be about the relative power of two employees you encountered in the back office of a bank if one were gray haired, white, and male and the other young, black, and female.

Differences in power, derived from these ascribed characteristics, can also make coinquiry unsafe for the less powerful party. Similarities, especially across several indicators, can likewise provide important clues about the perceived utility of coinquiry. The closer I am, for instance, to my client in terms of age, socioeconomic status, work experience, and so on, the easier it is for the two of us to develop rapidly an appreciation of each other's worlds. This increases the chances of identifying each other as having something valuable to offer through a coinquiry process.

Technology.   *Technological factors* can affect the perceived safety of coinquiry by giving different amounts of power to two people through their positions in strategic work flows. Two managers may be equals in terms of their organizational ranks and statuses, for instance, as the marketing and production managers, respectively, of a small company. But if in that company's industry, the critical variables for organizational success are under production's control, the marketing manager might experience the production manager as considerably more powerful. Engaging in coinquiry with him or her about one's frustrations in responding to customer requests might be unsafe, if the marketing manager senses that the production manger will use information to make unilateral decisions about which customers to favor.

Informal Organization.   The *informal organization* that is shared by two people can affect their relationship in much the same way that formal organizational variables do. Especially in fairly stable work groups where members are not differentiated markedly in terms of their formal statuses; demographic variables, personalities, and positions in the work flow often interact to create an informal status hierarchy.[5] Individuals who emerge as informal leaders have more control over the distribution of social rewards and punishments—for example, praise, camaraderie, ostracism, and isolation. Concern over the use of these resources can have the same effect on some people as does the capacity to pull formal rank.

Likewise, demographic, personality, and work flow variables can interact to create informal cliques whose boundaries may inhibit interaction across their memberships. Such boundaries are often reinforced by invidious attributions and specific norms against interaction. At a minimum, they limit the degree to which members of different cliques are likely to view coinquiry as especially useful for satisfying personal needs. Cooperation in role may be the norm across all cliques but sharing of personal concerns about one's own role may be prescribed to interactions "among one's own kind."

Personality.   Each party's *personality*, of course, has a tremendous impact on any relationship. The relatively enduring qualities of an individual's thinking are the most direct forces shaping not only how one interprets the other variables we have discussed, but also how one acts in response to these interpretations.

As part of one's analysis, it is useful to consider two features that are likely to affect a person's choice of coping strategy. As I mentioned in Chapter One, these are sense of competence and identity. In an instrumental organization, one's sense of competence is an integral part of any judgment about how equal one is to other members. One may be new or old, highly or poorly educated, and one's job may be central or peripheral to the organization's success, but the assumption of equality can be supported if one is competent at one's job, regardless of these conditions.

While competence affects judgments about equality, clarity about one's identity affects judgments about stepping out of role. Individuals who have a clear sense of who they are, need to rely less on any role they play in their relations with others. Consequently, they can talk about their roles as fellow adults, without being threatened that the dialogue will lead to changes they cannot cope with.

The simplest way I have found to measure each of these variables is to ask a client to rate himself or herself on them. The literal responses might not always be true, but the total message tends to come through loud and clear.

Networks.   Exploring two individuals' personal networks facilitates the development of a summary picture of their relationship. By a *network*, here, I mean the pattern of significant relationships that two people have with other colleagues besides

[5]George C. Homans, *The Human Group* (New York: Harcourt, Brace and World, Inc., 1950), pp. 48-155.

themselves and that forms the context in which their particular relationship is embedded.

Typically, in the initial stages of an OD project one interviews most of these individuals and gathers enough data to make some summary statements about each party's network, as well as the rest of the characteristics just discussed. Useful insights can be gained from drawing a sociogram of the two parties' relationships indicating what one believes are their salient aspects. Figure 12–2 is an example of such an analysis, which I used in thinking about a difficult relationship between two physicians: Bill, a physician and department chairman, and Alex, an older physician in the same department who shared a particular medical subspecialty with Bill. (Please review the diagram carefully before reading further.)

George, Bill's superior, had hired Bill three years before, following the larger organization's decision to expand Bill's department. Bill had concluded shortly after his arrival that Alex was no longer breaking new ground in specialty B, which he knew well because it was also one of his own. He hired Peter a year later, essentially to take Alex's place. Alex was quite aware of this, but at the same time he admired Peter, who had done his residency at the same institution as he had. In fact, Peter's presence had

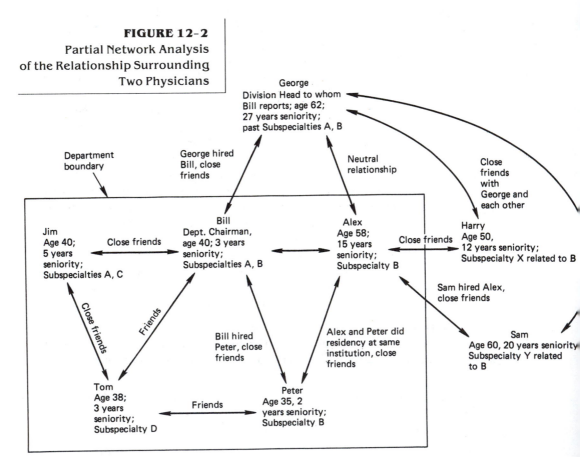

FIGURE 12-2
Partial Network Analysis
of the Relationship Surrounding
Two Physicians

rejuvenated Alex. The two men were collaborating on some new clinical research, which Sam and Harry, two of Alex's long-term friends, were also excited about.

At the time I entered the scene as a consultant on a development project not dissimilar to the South City project discussed in Chapter Two, Bill was doing everything he could to get Alex to leave the institution—for example, talking to George about Alex, referring his specialty B patients to Peter, associating closely with Jim, Tom, and Peter in running the department, and ignoring Alex whenever he could. Bill was convinced that Alex was simply riding on Peter's coattails. However, George (Bill's boss) had recently made it clear to Bill that Alex was still a well-respected member of the institution and would not be eased out. Thus, one of the tasks my colleagues and I faced was to help Bill and Alex develop a sufficiently cooperative relationship for the two of them to get along with each other for the foreseeable future.

We will not go into how we did this other than to note the utility of the network analysis as a diagnostic tool for summarizing some of the critical issues involved. Specifically, it helped to clarify the basic age and seniority split between Alex and the rest of the department. This went hand in hand with major differences in training and familiarity with the newest medical technology. The diagram also highlighted the status problems Bill was having from being organizationally superior as chairman to Alex but not influential enough to remove Alex because of Alex's older ties. Perhaps most important, it made it easy to identify Peter as a key resource for resolving Bill and Alex's differences. Peter's cooperation proved to be a major ingredient in helping the two men come to terms with each other, and eventually in Alex's developing satisfactory relationships between Alex, Tom, and Jim.

With this specific example in mind, it is now possible to consider the impact of the network surrounding a relationship on the prospects for coinquiry within it. Basically, one can view the network as a kind of selective amplifier. Power differences in a relationship can be amplified or attenuated by the characteristics of the other people each party associates with. Likewise, individual identities can be reinforced or attenuated. Thus, the same sets of personal qualities can promote or hinder coinquiry, depending on the larger pattern of relationships in which the two parties are embedded.

Analyzing the context of a client's relationships enables one to draw conclusions both about the pattern of forces working for and against coinquiry with particular co-workers, and the prospects for changing them. While one would like to assume that propitious avenues for change can always be found, this may not be the case. When several factors are negative with respect to any one relationship, one might choose to limit one's efforts to helping a client deal with his or her other relationships first, thereby enhancing this person's network to the point where some of the conditions affecting the more troublesome relationship begin to change. Assuming, however, that at least some promising avenues can be identified, the next step is to model the coinquiry process.

Modeling

Modeling the coinquiry process with a client in a way that will maximize the latter's learning requires the development of mutual trust and respect. Initial diagnostic interviews often provide spurious data because these conditions have yet to develop. However, even in these interviews one can demonstrate a commitment to learn about and appreciate the client's world in ways that are likely to get the relationship off to a good start. Such behaviors might include: listening empathically and letting the client know you understand what he or she is saying; expressing curiosity about the client's perspective on important issues such as organization policy; sincere, affective acknowledgment of the trials and tribulations that the client does care to share, and willingness to help the client articulate difficult issues; and, in general, using a helping oriented quasi-therapeutic approach in conducting these interviews.

The establishment of trusting relationships during the initial diagnostic phase can set the stage for more revealing conversations as data are fed back and subsequent interventions are designed and implemented. But the really important contacts are usually initiated by particular clients on an individual basis. Sometimes they are direct requests for help, but often the ways in which these invitations are made are easy to overlook or ignore—for example, a passing comment in the hallway, an invitation to stay and chat around some trivial issue after a meeting, a polite call to a consultant's office regarding a minor technicality and followed by an expression of interest in discussing more serious issues if the consultant's response is friendly, even a propensity to engage with the consultant more intensely than others in a meeting in order to test out the latter's interest.

If the consultant is to use role therapy as an important technique, these are the kinds of nuances that have to be spotted early and followed up. People use them as innocuous tests to see whether the consultant is really interested in their problems and, simultaneously, as veiled acknowledgments that the consultant may be worth listening to.

Once the client has invited the consultant into a meaningful dialogue, the process of appreciating the client's world needs to be continued. The consultant needs to become the client's ally, viewing the world from his or her perspective, understanding the choices the client has made to behave in particular ways, and acknowledging the frustrations the client is facing. This, in essence, is the first step in modeling the coinquiry process. No one wants to share personal issues with someone who is not making an honest attempt to understand and appreciate him or her.

During this process, the consultant also helps the client to articulate his or her envisioned roles and to sharpen the contrasts between this and what has actually been happening. For example, the consultant might participate in a dialogue such as the following:

Consultant: So you got into this meeting with Harry and found yourself getting mad because he was not willing to tell you what Jim had said about your project. Does this mean that you expect Harry to confide in you on all matters related to the project?

Ms. Smith: No, not necessarily all matters he finds out about. But Harry knows Jim's view is important to me, and that I would have a difficult time getting the project aproved if Jim were not supporting it.

Consultant: So in cases such as this, you do expect Harry to confide in you.

Ms. Smith: That's right. I guess I see him as my link with Jim, and I am really vulnerable when he doesn't do this for me.

Note that nothing has been resolved thus far. The initial task is simply to help the client sort out her thinking so that she can see her relationships with others in broader, more systemic terms.

The next step is perhaps more difficult. The consultant's objective now is to use this style of analysis to help the client think about how other actors in his or her role set might explain their own behavior. The discussion above might continue along the following lines:

Consultant: Why do you suppose Harry did not tell you what Jim had said? Do you think he's playing games with you?

Ms. Smith: That's certainly how I felt at the time. Though, in retrospect, I find this hard to believe. He's always treated me fairly and I don't see how his interests would be served by keeping Jim's view to himself.

Consultant: What kind of relationship does he have with Jim?

Ms. Smith: I think they're close. They interned together, joined the staff at the same time, and always seem to agree on important issues.

Consultant: I was just thinking that maybe Jim asked Harry not to discuss his views with you. Does that make any sense?

Ms. Smith: Well, that's possible. Come to think of it, Jim will have to engineer this thing pretty carefully if he is for me. One of my colleagues has another project that could use Jim's support, and if I acted even inadvertently as if Jim were behind me, I could set off a pretty crazy set of dynamics for both Jim and Harry to cope with. It's possible that both Jim and Harry thought it best not to discuss this with me.

Getting this far with any issue that is important to the client sets the stage for the third step in the modeling process. This involves bringing the client's attention to his or her reaction and making a pitch for coinquiry:

Consultant: I'd like to return to your conversation with Harry. Could you tell me what happened after you realized that he wasn't going to tell you Jim's position on your project? I know you got mad, but what did you do then?

Ms. Smith: Oh, I changed the subject. We ended up having a row about a really trivial issue.

Consultant: This may sound like a stupid question, but why didn't you just ask Harry point blank about where Jim was on your project?

Ms. Smith: Well, we don't have the kind of relationship where I can do that. It's got to sort of come out naturally. Harry has no real obligation to tell me these things. And he's so important to me that I don't want to do anything to upset the apple cart.

Consultant: Does anyone have such an obligation to you?

Ms. Smith: Officially, I guess Jim does. But I don't know him all that well, so I rely on Harry to tell me which way the wind is blowing. My dealings with Jim are pretty perfunctory. By the time I see him I already know what he's going to say.

Consultant: I wonder if there is a way we can think of for you to get to know Jim a little better.

The example we have been using might make it look as if modeling coinquiry was pretty straightforward. Thus, there is little wear and tear on the consultant. Sometimes it is, especially after a strong relationship has been established between the client and the consultant. Often, however, another element enters the picture.

Even though clients may see a consultant as a potentially helpful person, they may not anticipate that the consultant will encourage them to abandon past ways of behaving that they have become strongly attached to and try out new behaviors that may seem threatening. When this happens, the clients find themselves in the same bind with their helper, the consultant, as they do with their regular co-workers. There is a mismatch between their envisioned roles (expecting to work with the consultant to resolve their problems without encountering frustration, pain, and anxiety) and what they are experiencing in their interaction with the consultant. Quite naturally, clients respond in the ways they know and like best, and thus the consultant becomes the target of their favorite defenses.

The consultant's task in such instances is to recognize the situation for what it is and pursue the process of coinquiry to resolve it. The following is an example of such an attempt.

A consultant is having a conversation with the chairman of a medical department in a large health care center. He has been working with him and his department including physicians and support personnel for several months now. He has already engaged in an interview/feedback activity with the entire group, has followed this up with an open system planning session in which a sizeable agenda for the professional staff was created, and has begun to meet with this group on a weekly basis, acting as a process consultant to help them deal with these items. The progress of these sessions has been extremely slow.

However, by this time our consultant has also gotten to know each member of the group quite well, and is convinced that the difficulties are due at least in part to problems in the relationship between the chairman and two of his colleagues. He has witnessed several occasions in which the following scenario is played out. An agenda item is raised for discussion that the members have identified previously as requiring collaborative analysis and a high level of acceptance regarding its resolution, even though the chairman will have the final say. The chairman takes a minor role in the conversation, but two particular members of the group are quick to take distinct positions about what should be done. The consultant's process comments about remaining at an analytical level and avoiding closure until at least several options have been explored are ignored. At the same time, the chairman refuses to make a direct response to the options offered. The conversation continues without benefit of programmatic assessment until the chairman ends it by either tabling the issue or calling for further analysis. Another agenda item is raised and if the two members respond as they did before, the rest of the scenario is repeated.

The consultant's interpretation of this scenario is that the chairman is playing cat-and-mouse with these two colleagues, essentially engaging in avoidance behavior. Prior conversations with him have revealed that he distrusts both of them, because he thinks they want a larger share of control over departmental affairs than he is willing to give. They are both valued members, however, and consequently he does not want to engage in a showdown that might damage his reputation, even though he would probably win. At the same time, he has chosen the tactic described above for dealing with this situation rather than try to clarify his reasons for not giving these colleagues more influence and striving for mutual agreements that all three parties can live with. The consultant has requested this meeting with the intent of discussing the impact of the chairman's behavior on the group and to see whether he and the chairman can arrive at a more positive way of dealing with the latter's concern.

After the usual chitchat about the events of the day, the meeting begins in earnest when the consultant asks the chairman how he thinks the weekly meetings are going. The chairman responds by venting his frustrations regarding the two members, of which the consultant is already well aware. The consultant suggests that the meetings might go further if the chairman were to let events run their own course. In the initial planning for these sessions, it had been agreed that members would take turns at running them, guiding the group to a conclusion, subject to the chairman's veto. Since the chairman had ultimate control in any case, what could be lost by supporting this process?

After a long pause, the chairman responds by saying that he is thinking about closing down the OD project. He is highly frustrated with what is happening and is beginning to be convinced that he is simply not ready to buy into the consultant's approach. Things just do not seem right for continuing to work at this time.

After an equally long pause, the consultant responds. He begins by summarizing what the client has just said to make sure that he has understood, and the chairman confirms his interpretation. The consultant then says, "Aren't you doing the same thing with me that you have been doing in the meetings with George and Bill? It seems to me that every time they take the initiative on issues you feel uncomfortable about, you let them talk for awhile and then prevent a resolution from being reached by shelving further discussion, or calling for additional analysis, or avoiding a direct confrontation by saying you are not ready to make a decision yet."

The chairman becomes flustered and quietly admits that this is exactly what has happened. In the ensuing conversation he talks about how he deals with a great many issues in this way. The two discuss how successful this activity is and agree that the disadvantages often outweigh the gains. They return to the problem of managing the meetings and clarify how the chairman's willingness to let the conversation take its course until some clear alternatives have been established, examined, and the total group's views made known, need not be considered as a sign that he is giving away his control. The group's problem-solving activities can be used to help him think out his own alternatives.

Identifying a client's role reaction behavior when it is played out on oneself, and using coinquiry to deal with it, can be difficult for at least two reasons. First, it is hard to spot or treat objectively when it plays into one's own bad habits. While a consultant may espouse coinquiry, like any other human being he or she is probably well schooled in all four strategies and does not always choose the ideal. Thus, a consultant who is worried about finances may find it easy to deny that a client is using him or her to manipulate others, or the consultant may redefine his or her role to adapt to this behavior. Coinquiry is a two-way street, and if one is going to try to influence others to use it, one has to use it oneself.

Second, confronting clients with aspects of their here-and-now behavior that are not consistent with the collaborative mode can backfire if timed improperly. Clients may not trust a consultant sufficiently or rate this person's capacity to be helpful high enough to take the risks involved. Ultimately, the consultant can never know for sure whether these conditions exist in the clients' thinking. Thus, one must take a risk to get the process started. By the same token, unless the consultant is willing to take this risk at some point in time, success in introducing the coinquiry process may be permanently stymied.

Coaching

To the extent that a consultant is successful in modeling the coinquiry process for the client and the latter accepts it, the stage is set for helping the client practice it with colleagues. This can be a follow-up to or can start to take place during the modeling process itself. In fact, the activities of analysis, modeling, and coaching can all take place in the same conversation. *Coaching* refers to sustained attention toward helping the client practice coinquiry with others under the assumption that he or she knows and has experienced what it is all about. It can involve discussions of the kinds of concepts presented in this book or of any other frameworks in the therapeutic literature that parallel various aspects of this approach. At a minimum, it involves continued analysis and action planning with the client around attempts to deal with clients in a coinquiring manner.

For example, the client and consultant may plan a series of activities for the client to engage in with either the consultant present, as in group meetings, or absent, as in private conversations. The client, having attempted these activities, then meets with the consultant again to discuss what happened. This conversation may lead to new discoveries regarding the client's behavior, that of colleagues, or the behavior of the consultant. This, in turn, can lead to further modeling by the consultant for the client, or by the client for the consultant's benefit. More action planning results, and the cycle repeats itself until either party decides that the client no longer needs the consultant's help.

GUIDELINES FOR USING THE TECHNIQUE

Thus far, we have established that role therapy is a technique for inducing organization members to engage in coinquiry. Coinquiry is one of several strategies that people use to deal with differences between how they envision their roles prior to interaction with each other and what they actually experience during this interaction. It is the preferred behavior in Organization Development activities, because it alone involves and encourages the development of collegial relationships.

We have also noted that implementing the technique involves the consultant in three overlapping and mutually interdependent activities. These are: (1) analyzing the client's envisioned and experienced role behavior, the differences between the two, how the client currently deals with these differences, and the forces contributing to this coping style; (2) modeling coinquiry in one's relationship with the client as a way of demonstrating its positive effects and how they are achieved; and (3) coaching the client in initial attempts at coinquiry with others and providing a source of emotional and cognitive support during this process.

Finally, we have indicated that role therapy is not guaranteed to work all the time. While it can be conceived as a helping process that has the best interests of the client and the organization in mind, it is equally true to say that it is an influence attempt that is rooted in a particular set of values. People may reject it because they hold different values or because they consider the consultant an inappropriate partner for attempting to explore and enact these values.

We conclude this chapter with the following guidelines for enhancing one's chances of using the technique successfully.

> 1. Stick to analyzing and appreciating the client's role behavior early in the relationship. Avoid the temptation to coach the client until a firm relationship has been established and mutually shared goals have been agreed to.

Consultants who are new to role therapy tend to see the problem-solving and action planning aspects of the technique as the most exciting. However, neither of these activities is likely to bear much fruit unless a firm foundation has been laid out. It is important to remember that clients are likely to see the consultant initially as just another role player, to be dealt with and defended against like anyone else. They have a vision in mind of how they ought to behave with the consultant, and vice versa, which they will want to play out. The primary task of the consultant is to appreciate the clients' thinking in this regard and to help them, the clients, identify the directions they want to take through the relationship.

This involves analysis aimed at problem definition, not problem solving or action planning. It also involves helping the client appreciate his or her problems and frustrations. The more the consultant can facilitate this, the more he or she becomes a different kind of person to the client, someone who more truly understands and accepts the client's view of the world and the experiences that have created it. The consultant develops potency in the eyes of the client, in a sense, by being even better than the client at articulating and appreciating the latter's problems.

The more clients believe that the consultant really understands and appreciates their problems, the more likely they are to consider seriously any approaches the consultant might suggest to treat them. They may not believe the consultant's approach is better than theirs, but the fact that the consultant was able to help them articulate the problems themselves so well may suggest that there is something to be gained from the consultant's perspective.

   2.   Work toward a definition of *what* is the problem, not *who* is the problem.

The behaviors of denial, avoidance, and adaptation all contain the underlying assumption that, if something goes wrong and others find that a person is not acting in a way that all of them can accept as legitimate, it is the person who is the problem and not the role. To practice denial is essentially to bluff the discrepancy so that one, and by implication others, cannot communicate disapproval. The essence of avoidance is to create behaviors in others that at least prevent them from recognizing a discrepancy of which the self is aware. Adaptation is the private recognition that there is a discrepancy and that one is at fault and, therefore, must adjust one's behavior so as to minimize others' experience of this condition. In all three cases, the person is the figure whose behavior is problematic. The role is the blameless ground.

Coinquiry, by contrast, proceeds under the assumption that one's role, as one or others have defined it, may be just as much of a problem as the person. The task is to discover what behaviors are appropriate to achieve certain shared objectives, on the one hand, while recognizing and protecting commonly accepted personal prerogatives, on the other.

To induce this kind of analysis, clients need to feel that they do not have to be self-protective. This can happen if clients envision the changes to be aimed for as lying largely within the way they work with others, not in removing people from the system or punishing them for past behaviors. Thus, in working with them, it is useful to try to define *what* is the problem in systemic terms (in the way people work together) and to downplay problem definitions that single out a particular person as the source of their concerns.

This is not to deny that particular people, due to their character, habits, and/ or personal objectives, are sometimes major problem creators. Rather, it is to suggest that defining the problem in this way heightens preoccupation with self-protection that, in turn, encourages continued use of the other behavioral alternatives and discourages coinquiry.

   3.   Use external data first—for example, the client's personal reminiscences or interview/feedback material—in the analysis process. If you are not satisfied with the results, move to process comments on your on-the-spot interaction, and only then, if need be, to your personal experience of the client and his or her colleagues.

In trying to get a client to come to grips with a particular issue, the least intrusive intervention that does the job is the easiest to manage. This also allows one to check one's own thinking as vigorously as possible before plunging ahead. The objective is to let the client face an issue without creating so much anxiety that he or she will maintain old coping strategies or rupture the relationship rather than pursue the analysis once started.

The personal experiences of clients as they report them to you are the most benign to work with, since the clients can always elaborate on them to confuse the issue if they do not want to deal with it.

Data generated through some sort of collaborative analysis such as an interview/feedback activity are slightly more potent, since they are not under the clients' immediate control. They may deny the relevance and validity of these data at first, but if clients experience your acceptance of their right to do this, they are also likely to return to some of the data that they find disconcerting but are willing to deal with. If the consultant is helpful here, the chances of successfully introducing even more sensitive issues in these data are increased.

Once your relationship is well established, or indeed, if the relationship is already in danger, it might be appropriate to point to on-the-spot behavior, such as we have described earlier. As noted in the example above, this took place at an advanced level of consultant/client relationship. It was both a critical intervention in the project and a major test of the relationship itself.

Finally, the consultant's personal disclosures of past experiences with the client and his or her colleagues can be extremely powerful tools for change. For example, in addressing a client's denial behavior, the consultant may point to a specific instance that the consultant witnessed in which the client refused to recognize failure to meet an obligation. Unless the relationship is a strong one, the result could very easily be further denial or a complete rejection of the consultant as an alternative to accepting these data and exploring with the consultant why this happened.

> 4. Conceive of the overall balance of power in your relationship as moving from collaboration to probably a high degree of directiveness on your part, back to collaboration, to (near the end) considerable directiveness on the client's part.

Successful role therapy relationships proceed along these lines. The initial shift to directiveness by the consultant tends to come when the client chooses to trust the consultant and raises issues that he or she finds especially difficult to cope with. Success depends on the consultant's anticipation of this event and on helping to precipitate its occurrence only after gaining some clear data based on ideas on how to be helpful. The movement back to collaboration comes when the client experiences some success in following these suggestions and feels the need for less support. If success continues, this leads naturally to a point where the client has enough to work on to be selective about what he or she wants to do, and thus invites the consultant's entry in accordance with his or her own priorities. New crises, of course, can cause the cycle to be repeated. In some degree, the same pattern occurs in single conversations as well.

> 5. Accept the fact that your appreciation of the client will always be selective. Some of your goals will inevitably be incompatible with his or hers. Recognize this to yourself and share your differences with your client when they involve important values. Be your own best consultant and refrain from airing such differences when they are petty.

All client/consultant relationships remain ambivalent. None of us ever likes or accepts every aspect of our clients, nor do we always find their goals laudable. No doubt, the same is true regarding clients' views of their consultants. But, provided the balance is on the positive side for both parties, the dissonance this creates in the relationship provides added leverage for change. It makes both sides clarify their own choices about how they do want to collaborate. It cements commitment to these choices as justification for continuing the relationship in the face of the differences that do exist.

Behaviorally, the obligation of the consultant is twofold. First, one must curb one's own depreciation of the client to those aspects of this person's behavior and thinking that are inconsistent with one's highest values, and be open about these values as they relate to a client's objectives at the beginning of the relationship. Second, one must help the client interpret others' depreciation in terms of his or her highest values and help clarify and confront the differences between the client's and these people's goals. This is often a difficult task. We have to discount the pettiness in ourselves and others, and help our clients do the same. And the confrontations we help to create over goals may lead people to change their careers or groups to disband. The results are worth it, however, because they represent the baseline conditions that have to be clarified in order to prevent the collaborative approach from becoming a sham.

This discussion of guidelines for using the technique concludes our treatment of role therapy as a methodology for building collegial relationships and also marks the end of our exposition of the theory and technique of organization development in general. A postscript follows with suggestions for what one might do next as a prospective OD practitioner.

POSTSCRIPT

Role therapy along with techniques for developing task forces and engaging in process consultation are only the beginning of a long list of more focused intervention strategies that one can use to follow up an organizational analysis. Third-party consultation, role negotiation, task team development, intergroup mirroring, open systems planning, job enrichment, role analysis, career pathing, T-groups, and all forms of off-site workshops and retreats are just some of the many possibilities available today.[1] I chose to focus on these three because they represent some of the most basic ways to proceed after an analysis has been completed, and most other techniques can be chosen with clients in the context of task force work, and/or the opportunities that arise during process consultation, and/or role therapy.

Few of the techniques we have not covered, I believe, are any more advanced intellectually or more demanding in terms of interpersonal skills than those we have. They simply fit more specific client needs and therefore are more appropriate for specialized texts, articles, and readers. More important, all of them rely on a careful prior analysis and an underlying philosophy if they are to be used to good effect.

OD IN EVERYDAY LIFE

I began this book with the position that the essence of OD lies in the pursuit of some basic social values. These values do not point to a single best way to behave under all conditions, but they do suggest patterns of behavior that are both revered by our broader culture and highly underutilized in organizational settings. OD succeeds by modeling these values for clients in the context of action research projects on current organizational issues.

[1]For an overview of the many types of OD interventions used today, see Wendell L. French and Cecil H. Bell, *Organization Development*, 2nd ed. (Englewood Cliffs, N.J.: Prentice-Hall, Inc., 1978).

The topics we have covered have been intended to provide you, the reader, with both a kind of vicarious experience in the OD process and the necessary concepts and techniques for trying it out on your own. While we have discussed most of the material from the viewpoint of someone in a formal consulting role, very little stands in the way of using any of the techniques covered in any organizational role that involves working with more than a few people.

Every encounter with a member of an organization, be it one's own or another, provides opportunities for scouting, entry, and contracting around action research objectives. Almost any project that requires interaction with other people, and especially with other members of one's own organization, is amenable to collaborative analysis.

Programmatic interview and feedback activities can, of course, be overdone, just as can any other technique. But what is noteworthy is how few managers have bothered to try this approach even once. The natural tendency in our current managerial culture is to view every assignment as an individual effort. The possibilities of turning even a small proportion of most project assignments into truly collaborative efforts are immense.

Likewise, there are frequent opportunities for most managers to try out OD-oriented approaches in task force activities, routine meetings, and calls for personal advice from co-workers. What stands in the way, most often, is not the lack of opportunities but the awareness of how one might proceed.

NEXT STEPS IN EXPLORING THE FIELD

For those readers who find this book's approach intriguing, the next logical step is to try out its techniques in the context of daily work, whatever it may be. Depending upon the organizational culture one lives within, this may be very easy or extremely difficult. By doing this, however, one can discover how important the material really is to one's own life interests. Pursuing OD values is typically not an easy matter, and even small-scale attempts can create unanticipated resistance in one's colleagues. An important aspect of becoming an OD practitioner is developing a sense of comfort and conviction in meeting such resistance.

Three other activities can be done concomitantly. First, it is very helpful to find other colleagues who are interested in the field, to share ideas with them, and, where possible, work together on projects. While numerous OD organizations exist for helping one do this, fellow organization members are likely to provide the most help and to have the greatest understanding of one's personal situation. Second, unless one has already had considerable training in counseling and group dynamics, further training in these areas is almost imperative. Third and finally, the literature on OD is growing rapidly. While its quality varies markedly, extensive reading in the field is a useful way to test one's interest further and to begin to integrate the multiple perspectives the field has to offer. The value-oriented approach this book has taken is sympathetic to many writings but less so to others. Thus, it can serve as a reference point for developing one's own perspective.

This last point is probably the most important for the new practitioner. OD is not a well-integrated field with strong traditions to bolster its techniques and clear directions for future development. To enter the field of OD is not to pursue a well-recognized identity, as one would in going into medicine, law, or even business. The field today is more like an impressionist painting, with the figures discernible but not clear. Likewise, people who become known as OD practitioners tend to be known as unique individuals rather than as members of a distinct group. They are rarely experienced as interchangeable, and they rarely appeal to exactly the same clientele.

Thus, to become an OD practitioner is to discover one's own qualities as a helpful human being and a shaper of organization life, just as to practice OD is to commit oneself to making it possible for others to do the same.

BIBLIOGRAPHY

Banaka, William H., *Training in Depth Interviewing*. New York: Harper and Row, 1971.

Bandler, Richard, and John Grinder, *The Structure of Magic I*. Palo Alto, Calif.: Science and Behavior Books, Inc., 1975.

Beckhard, Richard, *Organization Development: Strategies and Models*. Reading, Mass.: Addison-Wesley Publishing Co., 1969.

Beckhard, Richard, and Reuben T. Harris, *Organizational Transitions: Managing Complex Change*. Reading, Mass.: Addison-Wesley Publishing Co., 1979.

Beer, Michael, Corning Glass Works (A) 9-477-024. Boston, Mass.: HBS Case Services, Harvard Business School, 1978.

Beer, Michael, Corning Glass Works (B) (revised 7/78) 9-477-073. Boston, Mass.: HBS Case Services, Harvard Business School, 1977.

Beer, Michael, Corning Glass Works (C) 9-477-074. Boston, Mass.: HBS Case Services, Harvard Business School, 1978.

Bennis, Warren G., *Organization Development: Its Nature, Origins, and Prospects*. Reading, Mass.: Addison-Wesley Publishing Co., 1969.

Blake, Robert R., and Jane Srygley Mouton, *The Managerial Grid Laboratory Seminar Materials*. Austin, Tex.: Scientific Methods, Inc., 1962.

Blake, Robert R., and Jane Srygley Mouton, "An Overview of the Grid," in *Training and Development Journal*. The American Society for Training and Development, Inc., May 1975, pp. 29-37.

Bradford, Leland P., Jack R. Gibb, and Kenneth D. Benne, *T-Group Theory and Laboratory Method*. New York: John Wiley and Sons, Inc., 1964.

Burke, W. Warner, and Harvey A. Hornstein, *The Social Technology of Organization Development*. Fairfax, Va.: Learning Resources Corporation, 1972.

Burke, W. Warner, and Warren H. Schmidt, "Management and Organization Development: What Is the Target of Change," in *Personnel Administration*. Chicago, Ill.: International Personnel Management Association, March-April 1979, pp. 44-57.

Burns, Tom, and G. M. Stalker, *The Management of Innovation*. London: Tavistock Publications, 1961.

Cameron-Bandler, Leslie, *They Lived Happily Ever After*. Cupertino, Calif.: Meta Publications, 1978. See especially pp. 174-80.

Delbecq, Andre I., Andrew H. Van de Ven, and David H. Gustafson, *Group Techniques for Program Planning: A Guide to Nominal Group and Delphi Processes*. Glenview, Ill.: Scott, Foresman and Company, 1975.

Erickson, Eric H., *Childhood and Society*. New York: W.W. Norton Company, 1950. See especially pp. 263-66.

French, Wendell L., and Cecil H. Bell, Jr., *Organization Development*. Englewood Cliffs, N.J.: Prentice-Hall, Inc., 1973.

French, Wendell L., and Cecil H. Bell, Jr., *Organization Development: Behavioral Science Interventions for Organization Improvement*. 2nd ed. Englewood Cliffs, N.J.: Prentice-Hall, Inc., 1978.

French, Wendell L., Cecil H. Bell, Jr., and Robert A. Zawacki, *Organization Development: Theory, Practice, and Research*. Dallas, Tex.: Business Publications, Inc., 1978.

French, John R. P., and Bertram Raven, "The Bases of Social Power," in *Group Dynamics*, 3rd ed. New York: Harper and Row, 1968, pp. 259-69.

Frohman, Mark A., Marshall Shashkin, and Michael J. Kavanagh, "Action-Research as Applied to Organization Development," in *Organization and Administration Sciences*, Vol. 7, Numbers 1 and 2, Spring/Summer 1976.

Galbraith, Jay R., "Organization Design: An Information Process View," in *Interfaces*, Vol. 4, Number 3, May 1974, pp. 28-36.

Goffman, Erving, *Interaction Ritual*. Garden City, New York: Anchor Books, 1967.

Harrison, Roger, "Choosing the Depth of Organizational Intervention," in *The Journal of Applied Behavioral Science*, Vol. 2, Number 6, pp. 182-202.

Hershey, P., and K. Blanchard, *Management of Organizational Behavior*. Englewood Cliffs, N.J.: Prentice-Hall, Inc., 1972.

Homans, George C., *The Human Group*. New York: Harcourt, Brace and World, Inc., 1950.

Johnson, Harry M., *Sociology: A Systematic Introduction*. New York: Harcourt, Brace and World, Inc., 1960.

Kotter, John P., *Organizational Dynamics: Diagnosis and Intervention*. Reading, Mass.: Addison-Wesley Publishing Co., 1978.

Kotter, John P., *Power in Management*. New York: AMACOM, 1979.

Kotter, John P., Leonard A. Schlesinger, and Vijay Sathe, *Organization: Text, Cases, and Readings on the Management of Organizational Design and Change*. Homewood, Ill.: Richard D. Irwin, Co., 1979.

Lawrence, Paul R., and Jay W. Lorsch, *Developing Organizations: Diagnosis and Action*. Reading, Mass.: Addison-Wesley Publishing Co., 1969.

Lawrence, Paul R., and Jay W. Lorsch, *Organization and Environment: Managing Differentiation and Integration*. Boston, Mass.: Division of Research, Graduate School of Business Administration, Harvard University, 1967.

Levinson, Harry, *Organizational Diagnosis*. Cambridge, Mass.: Harvard University Press, 1972.

Lippit, Gordon L., *Organization Renewal*. New York: Appleton-Century-Crofts, 1969.

Lorsch, Jay W., "A Note on Organization Design," 9-476-094. Boston, Mass: HBS Case Services, Harvard Business School, 1975.

Lorsch, Jay W., and John Morse, *Organizations and Their Members: A Contingency Approach*. New York: Harper and Row, 1974.

Nadler, David A., *Feedback and Organization Development: Using Data-Based Methods*. Reading, Mass.: Addison-Wesley Publishing Co., 1977.

Nadler, David A., and Michael T. Tushman, "A Model for Diagnosing Organizational Behavior," in *Organizational Dynamics*. New York: AMACOM, Autumn 1980.

Neilsen, Eric H., "Reading Clients' Values from Their Reactions to an Interview/Feedback Process," in *The Academy of Management Proceedings 1978*. Wichita, Kansas: Academy of Management, 1978, pp. 308-12.

Neilsen, Eric H., "The Human Side of Growth," in *Organizational Dynamics*. New York: AMACOM, Summer 1978, pp. 61-80.

Neilsen, Eric H., and Suresh Srivastva, "Role Therapy as a Modal Intervention in Health Care Organizations," in *Organizational Development in Health Care Organizations*, Newton Margulies and John D. Adams (eds.). Reading, Mass.: Addison-Wesley Publishing Co., 1982. See especially pp. 331-56.

Parsons, Talcott, "General Theory in Sociology," in *Sociology Today: Problems and Prospects*, Robert K. Merton, Leonard Broom, and Leonard S. Cottrell, Jr. (eds.), Vol. I. New York: Harper and Row, 1959, pp. 3-38.

Pfeffer, Jeffrey, *Power in Organizations*. Marshfield, Mass.: Pitman Publishing, Inc., 1981.

Rogers, Carl R., and Richard E. Farson, *Active Listening*. Chicago: Industrial Relations Center, The University of Chicago, 1957.

Rogers, Carl R., *On Becoming a Person*. Boston, Mass.: Houghton Mifflin Co., 1962.

Schein, Edgar H., *Process Consultation: Its Role in Organization Development*. Reading, Mass.: Addison-Wesley Publishing Co., 1969.

Schmuck, Richard, and Matthew Miles, *Organization Development in Schools*. Palo Alto, Calif.: National Press Books, 1971.

Schutz, William, *FIRO: A Three Dimensional Theory of Interpersonal Behavior*. New York: Holt, Rinehart and Co., 1958.

Seiler, James A., *Systems Analysis in Organizational Behavior*. Homewood, Ill.: Irwin-Dorsey, 1967.

Thelen, Herbert A., *Dynamics of Groups at Work*. Chicago, Ill.: University of Chicago Press, 1954.

Thompson, James D., *Organizations in Action*. New York: McGraw-Hill Book Co., 1967.

Weisbord, Marvin (Senior Vice President—Block Petrella Weisbord, Ardmore, Pa.), "The Organization Development Contract," in *Organization Development Practitioner*, Vol. 5, Number 2. Plainfield, N.J.: National OD Network, 1973, pp. 1-4.

Woodward, Joan, *Management and Technology*. London: Her Majesty's Printing Office, 1958.

Zaleznik, A., C. R. Christensen, and F. J. Roethlisberger, *The Motivation, Productivity, and Satisfaction of Workers: A Prediction Study*. Boston, Mass.: Division of Research, Harvard Business School, 1958.

INDEX

A

Action implementation, at South City Chemical, 50-55

Action planning:
  at South City Chemical, 48-50
  transition from feeding back data, 217-19
    categorizing problems for action, 219
    modified nominal group technique, 218
  types of follow-up activities, 220

Action research:
  analysis model (*see* Organizational analysis)
  as an approach to OD, 93, 105-11

Active listening:
  in developing collegial relationships, 75
  guidelines for, 173-75
  and maintenance of self-concept, 171-73
  in process consultation, 234

Analyzing data:
  developing a shared analysis, 198-99
  at Northern Medical, 5-11
  in preparing a quotation package, 204
  at South City Chemical, 41-54
  see also Organizational analysis

B

Banaka, William, 76, 156, 159, 160
Bandler, Richard, 161, 162, 164, 165, 167, 168
Beckhard, Richard, 1, 113

Beer, Michael, 102, 105
Bell, Cecil, 2, 105, 267
Benne, Kenneth, 94
Bennis, Warren, 1
Blake, Robert, 96, 97
Blanchard, 97
Bradford, Leland, 94
Bridging experience and language, 161-71
  human modeling processes, 161-62
  the Meta-model, 162-67
    caveat to the Meta-model in OD, 167
    representational awareness, 167-71
    sample client-consultant dialogue, 169-71
Broom, Leonard, 114
Burke, Warner, 2, 139, 141
Burns, Tom, 99

C

Cameron-Bandler, Leslie, 162, 167
Cartwright, Dorwin, 57
Case Western Reserve University, 32, 33
Christensen, C. Roland, 237
Client-consultant interaction:
  collaboration during entry, 146-47
  conflict, 73-74
  dimensions of, 154-55
  the doctor-patient model, 146
  four kinds of interaction (figure), 155
  the purchase model, 146